Study Guide to Accompany

Fundamentals of Nursing

THE ART AND SCIENCE OF NURSING CARE

FOURTH EDITION

Study Guide to Accompany

Fundamentals of Nursing

THE ART AND SCIENCE OF NURSING CARE

FOURTH EDITION

Carol Taylor, CSFN, RN, MSN, PhD
Director, Center for Clinical Bioethics
Assistant Professor, Nursing
Georgetown University
Washington, DC

Carol Lillis, RN, MSN
Interim Dean
Allied Health and Nursing
Delaware County Community College
Media, Pennsylvania

Priscilla LeMone, RN, DSN, FAAN
Associate Professor and Director/Undergraduate Program
Sinclair School of Nursing
University of Missouri-Columbia
Columbia, Missouri

Marilee LeBon, BA
Journalist
Mountaintop, Pennsylvania

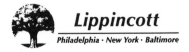
Lippincott
Philadelphia · New York · Baltimore

Ancillary Editor: Doris Wray
Senior Project Editor: Erika Kors
Senior Production Manager: Helen Ewan
Senior Production Coordinator: Mike Carcel
Design Coordinator: Brett MacNaughton
Manufacturing Manager: William Alberti

Fourth Edition

ISBN 0-7817-2285-3

Any procedure or practice described in this book should be applied by the health care practitioner under appropriate supervision in accordance with professional standards of care used with regard to the unique circumstances that apply in each practice situation. Care has been taken to confirm the accuracy of information presented and to describe generally accepted practices. However, the authors, editors, and publisher cannot accept any responsibility for errors or omissions or for any consequences from application of the information in this book and make no warranty, express or implied, with respect to the contents of the book.

Every effort has been made to ensure drug selections and dosages are in accordance with current recommendations and practice. Because of ongoing research, changes in government regulations, and the constant flow of information on drug therapy, reactions, and interactions, the reader is cautioned to check the package insert for each drug for the indications, dosages, warnings, and precautions, particularly if the drug is new or infrequently used.

Preface

Marilee LeBon, in close consultation with the authors of the fourth edition of *Fundamentals of Nursing: The Art and Science of Nursing Care,* has carefully developed these student learning guides. We recognize that beginning students in nursing must learn an enormous amount of information and skills in a short period of time. The questions in the learning guides, arranged by chapter, are structured to help you integrate and begin to apply the knowledge in the practice of nursing. Each chapter includes the following sections:

- *Chapter Overview:* This section, placed at the beginning of each chapter of the study guide, summarizes the material in the corresponding textbook chapter.
- *Learning Checklist:* This section refers to the learning objectives listed at the end of each textbook chapter. The objectives are written so that you can focus your study time on the critical elements of each chapter and structure your learning to gain essential information.
- *Exercises:* The exercises in each chapter group similar types of questions together to help you in learning the information in a variety of different formats. The types of questions included will follow the same format in each study guide chapter. Please note that not all of these types of questions will be found in each study guide chapter. The format is:

  Matching Questions
  Multiple Choice Questions
  Correct the False Questions
  Completion Questions
  Critical Care Questions
  Patient Care Studies

The Guide to Critical Thinking and Developing Blended Skills, which is new to this edition, offers an exciting and practical means to challenge the assumptions you bring to nursing and to "stretch" your application of new theoretical concepts. The Patient Care Studies in the clinical nursing care chapters provide a unique opportunity for you to "encounter" an actual patient and to use the nursing process to assess and diagnose the patient's need for nursing and to meet these needs.

The answers to the questions are included in the back of the book so that you can immediately assess your own learning as you complete each study guide.

We hope you find this study guide to be helpful and enjoyable and we wish you every success as you begin the exciting journey toward becoming a nurse.

Carol Taylor
Carol Lillis
Priscilla LeMone
Marilee LeBon

Contents

UNIT I
Foundations of Nursing Practice

1 Introduction to Nursing   3
2 Health of the Individual, Family and Community   8
3 Culture and Ethnicity   12
4 Health and Illness   17
5 Theoretical Base for Nursing Practice   21
6 Values and Ethics in Nursing   25
7 Legal Implications of Nursing   31

UNIT II
Promoting Health Across the Life Span

8 Developmental Concepts   39
9 Conception Through Young Adult   45
10 The Aging Adult   51

UNIT III
Community-Based Settings for Patient Care

11 Community-Based Healthcare   57
12 Continuity of Care   63
13 Home Healthcare   67

UNIT IV
The Nursing Process

14 Blended Skills and Critical Thinking
   Throughout the Nursing Process   73
15 Assessing   79
16 Diagnosing   83
17 Planning   88
18 Implementing   94
19 Evaluating   98
20 Documenting, Reporting, and Conferring   102

UNIT V
Roles Basic to Nursing Care

21 Communicator   109
22 Teacher and Counselor   116
23 Leader, Researcher, and Advocate   122

UNIT VI
Actions Basic to Nursing Care

24 Vital Signs   129
25 Health Assessment   135
26 Safety   143
27 Asepsis   149
28 Medications   155
29 Perioperative Nursing   164

UNIT VII
Promoting Healthy Psychological Responses

30 Self-Concept   173
31 Stress and Adaptation   180
32 Loss, Grief, and Dying   186
33 Sensory Stimulation   192
34 Sexuality   198
35 Spirituality   205

UNIT VIII
Promoting Healthy Physiologic Responses

36 Hygiene   213
37 Skin Integrity and Wound Care   221
38 Activity   229
39 Rest and Sleep   239
40 Comfort   247
41 Nutrition   257
42 Urinary Elimination   266
43 Bowel Elimination   274
44 Oxygenation   283
45 Fluid, Electrolyte, and Acid-Base Balance   292
   Answer Key   303

UNIT I

Foundations of Nursing Practice

CHAPTER 1

Introduction to Nursing

CHAPTER OVERVIEW

- Nursing has always involved caring. The role of the nurse as caregiver has been present since early civilization.

- Definitions of nursing have changed and expanded through time in response to societal needs and the social and political structure in which nursing has existed.

- The base for nursing practice and nursing education as we currently know it was established by Florence Nightingale, who positively influenced healthcare standards, nursing practice, nursing education, and women's rights.

- Nursing education in North America has changed from service-oriented hospital training schools to educational programs primarily offered in colleges and universities.

- The roles, functions, and professional status of nursing have been defined and described by ICN, ANA, and CAN. In all definitions, the central focus of nursing is the person receiving care.

- Nursing is an emerging profession and discipline. It is a practice that applies knowledge through specialized skills, upholds standards developed by and for the profession, develops theories and conducts research, and uses the nursing process to give individualized and holistic care.

■ Learning Checklist

Review the learning checklist at the end of the chapter in your textbook and be sure you can meet each objective.

■ Exercises

MATCHING

Match the aims of nursing, listed in Part A, with the nursing action that would accomplish these aims, listed in Part B. Answers may be used more than once.

PART A

a. promoting health
b. preventing illness
c. restoring health
d. facilitating coping

PART B

1. __a__ Increase student awareness of sexually transmitted diseases by distributing informational pamphlets at a college health center.

2. _____ Perform diagnostic measurements and examinations in an outpatient setting.

3. _____ Facilitate decisions about lifestyles that would enhance the well-being of a teenager.

4. _____ Provide community programs and resources that encourage healthy eating habits and regular exercise.

5. _____ Teach a patient and his family how to live with diabetes.

6. _____ Teach a class on the nutritional needs of pregnant women.

7. _____ Change the bandages of a patient who has undergone heart surgery.

8. _____ Assist a patient and his family to prepare for death.

9. _____ Provide counseling for the family of a teenager with an eating disorder.

10. _____ Serve as a role model of health for your patients by maintaining a healthy weight.

11. _____ Start an intravenous line for a malnourished elderly person.

12. _____ Help a person with paraplegia learn how to use a wheelchair.

CORRECT THE FALSE STATEMENTS

Circle the word true or false that follows the statement. If the word false has been circled, change the underlined word/words to make the statement true. Place your answer in the space provided.

1. A *nurse practice act* is a law that regulates the practice of nursing.

   True   False   _____

2. The ANA defines *continuing education* as those professional development experiences designed to enrich the nurse's contribution to health.

   True   False   _____

3. The legal right to practice nursing is termed *professional standards*.

   True   False   _____

4. When nurses complete a diploma, associate degree, or baccalaureate program, they become licensed as a *licensed practical nurse*.

   True   False   _____

5. In early civilizations influenced by the theory of animism, *the role of physician and nurse were interchangeable*.

   True   False   _____

6. The *ANA*, founded in 1899, was the first international organization of professional women, with nurses from both the United States and Canada as charter members.

   True   False   _____

7. All nursing actions focus on *the orders of the physician*.

   True   False   _____

8. *Practical nursing* was developed to prepare nurses to give bedside nursing care to patients.

   True   False   _____

9. When the major goals of healthcare—promoting, maintaining, or restoring health—can no longer be met, *the nurse's duties are terminated*.

   True   False   _____

10. Nursing has evolved through history from a technical service to a *knowledge-centered process* that allows maximizing of human potential.

    True   False   _____

MULTIPLE CHOICE

Circle the letter that corresponds to the best answer for each question.

1. Which of the following statements most clearly defines the role of the nurse in the early Christian period?

   a. The nurse was viewed as a slave carrying out menial tasks based on the orders of the priest-physician.

   b. Women called deaconesses made the first organized visits to the sick and members of male religious groups gave nursing care and buried the dead.

   c. The nurse was usually the mother who cared for her family during sickness by providing physical care and herbal remedies.

   d. Women who had committed crimes were recruited into nursing in lieu of serving jail sentences.

2. Which of the following nursing advocates elevated the status of nursing to a respected occupation, improved the quality of nursing care, and founded modern nursing education?

   a. Jane Addams

   b. Clara Barton

   c. Dorothea Dix

   d. Florence Nightingale

3. Which of the following statements is an accurate description of nursing's role, according to the ANA Committee on Education?

   a. Nursing is a profession dependent upon the medical community as a whole.

   b. It is the role of the physician, not the nurse, to assist patients in understanding their health problems.

   c. It is the role of nursing to provide services that contribute to the health and well-being of the people.

   d. The essential components of professional nursing care are strength, endurance, and cure.

4. The various definitions of nursing provided in this chapter conclude that the central focus of nursing is based on which of the following?
   a. the care provided by the nurse
   b. the patient receiving care
   c. the nurse as the caregiver
   d. nursing as a profession

5. Who established the Red Cross in the United States in 1882?
   a. Clara Barton
   b. Dorothea Dix
   c. Jane Addams
   d. Florence Nightingale

6. When a nurse helps a patient make an informed decision about his/her own health and life, which of the following nurse's roles has been performed?
   a. advocate
   b. counselor
   c. caregiver
   d. communicator

7. Which of the following developments had the greatest influence on the development of nursing as a profession since the 1950s?
   a. Large numbers of women began to work outside the home, asserting their independence.
   b. Nursing practice was broadened to include practice in a wide variety of healthcare settings.
   c. Male dominance in the healthcare profession slowed the progress of professionalism in the nursing practice.
   d. Hospital schools were established to provide more easily controlled and less expensive staff for the hospital.

8. Learning how to use a new piece of hospital equipment would most likely occur in which type of educational setting?
   a. continuing education
   b. graduate education
   c. in-service education
   d. undergraduate studies

9. Which of the following nursing education programs attracts more men, minorities, and nontraditional students and prepares nurses to give care to patients in structured settings?
   a. diploma in nursing
   b. associate degree in nursing
   c. baccalaureate degree in nursing
   d. graduate education in nursing

10. Which of the following is used by the nurse to identify the patient's healthcare needs and strengths and to establish and carry out a plan of care to meet those needs?
    a. nursing standards
    b. nursing orders
    c. nursing practice acts
    d. nursing process

COMPLETION

Nursing has been defined in many ways, but there are essential elements present in most thoughtful perspectives. Use your own words to expand the following short definitions of nursing.

1. Nursing is caring. _____
   _____
   _____

2. Nursing is sharing. _____
   _____
   _____

3. Nursing is touching. _____
   _____
   _____

4. Nursing is feeling. _____
   _____
   _____

5. Nursing is listening. _____
   _____
   _____

6. Nursing is accepting. _____

_____

_____

7. Nursing is respecting.

_____

_____

8. Give an example in which a nurse may
   incorporate the following broad aims of nursing
   into a nursing care plan for a patient undergoing
   diagnostic tests for lung cancer, who smokes two
   packs of cigarettes a day.

   a. Promoting wellness: _____

   _____

   _____

   b. Preventing illness: _____

   _____

   _____

c. Restoring health: _____

_____

_____

d. Facilitating coping: _____

_____

_____

*Complete the following table with the correct word or phrase to differentiate
among the nursing roles that are listed.*

Title	Education/Preparation	Role Description
EXAMPLE Nurse Researcher	Advanced degree	Conducts research relevant to nursing practice and education
9. Nurse Midwife		
10. Nurse Practitioner		
11. Nurse Anesthetist		
12. Nurse Administrator		
13. Nurse Entrepreneur		

Complete the following table describing the role of medicine and the role of the nurse in the listed time periods.

Timeline	Role of Medicine in Society	Role of Nurse in Society
14. Precivilization (Theory of Animism)		
15. Beginning of civilization		
16. Beginning of 16th century		
17. 18th–19th century		
18. World War II		
19. 1950s to present		

20. List the criteria that define the following concepts.

    a. A profession: _____

    b. A discipline: _____

21. Describe how the following issues are affecting nursing in transition.

    a. Technological advances: _____

    b. Nursing actions: _____

GUIDE TO CRITICAL THINKING AND DEVELOPING BLENDED SKILLS

1. Think of nursing situations in which the nurse involved promoted each of nursing's aims.

    a. Describe an instance of each:

    Promoting health _____

    Preventing illness _____

    Restoring health _____

    Facilitating coping _____

    b. Describe the factors that might warrant a particular nursing aim in each case.

    c. How would you evaluate if your nursing aims were successful?

2. Research a historical figure in nursing that you respect and admire. Write a potential nursing philosophy that would best express this person's nursing goals. Then interview a modern-day nurse about his/her nursing philosophy. See how the two philosophies differ. Form your own nursing philosophy based on your results.

CHAPTER 2

Health of the Individual, Family, and Community

CHAPTER OVERVIEW

- Basic human needs are common to all people and are essential to health and survival. Many needs are met through a person's social environment, specifically the person's family and community.

- Maslow's hierarchy of basic human needs describes five levels of needs: (1) physiologic, (2) safety and security, (3) love and belonging, (4) self-esteem, and (5) self-actualization.

- Physiologic needs have the highest priority and are the base of the hierarchy. These needs include oxygen, food, water, temperature, elimination, sexuality, physical activity, and rest.

- Safety and security needs include a physical component, involving protection from potential or actual harm, and an emotional component, including trust and freedom from fear.

- Love and belonging needs include both giving and receiving love, and having a sense of belonging to others.

- Self-esteem needs focus on a person's feeling good about himself or herself and believing that others also hold that person in high regard.

- Self-actualization needs are the highest level of need and are met when a person achieves his or her potential.

- The family, the basic social unity of society, serves as a buffer between the needs of society and the needs of individual members. Many different family structures (or forms) exist, but all families carry out the same functions: physical, economic, reproductive, affective and coping, and socialization.

- The family life cycle has definite stages and developmental tasks.

- Family-centered nursing care incorporates basic human needs, family concepts, and risk factors into nursing interventions to promote wellness.

- The community provides an environment that is an integral component of individual needs and family functions. Holistic nursing care integrates community risk factors and influences in all healthcare settings.

■ Learning Checklist

Review the learning checklist at the end of the chapter in your textbook and be sure you can meet each objective.

■ Exercises

MATCHING

Match Maslow's basic human needs, listed below in Part A, with the appropriate example, listed in Part B. Some answers will be used more than once.

PART A

a. physiologic needs

b. safety and security needs

c. love and belonging needs

d. self-esteem needs

e. self-actualization needs

PART B

1. _____ A nurse invites a patient's estranged son to visit him.

2. _____ A nurse attains a master's degree in nursing by going to school in the evening.

3. _____ A nurse washes her hands and puts on gloves before inserting a catheter in a patient.

4. _____ A home care practitioner requests a quiet environment so her elderly patient can get some rest.

5. _____ A nurse counsels an overweight teenager on proper nutrition.

6. _____ A nurse refers a patient's spouse to an Alanon group meeting.

7. _____ A student nurse takes a course in communications to improve her ability to relate to patients.

8. _____ A nurse administers pain medication to a postoperative patient.

Match the correct risk factor category listed in Part A with the appropriate example of family risks listed in Part B. Some answers will be used more than once.

PART A

a. lifestyle

b. social/psychologic

c. environmental

d. biologic

PART B

9. _____ A child with severe birth defects is born into a family.

10. _____ A teacher reports to a teenager's parents that drugs have been found in their son's locker.

11. _____ A recently divorced single parent of a 2-year-old child must return to work, but cannot find adequate child care on her budget.

12. _____ Two families are forced to live together in cramped conditions to make ends meet.

13. _____ Families in a city ghetto area fear walking to school and work because of gang activity on their street.

14. _____ An older adult living with her son's family cannot tolerate what she feels is inadequate discipline of her grandchildren.

15. _____ A 13-year-old girl in her first trimester of pregnancy admits that she was under the impression that she couldn't become pregnant her "first time."

16. _____ A family vacationing in Mexico becomes ill after drinking the local water.

17. _____ A couple learns that their infant has sickle cell anemia.

18. _____ A five-year-old girl accuses her uncle of "touching her inappropriately."

19. _____ A 3-month-old infant fails to thrive owing to malnutrition.

20. _____ A woman whose mother died of breast cancer finds a lump in her breast during her monthly breast examination.

MULTIPLE CHOICE

Circle the letter that corresponds to the best answer for each question.

1. Which of the following needs has the highest priority?

   a. the need to be loved by someone

   b. the need to be the best nurse you possibly can

   c. the need to live in a safe environment

   d. the need for oxygen to relieve respiratory distress

2. Which of the following theorists identified stages of the family cycle and critical family developmental tasks?

   a. Duvall

   b. Erickson

   c. Maslow

   d. Johnson

3. A change in body image, such as the loss of a body part, may affect which of the following types of human needs?

   a. love and belonging needs

   b. safety and security needs

   c. self-actualization needs

   d. self-esteem needs

4. Which of the following would be considered a community risk factor?

   a. A woman finds out that she is genetically inclined to develop crippling arthritis.

   b. An 80-year-old man is at risk for falls in his home because of clutter in his hallways and stairways.

   c. Children of a low-income family are kept inside the home on a sunny summer day due to lack of recreational opportunities in their neighborhood.

   d. A child is born with severe mental retardation.

5. Which of the following serves as a buffer between the needs of society and the needs of individual members?

   a. family

   b. community

   c. church

   d. parents

COMPLETION

1. Give an example of the following family functions and explain how each meets the needs of individual family members and society as a whole.

   a. Physical: _____

   _____

   _____

   b. Economic: _____

   _____

   _____

   c. Reproductive: _____

   _____

   _____

   d. Affective and coping: _____

   _____

   _____

   e. Socialization: _____

   _____

   _____

2. A first time mother-to-be is taken to the surgical unit for an emergency cesarean section. Her husband is nearby with a look of confusion and apprehension on his face. Give an example of how each of the following basic needs can be met by the nurse in caring for this couple.

   a. Physiologic needs: _____

   _____

   _____

   b. Safety and security needs: _____

   _____

   _____

   c. Love and belonging needs: _____

   _____

   _____

   d. Self-esteem needs: _____

   _____

   _____

   e. Self-actualization needs: _____

   _____

   _____

3. Describe how the following factors have changed the traditional family.

   a. Economic change: _____

   _____

   _____

   b. Increased career opportunities for women: _____

   _____

   _____

4. List three families you have dealt with in your life experience. Describe how each family differs from one another. Which families do you feel have been most effective in preparing members to meet individual, family, and community needs? Explain your choices.

   a. _____

   _____

   _____

   b. _____

   _____

   _____

   c. _____

   _____

   _____

GUIDE TO CRITICAL THINKING AND DEVELOPING BLENDED SKILLS

1. Volunteer some of your time at a local homeless shelter or any other service-oriented organization. Identify the individual immediate and long-term needs of the individuals served. Make a list of these needs in order of importance. What can be done to help promote health in these individuals? Explain how you could attempt to provide the following basic needs for the individuals served:

   a. Physiologic needs _____

   b. Safety and security needs _____

   c. Love and belonging needs _____

   d. Self-esteem needs_____

   e. Self-actualization needs _____

2. Review the lifestyles of some of your favorite TV drama characters. Identify the risk factors of the main characters involved. Give an example of a character at risk for:

   a. Lifestyle _____

   b. Social/psychologic_____

   c. Environmental_____

   d. Biologic_____

3. Describe an appropriate nursing response for each example noted above.

   _____

   _____

   _____

   _____

   _____

CHAPTER 3

Culture and Ethnicity

CHAPTER OVERVIEW

- Culture is the set of values, beliefs, and traditions held by a specific social group that is learned and handed down from generation to generation.

- One's culture guides behavior, is transmitted primarily through language, and can be adapted over time.

- Ethnic groups are made up of people who share common and unique cultural and social beliefs and social patterns.

- Stereotyping, which occurs when the assumption is made that all members of a culture or ethnic group are alike, often is practiced by the dominant group about a minority group in a culture.

- As members of a minority group live within a dominant group, cultural characteristics often are lost through assimilation.

- A wide variety of cultural and ethnic characteristics affect transcultural nursing care. These characteristics include family member roles, communications, nutrition, and income levels.

- Poverty has a major influence on health and illness, affecting health-related behaviors. This issue is made even more complex because of the increased number of families headed by single women, of older people, and of homeless families.

- Certain physiologic and psychologic characteristics that are found in specific cultural and ethnic groups are risk factors for illness.

- As part of the healthcare system, which has its own values and behaviors, nurses must be aware of the tendency of healthcare professionals toward cultural imposition and ethnocentrism.

- Guidelines for transcultural nursing care help the nurse accept the values, beliefs, and behaviors of others. Holistic nursing care requires that cultural influences and factors be integral components of an individualized plan of care.

- When nurses provide transcultural care, they demonstrate cultural sensitivity by recognizing and respecting cultural diversity.

■ Learning Checklist

Review the learning checklist at the end of the chapter in your textbook and be sure you can meet each objective.

■ Exercises

MATCHING

Match the term in Part A with the correct definition listed in Part B.

PART A

a. culture

b. minority groups

c. dominant group

d. ethnicity

e. subculture

f. cultural assimilation

g. cultural blindness

h. cultural imposition

i. race

j. stereotyping

k. cultural conflict

l. ethnocentrism

PART B

1. _____ A large group of people who are members of a larger cultural group, but have certain characteristics not common to the larger culture.

2. _____ When one assumes that all members of a culture or ethnic group act alike.

3. _____ The sense of identification that a cultural group has collectively, based on the group's common heritage.

4. _____ A set of values, beliefs, and traditions handed down from generation to generation.

5. _____. The loss of cultural characteristics that make minority groups different due to living within a dominant group.

6. _____ A group that has some physical or cultural characteristic that identifies the people in it as different; the group may believe that they are discriminated against because of that characteristic.

7. _____ Occurs when one ignores differences in cultures and proceeds as though they do not exist.

8. _____ A classification of people according to physical characteristics, such as skin pigmentation, body stature, facial features, and hair texture.

9. _____ The group within the culture that has the authority to control the value system and determine the rewards of the system.

10. _____ The belief that everyone should conform to the majority belief system.

11. _____ The idea that one's own ideas, practices, and beliefs are the best, are superior, or are the most preferred to those of others.

Match the disease listed in Part A with its definition listed in Part B.

PART A

a. sickle cell anemia

b. G6PD deficiency

c. Tay-Sachs disease

d. thalassemia

e. gout

f. sarcoidosis

g. keloid formation

h. lactase deficiency

i. cystic fibrosis

PART B

12. _____ Overgrowth of connective tissue occurring during the healing process.

13. _____ A genetic disorder that affects the hemoglobin RBCs. The production of alpha or beta globin chains is defective.

14. _____ Excess quantities of uric acid found in blood are deposited in joints and cartilage.

15. _____ The shape of the red blood cells causes them to break down more rapidly than normal shaped RBCs.

16. _____ A devastating hereditary disorder affecting people of Eastern European Jewish descent, resulting in short life span of victim.

17. _____ The formation of multiple tubercles or nodules on various parts of the body.

18. _____ Sex-linked deficiency of an enzyme normally found in red blood cells causing red blood cells that are unable to maintain cell membrane.

19. _____ Intolerance to milk and milk products.

Place the letter of the ethnic group affected by the following disorders on the line provided. Some disorders will have more than one ethnic group.

a. African heritage

b. Native American

c. Mediterranean background

d. East European Jewish descent

e. Asian

f. Hispanic

g. Hawaiian

20. _____ keloid formations

21. _____ lactase deficiency

22. _____ sickle cell anemia

23. _____ Tay-Sachs disease

24. _____ G6PD deficiency

25. _____ thalassemia

26. _____ sarcoidosis

27. _____ gout

Match the cultural group listed in Part A with its concept of health listed in Part B.

PART A

a. Native American

b. Black/African-American

c. Cambodian

d. Chinese American

e. Gypsies (Roma)

f. Hmong

g. Mexican-American

h. Puerto Rican

i. Samoan

j. Vietnamese

PART B

28. _____ Absence of mental, spiritual, or physical discomforts as well as not being too thin and being clean are perceived as healthy.

29. _____ Traditional health beliefs are holistic and health oriented.

30. _____ Principles of harmony and balance within self. Overweight is a positive sign of good economic status and contentment.

31. _____ Being healthy is seen as being in equilibrium. Health needs to be individually maintained but is influenced by family and community.

32. _____ Maintaining feelings of well-being, ability to fulfill role expectations, freedom from pain and excessive stress.

33. _____ Holistic approach, including aspects of body, mind, and spirit. Includes relationships with family, environment, and spiritual world.

34. _____ Maintaining balance between Yin and Yang influences in the body and in the environment.

35. _____ Being able to perform expected routines and duties.

36. _____ Maintaining moral purity, keeping upper and lower body separate, and practicing good behavior. Good health, prosperity, large families, and good appearance are intertwined.

MULTIPLE CHOICE

Circle the letter that corresponds to the best answer for each question.

1. The use of eye contact varies from culture to culture. Which of the following assumptions may be accurate when eye contact is used as nonverbal communication by different cultural groups in the following situations?

    a. A Native American stares at the floor during conversations with the nurse. *Assumption:* He is embarrassed by the conversation.

    b. A Hasidic Jewish male listens intently to a male physician making direct eye contact, but refuses to make eye contact with a female nursing student. *Assumption:* Jewish males consider females inferior to males.

    c. A Muslim-Arab woman refuses to make eye contact with her male nurse. *Assumption:* She is being modest.

    d. An African-American male rolls his eyes when asked how he copes with stress in the workplace. *Assumption:* He may feel he has already answered this question and has become impatient.

2. Which of the following statements about food accurately reflects foods that are edible for various cultural groups?

    a. Some Asian, Hispanic, and Seventh-Day Adventist religious beliefs prohibit the consumption of pork.

    b. Patients following a vegetarian diet will generally include chicken on their menu.

    c. Vietnamese patients will not eat beans.

    d. French patients consider corn to be animal feed.

3. Nursing is a subculture of which of the following larger cultures in our society?

    a. healthcare providers

    b. organizations of nurses

    c. institutions

    d. healthcare systems

4. An African-American patient complains of gas after consuming a bedtime snack of cheese and crackers. This may be a symptom of which of the following conditions?

    a. lactase deficiency

    b. keloid formation

    c. thalassemia

    d. G6PD deficiency

5. Which of the following best describes the type of health promotion practiced by the Vietnamese?

    a. One should eat a diet balanced with Yin and Yang foods and maintain harmony with friends and family.

    b. Health promotion encompasses physical, spiritual, emotional, and social factors. One should consume lots of fresh vegetables, fruit, fish, and meat and stay clean and warm.

    c. Proper diet, proper behavior, and exercise in fresh air are prescriptions for maintaining health.

    d. Illness is seen as preventable; nutrition is important, but not physical activity.

6. If a patient refuses to allow the nurse to draw blood for a test because he believes blood is the body's life force and cannot be regenerated, it is likely that he belongs to which of the following ethnic groups?

a. Hispanic-Puerto Rican

b. Asian

c. Hispanic-Mexican

d. African-American

7. Which of the following statements would best apply to Native American cultures?

a. The family is not expected to be part of the nursing care.

b. Direct eye contact is preferred when speaking to healthcare professionals.

c. A low tone of voice is considered respectful.

d. Careful notes are kept regarding their home care and medications.

8. In which of the following ethnic groups would folk-healing practices and home remedies be used by some families for particular illnesses?

a. African-American

b. White middle class

c. Asian

d. Jewish descent

9. A 79-year-old Native American woman is placed in a nursing home by her son, who is no longer able to care for her. She appears disoriented and complains of the "bright lights and constant activity." It would be likely that her feelings are a result of which of the following conditions?

a. culture assimilation

b. culture disorientation

c. culture blindness

d. culture shock

COMPLETION

1. How would you advise impoverished patients who are not meeting their healthcare needs due to the following conditions:

a. Lack of transportation to healthcare clinic/hospital/doctor's office: _____

_____

_____

b. Living in overcrowded conditions; absence of running water or adequate sanitation:

_____

_____

c. Use of drugs or alcohol to escape reality of situation: _____

_____

_____

2. Explain how cultural factors may affect the interaction of a nurse with a patient in the following situation: A nurse attempts to perform a nursing history on an Appalachian woman admitted to the hospital with chest pain.

a. Patient refuses to answer healthcare questions and refers to her "granny" woman as a source of information: _____

_____

_____

b. Patient's extended family is present during the interview and answers each question before the patient has a chance to speak: _____

_____

_____

c. Patient states that she has always taken a special herb prepared by her folk healer to alleviate her chest pains. She states that she does not trust modern medications: _____

_____

_____

3. Using the *Transcultural Assessment: Health-Related Beliefs and Practices* located in your textbook, assess the health-related beliefs of a patient of a different culture. How do this patient's beliefs differ from yours? What nursing actions could you take to help this patient express and practice their beliefs?

Patient/culture/medical condition: _____

_____

Health-related beliefs: _____

_____

_____

How my beliefs differ: _____

_____

_____

Nursing actions for patient: _____

_____

_____

4. List four transcultural assessments that should be considered when caring for non–English-speaking patients.

   a. _____

   b. _____

   c. _____

   d. _____

5. Explain why the following groups of people are at high risk for living in poverty.

   a. Families headed by single women: _____

   _____

   b. Older adults: _____

   _____

   c. Future generations of those now in poverty: ____

   _____

   _____

6. How would you define poverty and its effects on healthcare? _____

   _____

   _____

GUIDE TO CRITICAL THINKING AND DEVELOPING BLENDED SKILLS

1. How would you respond to the individual nursing needs of the following patients:

   a. A Jewish male refuses to let a female nurse perform a nursing history and asks for a male doctor to examine him instead.

   b. An African-American female, age 13, delivers her first baby. She tells you she had an abortion, but is ready for this new baby.

   c. An Asian-American who speaks halting English brings his grandfather (who speaks no English), to the ER. The grandfather presents with the warning signs of MI.

2. Interview fellow classmates and friends representing different cultures to determine how they respond to an illness in the family. Ask them what home remedies they use for the common cold. Identify any risk factors they may have for serious illness, including culturally related diseases.

CHAPTER 4

Health and Illness

CHAPTER OVERVIEW

- Health and illness are relative processes, defined by each person. Wellness, or the achievement of maximum function and strength, is possible even when a person has been diagnosed as being ill.

- Health and illness relationships and interaction can be described by the use of models such as the health–illness continuum, high-level wellness model, agent–host–environment model, and health-belief model.

- Wellness levels are influenced by the dimensions that compose the whole person, by needs, and by self-concept. These factors are interrelated and affect actual and potential health–illness status and behaviors.

- People at risk for an illness can be identified through a health-risk appraisal. If a person is identified at risk for illness, nurses can promote lifestyle practices that support health.

- Acute illnesses occur rapidly, have a relatively short time span, and may be either self-treated or require medical intervention. The person with an acute illness progresses from the onset of symptoms to recovery through certain definite stages.

- Chronic illnesses more often have a slow onset, cause permanent damage, and require long-term medical care. The increasing number of older adults, accompanied by an increase in chronic illnesses, means that nursing care of the chronically ill will become even more important in the 21st century.

- Nursing care for patients in both health and illness must include their family members. Illness results in altered expectations and reactions from family members.

- Nurses carry out wellness promotion activities on primary, secondary, and tertiary levels.

■ Learning Checklist

Review the learning checklist at the end of the chapter in your textbook and be sure you can meet each objective.

■ Exercises

MATCHING

Match the risk factors listed in Part A with their appropriate examples listed in Part B. Answers may be used more than once.

PART A

a. age

b. genetic composition

c. physiologic factors

d. health habits

e. lifestyle

f. environment

PART B

1. _____ A mother and her school-age child are concerned about increasing gang-related violence in their neighborhood.

2. _____ A teenager who is a new driver is admitted to the ER with multiple fractures after wrecking his car.

3. _____ A woman with multiple sex partners tests positive for HIV.

4. _____ A woman is worried about breast cancer because it "runs in the family."

5. _____ An overweight executive presents with high blood pressure.

6. _____ An alcoholic male develops a liver abscess.

7. _____ A patient tells you his father died of colon cancer.

8. _____ A smoker develops a chronic cough.

9. _____ A toddler presents with a mild concussion following a fall.

10. _____ A pregnant woman has toxemia in her fifth month.

11. _____ A 40-year-old man has a father and brother who died of heart attacks at an early age.

12. _____ An elderly man fractures a hip and ankle bone when falling down a flight of stairs in his home.

Match the model of health and illness listed in Part A with the correct definition in Part B.

PART A

a. agent–host–environment model

b. health-belief model

c. health–illness continuum

d. high-level wellness model

e. health promotion model

PART B

13. _____ This model views health as a constantly changing state, with high-level wellness and death being on opposite ends of a graduated scale.

14. _____ Halbert Dunn's model of health based on a person functioning to maximum potential while maintaining balance and a purposeful direction in the environment.

15. _____ This model, developed by Leavell and Clark for use in community health, is helpful for examining the causes of disease in an individual by looking at and understanding risk factors.

16. _____ Rosenstock's model of health based on three components of disease perception: (1) perceived susceptibility to a disease, (2) perceived seriousness of a disease, and (3) perceived benefits of action.

17. _____ This model, developed by Pender, illustrates the multidimensional nature of persons interacting with their environment as they pursue health.

MULTIPLE CHOICE

Circle the letter that corresponds to the best answer for each question.

1. Immunizing children against measles is an example of which of the following levels of preventive care:
   a. primary
   b. secondary
   c. tertiary

2. Referring an HIV-positive patient to a local support group is an example of which of the following levels of preventive care?
   a. primary
   b. secondary
   c. tertiary

3. In which of the following stages of acute illness does the patient decide to accept the diagnosis and follow the prescribed treatment plan?
   a. stage 1
   b. stage 2
   c. stage 3
   d. stage 4

4. Which of the following best describes a period of remission in a patient with a chronic illness?
   a. The symptoms of the illness reappear.
   b. The disease is no longer present.
   c. New symptoms occur at this time.
   d. Symptoms are not experienced.

5. During the recovery and rehabilitation stage of illness, the person who is ill is expected to do which of the following?
   a. give up the dependent role
   b. assume a dependent role
   c. seek medical attention
   d. recognize symptoms of illness

6. Needs are an integral part of each person's human dimension. Which needs are met when a person feels a sense of belonging to a group or community and being loved by others?
   a. spiritual needs
   b. sociocultural needs
   c. intellectual needs
   d. emotional needs

COMPLETION

1. Describe how your own self-concept has been influenced by the following factors:

   a. Interpersonal interactions: _____

   _____

   _____

   b. Physical and cultural influences: _____

   _____

   _____

   c. Education: _____

   _____

   _____

   d. Illness: _____

   _____

   _____

2. Compare and contrast the two types of illnesses listed below:

   a. Acute illness: _____

   _____

   _____

   b. Chronic illness: _____

   _____

   _____

   _____

3. Give an example that represents each of the following factors that influence health. For example:

   Physical dimension: An older adult must learn to live with and control his diabetes.

   a. Physical dimension: _____

   _____

   _____

   b. Emotional dimension: _____

   _____

   _____

   c. Intellectual dimension: _____

   _____

   _____

   d. Environmental dimension: _____

   _____

   _____

   e. Sociocultural dimension: _____

   _____

   _____

   f. Spiritual dimension: _____

   _____

   _____

   _____

4. Describe where you personally fit on the health-illness continuum and why: _____

   _____

   _____

   _____

5. List two examples of nursing actions which would be performed at each of the following levels of preventive care.

   a. Primary preventive care: _____

   _____

   _____

   b. Secondary preventive care: _____

   _____

   _____

   c. Tertiary preventive care: _____

   _____

   _____

   _____

6. Describe Dunn's processes (high-level wellness health model) that are a part of each individual's perception of their own wellness state and help that person know who and what he/she is.

   a. Being: _____

   b. Belonging: _____

   c. Becoming: _____

   d. Befitting: _____

GUIDE TO CRITICAL THINKING AND DEVELOPING BLENDED SKILLS

1. Identify and compare the factors affecting the health and illness of the following patients:

   a. A 39-year-old pregnant woman who has been in good health throughout her pregnancy is admitted to the OB unit for vaginal bleeding in her sixteenth week of pregnancy. Her husband is at her bedside.

   b. A 20-year-old woman in her 23rd week of pregnancy, who is addicted to crack cocaine, is brought to the ER by her boyfriend. She is having contractions.

   Determine the nurse's role in assisting these patients and their families.

2. Interview two patients: one who has recently experienced an acute illness and one who is chronically ill. Identify the individual health risk factors, basic human needs, and self-concepts of each patient. Explore and compare the different ways acute and chronic illnesses affect patients and their families.

CHAPTER 5

Theoretical Base for Nursing Practice

CHAPTER OVERVIEW

- Nursing is a combination of a body of knowledge and the application of that knowledge through nursing practice.

- Large bodies of knowledge organize and structure both facts and events into philosophies, concepts, and theories. These bodies of knowledge are then put into action by a process. In nursing, this is the nursing process.

- Nursing theories provide for the improvement of nursing practice through nursing research.

- Florence Nightingale's philosophy and theory of nursing provided the base for modern nursing.

- Nursing theory describes or explains nursing and usually includes the concepts of person, environment, health, and nursing.

- Nursing theories are often based on other processes and theories, including general systems adaptation and human development.

- Changes in society during the 20th century led to improvement and advances in nursing education, nursing research, and nursing practice.

- Nursing theory provides rationale for nursing actions, gives direction to all aspects of nursing, improves communications, and provides autonomy for the profession of nursing.

- Individual theories and conceptual models provide an organizing framework that can be applied to nursing practice.

■ Learning Checklist

Review the learning checklist at the end of the chapter in your textbook and be sure you can meet each objective.

■ Exercises

MATCHING

Match the term in Part A with the correct definition listed in Part B.

PART A

a. adaptation theory

b. general systems theory

c. philosophy

d. concept

e. theory

f. process

g. developmental theory

h. nursing theory

i. system

j. knowledge system

PART B

1. _____ The action phase of a conceptual framework; a series of actions, changes, or functions that bring about a desired goal.

2. _____ The study of wisdom, fundamental knowledge, and the processes used to develop and construct our perceptions of life.

3. _____ A set of interacting elements, all serving the common purpose of contributing an overall goal.

4. _____ Differentiates nursing from other disciplines and activities in that it serves the purposes of describing, explaining, predicting, and controlling desired outcomes of nursing care practices.

5. _____ Abstract impressions from the environment organized into symbols of reality; describes objects, properties, and events, and the relationships among them.

6. _____ A statement that explains or characterizes an action, occurrence, or event that is based on observed facts, but lacks absolute or direct proof.

7. _____ Emphasizes relationships between the whole and the parts and describes how parts function and behave.

8. _____ Defines a continuously occurring process that effects change and involves interaction and response.

9. _____ Outlines human growth as a predictable and orderly process beginning with conception and ending with death.

Match the nursing theorist in Part A with the central theme of the theory listed in Part B.

PART A

a. Dorothy E. Johnson

b. Imogene M. King

c. Madeline Leininger

d. Myra E. Levine

e. Betty Neuman

f. Dorothea E. Orem

g. Hildegard E. Peplau

h. Martha E. Rogers

i. Sister Callista Roy

j. Jean Watson

PART B

10. _____ Self-care deficit theory of nursing

11. _____ Behavioral systems model

12. _____ Adaptation model

13. _____ Theory of goal attainment

14. _____ Philosophy of science and caring

15. _____ Cultural care theory

16. _____ Theory of unitary human beings

17. _____ Four conservation principles theory of nursing

18. _____ Healthcare systems model

MULTIPLE CHOICE

Circle the letter that corresponds to the best answer for each question.

1. Which of the following statements accurately describes a characteristic of a *theory*?

   a. A theory is based on facts and contains absolute or direct proof.

   b. A theory is a single statement or concept that gives meaning to a series of events.

   c. Theories cannot be tested or changed.

   d. A theory is a group of concepts that form a pattern of reality.

2. When a nursing theorist identifies a specific idea or action and then makes conclusions about general ideas, he/she is using which of the following methods?

   a. inductive reasoning

   b. nursing process

   c. deductive reasoning

   d. general systems theory

3. Which of the following theories is based on the breaking down of whole things into parts and then learning how these parts work together as a whole?

   a. adaptation theory

   b. developmental theory

   c. general systems theory

   d. psychosocial theory

4. Which of the following statements accurately describes a characteristic of a *system*?

   a. A system is an entity in itself and cannot communicate with or react to its environment.

   b. Boundaries separate systems from each other and from their environments.

   c. All systems are closed in that they do not allow energy, matter, or information to move between systems and boundaries.

   d. Each system is independent of its subsystems in that a change in one element does not affect other systems.

5. According to Eric Erikson's developmental theory, psychosocial development is accomplished through which of the following processes?

   a. socialization

   b. human needs

   c. heredity

   d. health status

6. Of the four common components in theories of nursing, which of the following should be the focus of nursing?
   a. environment
   b. health
   c. nursing
   d. person

7. Which of the following theorists believed that a person was a *biopsychosocial being* who is basically good?
   a. Imogene M. King
   b. Madeline Leininger
   c. Sister Callista Roy
   d. Jean Watson

8. According to *Levine's* theory of nursing, nursing practice should focus on which of the following?
   a. The art and science of a human-to-human care process with a spiritual dimension.
   b. The human and the complexity of his or her relationships with the environment.
   c. The balance within an individual, specific to the behavioral system, when illness occurs.
   d. The variables affecting human response to stressors, with primary concern for the total person.

9. Which of the following would best define the environment in *Orem's* self-care model?
   a. modern society's values and expectations
   b. all of the patterns that exist external to the individual
   c. the culture of each individual group, or society
   d. the healthcare system, including the nurse

10. According to *Neuman's* healthcare system, how would health be defined?
    a. maintenance of the unity and integrity of the patient
    b. a state of well-being that is mainly known and expressed in cultural meanings and ways
    c. levels of wellness or stable lines of defense
    d. a state or process of being or becoming an integrated and whole person

COMPLETION

1. Nursing theories are often based on and influenced by other broadly applicable processes and theories. Briefly describe the ideas and principles of the following theories that are basic to many nursing concepts.
   a. General systems theory: _____
   _____
   _____
   b. Adaptation theory: _____
   _____
   _____
   c. Developmental theory: _____
   _____
   _____

2. List four basic characteristics of nursing theories.
   a. _____
   b. _____
   c. _____
   d. _____

3. List three contributions to nursing theory credited to Florence Nightingale.
   a. _____
   b. _____
   c. _____

4. Explain how the following factors have influenced the nursing profession.
   a. Cultural influences on nursing: _____
   _____
   _____
   b. Educational influences on nursing: _____
   _____
   _____
   c. Research and publishing in nursing: _____
   _____
   _____

d. Improved communication in nursing: _____

_____

_____

e. Improved autonomy of nursing: _____

_____

_____

5. Using Table 5-1 in your textbook, give an example of how the person in the following example would be defined and an assessment structured according to each theorist's conceptual model.

Example: Mark Bohn is a 24-year-old recovering alcoholic. Following treatment in a rehabilitation facility, Mark is currently attending AA meetings every evening and meeting with a home healthcare counselor twice a week.

a. Johnson's behavioral systems model: _____

_____

_____

b. King's theory of goal attainment: _____

_____

_____

c. Leininger's cultural care theory: _____

_____

_____

d. Levine's four conservative principles theory of nursing: _____

_____

_____

e. Neuman's healthcare systems model: _____

_____

_____

f. Orem's self-care deficit theory of nursing: _____

_____

_____

g. Peplau's psychodynamic nursing: _____

_____

_____

h. Roger's theory of unitary human beings: _____

_____

_____

i. Roy's adaptation model: _____

_____

_____

j. Watson's philosophy and science of caring: _____

_____

_____

6. Which nursing theorist(s) best defines your own personal beliefs about nursing practice, and why?

_____

_____

_____

GUIDE TO CRITICAL THINKING AND DEVELOPING BLENDED SKILLS

1. Describe how three different theories of nursing would direct the nursing care (identification and management of health/nursing needs) of this family:

A 15-year-old girl who self-mutilates by cutting is admitted to the psych ward for evaluation. Her family is anxious about her behavior and worried about her prognosis. A teacher who reported the incident is close to the girl and asks to speak to the attending physician.

2. Write the eleven theories discussed in this chapter on a piece of paper along with a brief description of their basic tenets. (Refer to Table 5-1 in the textbook.) Interview your faculty, nurses you know, and classmates and have them rank the theories in order of importance based on their own system of beliefs. Ask each participant to give you an example of their own personal philosophy that they would like to incorporate into their nursing practices. Note which theory was most widely respected and determine its value to your own practice.

CHAPTER 6

Values and Ethics in Nursing

CHAPTER OVERVIEW

- Knowing whether to perform a nursing action ("should I?") is often as important as knowing how to perform the action.

- A value is a belief about worth that acts as a standard to guide behavior. Values influence beliefs about human needs, health and illness, the practice of health behaviors, and human responses to health and illness.

- Values are formed over a lifetime from information a person receives from the environment and from the family and culture. Common modes of value transmission are modeling, moralizing, laissez-faire, rewarding and punishing, and responsible choice.

- The American Association of Colleges of Nursing identified altruism, aesthetics, equality, freedom, human dignity, justice, and truth as essential values for the practicing nurse.

- Although it is important for nurses to respect the value orientations of others, not all values are equal. Nurses may find themselves morally obligated to respond to patient values likely to cause harm to the patient or others.

- Values clarification is a process by which people come to understand their own values and value system. The process of valuing is centered on choosing, prizing, and acting.

- Ethics offers the nurse a means to look at and evaluate alternative courses of right action using basic moral concepts and principles. It reduces the likelihood that nursing actions to resolve ethical problems will be based solely on intuition, opinions, and self-interest.

- Theories of ethics offer moral guides to action and to character. Nursing ethics is a distinct subset of bioethics. Nurse ethicists frequently use two popular theoretical and practical approaches to ethics, the principle-based approach and the care-based approach.

- Nurse advocates who are sensitive to the need to promote both patient autonomy (self-determination) and patient well-being may experience ethical conflict, but are more likely than other nurses to be successful in securing the patient's genuine best interest.

- The nursing codes of ethics (ICN, ANA, CAN) provide a framework for making ethical decisions and set forth professional expectations. They inform both nurses and society of the profession's primary goals and values. Codes are effective only when upheld by members of the profession.

- Ethical problems faced by nurses include moral dilemmas and moral distress.

- One of several processes for resolving ethical problems in nursing is the following five-step process: (1) assess the situation (gather data); (2) diagnose (identify) the ethical problem; (3) plan: identify options and explore the probable consequences of each, and use ethical reasoning to decide on a course of action that you can justify; (4) implement your decision; and (5) evaluate your decision.

- Nurses often serve on institutional ethics committees whose chief functions include education, policy formation, case review, and consultation.

■ Learning Checklist

Review the learning checklist at the end of the chapter in your textbook and be sure you can meet each objective.

■ Exercises

MATCHING

Match the term in Part A with the correct definition listed in Part B.

PART A

a. value

b. ethical agency

c. advocacy

d. values clarification

e. ethics

f. morals

g. ethical dilemma

h. value system

i. ethical distress

PART B

1. __g__ Two (or more) clear moral principles apply, but support mutually inconsistent courses of action.

2. _____ A process of discovery allowing a person to discover what choices to make when alternatives are presented and to identify whether or not these choices are rationally made or the result of previous conditioning.

3. __A__ A personal belief about worth that acts as a standard to guide one's behavior.

4. __F__ Personal or communal standards of right and wrong.

5. __I__ Ethical problem in which the person knows the right thing to do, but institutional constraints make it nearly impossible to pursue the right actions.

6. _____ A commitment to developing one's ability to act ethically.

7. __E__ A systematic inquiry into the principles of right and wrong conduct, or virtue and vice, and of good and evil as they relate to conduct.

8. __C__ The protection and support of another's rights.

Match the essential values of the professional nurse in Part A with the appropriate example given in Part B. Answers may be used more than once.

PART A

a. altruism

b. autonomy

c. human dignity

d. integrity

e. social justice

PART B

9. _____ The nurse provides honest information to a patient about his illness.

10. _____ The nurse learns another language to help her better understand her patients.

11. _____ The nurse provides privacy for an elderly patient.

12. _____ The nurse arranges for free vaccinations for the children of a couple with no insurance.

13. _____ The nurse documents nursing care accurately and honestly.

14. _____ The nurse honors the right of a cancer patient to refuse chemotherapy.

15. _____ The nurse becomes a mentor for the student nurses on her ward.

16. _____ The nurse refuses to discuss a patient's condition with a curious friend.

17. _____ The nurse plans nursing care together with her patient.

18. _____ The nurse attends professional meetings addressing public misconceptions about the nursing profession.

19. _____ The nurse reports an error made by an incompetent co-worker.

20. _____ The nurse plans individualized nursing care for her patients.

Match the mode of value transmission in Part A with the appropriate example listed in Part B. Answers may be used more than once.

PART A

a. modeling

b. moralizing

c. laissez-faire

d. rewarding and punishing

e. responsible choice

PART B

21. _____ A child receiving good grades in school is taken to a video arcade to celebrate.

22. _____ A child is encouraged by parents to explore all aspects of their own personal code of ethics.

23. _____ A child whose parents smoke decides to give it a try.

24. _____ A child is left to his own devices when confronted with moral issues.

25. _____ A child is taught by school and parents that premarital sex is sinful.

26. _____ A child is encouraged to interact with people of various cultures to explore different values.

27. _____ A child is sent to his room following an altercation with his sibling.

28. _____ A child learns to eat a healthy diet by following his parent's example.

29. _____ A child is allowed to determine his own bedtime.

MULTIPLE CHOICE

1. When a nurse is able to recognize that an ethical moment has occurred with a patient, she is experiencing which of the following ethical abilities?
   a. ethical responsiveness
   b. ethical reasoning
   c. ethical sensibility
   d. ethical valuing

2. A nurse who is caring for a new mother realizes that she is not prepared to go home with her newborn after a hospital stay of only 24 hours, but hospital policy dictates that the mother be discharged. This nurse may be faced with which of the following moral problems?
   a. ethical uncertainty
   b. ethical distress
   c. ethical dilemma
   d. ethical dissatisfaction

3. Which of the following principles applies to utilitarian action guiding theory?

   a. The rightness or wrongness of an action depends on the consequences the action produces.
   b. An action is right or wrong independent of the consequences it produces.
   c. An action is right or wrong depending on the process used to arrive at the action.
   d. The rightness or wrongness of an action is not dependent on the process used to arrive at the action.

4. Which of the following guidelines was developed by the American Hospital Association to enumerate the rights and responsibilities of patients while receiving hospital care?
   a. code of ethics
   b. patient bill of rights
   c. biomedical ethics
   d. hospital patient advocacy

5. Which of the following elements of ethical agency could be described as the cultivated dispositions that allow one to act as one believes one ought to act?
   a. ethical sensibility
   b. ethical responsiveness
   c. ethical character
   d. ethical valuing

6. When a nurse provides the information and support patients and their families need to make the decision that is right for them, he/she is practicing which of the following principles of bioethics?
   a. autonomy
   b. nonmaleficence
   c. justice
   d. fidelity

COMPLETION

1. Describe how you, as a nurse, would help the following patient to define her values and choose a plan of action using the steps listed in your text.

   A 36-year-old mother of a 10-year-old child with cystic fibrosis works during the day as a cashier and is going to school at night to study nursing. Her husband is a salesman who has constant overnight travel. The child needs more attention than the mother has time to supply, and the mother feels guilty for spending time to better herself. She cannot afford to hire a full-time caretaker for her child.

   a. Values clarification: _____

   _____

   _____

   b. Choosing: _____

   _____

   _____

   c. Prizing: _____

   _____

   _____

   d. Acting: _____

   _____

   _____

2. Identify four ethical issues confronted by nurses in their daily nursing practice. How would you deal with these issues in your own practice?

   a. _____

   _____

   _____

   b. _____

   _____

   _____

   c. _____

   _____

   _____

   d. _____

   _____

   _____

3. Briefly describe the five principles approach to doing bioethics and give an example of each.

   a. Autonomy: _____

   _____

   _____

   b. Nomaleficence: _____

   _____

   c. Beneficence: _____

   _____

   _____

   d. Justice: _____

   _____

   _____

   e. Fidelity: _____

   _____

   _____

4. Describe how a nurse might react in the situation described below according to the elements of ethical agency.

   Situation: You overhear a nurse on you ward discussing with her patient another patient's HIV status. This is not the first time this nurse has been indiscreet. You are afraid to confront the nurse because she is your superior and has been known to punish co-workers who displease her by assigning them the most difficult cases.

   a. Ethical sensibility: _____

   _____

   _____

   b. Ethical responsiveness: _____

   _____

   _____

   c. Ethical reasoning: _____

   _____

   _____

   d. Ethical accountability: _____

   _____

   _____

e. Ethical character: _____

_____

_____

f. Ethical valuing: _____

_____

_____

g. Transformative ethical leadership: _____

_____

_____

5. Describe how you as a nurse would act as an advocate for the following patients:

a. A newborn baby born addicted to crack cocaine whose mother wants to take him home: _____

_____

_____

b. A 12-year-old female who seeks a pregnancy test at a Planned Parenthood Clinic without her parent's knowledge: _____

_____

_____

c. A 15-year-old anorexic girl who refuses to eat anything during her hospital stay: _____

_____

_____

d. A 28-year-old male patient, who contracted AIDS from an infected male partner, who tells you that the other nurses have been avoiding him: _____

_____

_____

e. A 48-year-old mother, with emphysema, who refuses to quit smoking: _____

_____

_____

f. A 78-year-old woman, in a nursing home, dying of cancer, who asks you to help her "end the pain" through assisted suicide: _____

_____

_____

6. List the qualities you possess that you feel are most important in developing your own personal code of ethics: _____

_____

_____

7. Use the five-step model of ethical decision making listed in your text to resolve the following moral distress: You believe a homeless patient, diagnosed with high blood pressure, needs a psychologic workup. She appears confused and unable to care for herself or manage her medication. She is alternately withdrawn and combative. You suspect she may have early Alzheimer's disease. Your superiors insist she be discharged without further treatment, and you are told there is no room for her on the psych ward.

a. Assess the situation: _____

_____

_____

b. Diagnose the ethical problem: _____

_____

_____

c. Plan: _____

_____

_____

d. Implement your decision: _____

_____

_____

e. Evaluate your decision: _____

_____

_____

8. Give an example of an ethical problem that may occur between the following health personnel, patients, and institutions.

a. Nurse/patient: _____

b. Nurse/nurse: _____

c. Nurse/physician: _____

d. Nurse/institution: _____

GUIDE TO CRITICAL THINKING AND DEVELOPING BLENDED SKILLS

1. Describe how you would respond in an ethical manner to the requests of the following patients:

   a. A patient who is suffering from end-stage pancreatic cancer confesses to you that the only relief he can get from his intolerable pain is from smoking marijuana. He asks you to look the other way while he lights up a joint.

   b. The anxious father of a 17-year-old gay patient asks you to perform an HIV test on his son without his son's knowledge.

   c. A woman who presents with contusions and marks consistent with spousal abuse tells you in confidence that her husband pushed her down the steps. She asks you not to tell anyone. When her husband arrives he hovers over her in an obsessive and overly protective manner.

2. Describe what you would do in the following situations:

   a. A doctor asks you to falsify a report that he prescribed medicine contraindicated for a patient's condition.

   b. A nurse co-worker refuses to bathe an HIV-positive patient.

   c. Due to administrative cutbacks, there are not enough nurses scheduled to cover the critical care unit in which you work.

Share your responses with a classmate and explore the difference in your responses. What competencies and character traits promote ethical behavior?

CHAPTER 7

Legal Implications of Nursing

CHAPTER OVERVIEW

- As the roles and duties of the nurse have expanded, so has the legal accountability of the nurse.

- Laws are standards or rules of conduct established and enforced by the government of a society to protect the rights of the public. Laws may be constitutional, statutory, administrative, or common.

- Voluntary standards regulating nursing practice are developed and implemented by the nursing profession itself. These standards include the ANA standards of practice, professional standards for the accreditation of education and service programs, and certification standards.

- Legal standards are mandatory and are developed by legislative action controlling professional conduct. They include the nurse practice acts and rules and regulations of nursing.

- Credentialing is the process of ensuring and maintaining professional competence. Credentialing involves accreditation, licensure or registration, and certification.

- A nurse whose license is suspended or revoked because the nurse engaged in drug and alcohol abuse or other acts of unprofessional conduct is entitled to due process of law.

- Intentional torts for which the nurse may be liable include assault and battery, defamation of character, invasion of privacy, false imprisonment, and fraud.

- Every individual has the right to be free from invasion of person, and thus consent is needed for all diagnostic, treatment, or research procedures. The person performing the procedure is responsible for obtaining informed consent. Documenting the informed consent may be delegated to nursing.

- Negligence is defined as performing an act that a reasonably prudent person under similar circumstances would not do or as failing to perform an act.

- Legal safeguards for the nurse include understanding and fulfilling the terms of contracts with employers and employees, competent practice, thorough patient education, safe execution of physician orders, careful documentation, professional liability insurance, and participation in risk management programs.

- The patient's record should never be tampered with in an attempt to prepare a better defense.

- Competent practice includes respecting legal boundaries of nursing, following institutional procedures and policies, owning personal strengths and being aware of weaknesses, evaluating proposed assignments, keeping current, respecting patient rights and developing rapport with patients, providing careful documentation, and working with nursing management to develop and implement programs to improve quality care and decrease risks of patient injury.

- Student nurses are legally responsible for their own acts of negligence resulting in patient injury. They are held to the same standard of care that would be used to evaluate the actions of an RN.

- Nurses need to be knowledgeable about specific laws affecting nursing practice. These include laws regulating occupational health and safety, the National Practitioner Data Bank, reporting obligations, controlled substances, discrimination/sexual harassment, persons with disabilities, wills, and legislation related to dying and death.

■ Learning Checklist

Review the learning checklist at the end of the chapter in your textbook and be sure you can meet each objective.

■ Exercises

MATCHING

Match the type of tort, listed in Part A, with an example of the tort, listed in Part B.

PART A

a. assault

b. battery

c. slander

d. liability

e. invasion of privacy

f. false imprisonment

g. fraud

h. negligence

i. libel

PART B

1. _____ A nurse seeking a middle management position in long-term care claims to be certified in gerontologic nursing, which is not the case.

2. _____ A nurse tapes an interview with a patient without his knowledge.

3. _____ A nurse threatens to slap an elderly patient who refuses to clean up after herself.

4. _____ A nurse spreads a rumor that a patient is a compulsive gambler.

5. _____ A nurse forgets to replace an IV bag that is empty.

6. _____ A nurse uses restraints on a patient unnecessarily.

7. _____ A nurse physically attacks a patient who complains that she is not being cared for properly by the nurses.

8. _____ A nurse circulates a petition among her co-workers in an attempt to remove a co-worker from her unit who has engaged in inappropriate behavior with a patient. This behavior is described at the top of the petition.

Match the terms, listed in Part A, with their definitions, listed in Part B.

PART A

a. litigation

b. plaintiff

c. defendant

d. crime

e. credentialing

f. felony

g. tort

h. contract

i. testator

j. beneficiary

k. misdemeanor

l. precedent

PART B

9. _____ The person who makes a will.

10. _____ The exchange of promises between two parties.

11. _____ The process of a lawsuit.

12. _____ The case that first sets down the rule by decision.

13. _____ The one being accused in a lawsuit

14. _____ A wrong against a person or his or her property, considered to be against the public as well.

15. _____ Crimes that are commonly punishable with fines or imprisonment for less than 1 year, or with both, or with parole.

16. _____ The person or government bringing suit against another.

17. _____ A crime punishable by imprisonment in a state or federal penitentiary for more than 1 year.

18. _____ A wrong committed by a person against another person or his or her property which generally result in civil trials.

19. _____ A person who receives money or property from a will.

Match the type of law listed in part A, with an example of the law, listed in part B.

PART A

a. administrative law

b. common law

c. public law

d. private law

e. criminal law

f. constitutional law

g. statutory law

PART B

20. _____ Laws regulating relationships between individuals and the government

21. _____ Nurse practice acts

22. _____ Rules and regulations of boards of nursing

23. _____ Malpractice law

24. _____ Laws regulating relationships among people

25. _____ Laws involving murder, manslaughter, criminal negligence, theft, and illegal possession of drugs

MULTIPLE CHOICE

Circle the letter that corresponds to the best answer for each question.

1. A body of law that has evolved from accumulated judiciary decisions is known as which of the following?

    a. statutory law

    b. administrative law

    c. common law

    d. constitutional law

2. A nurse who misrepresents the outcome of a procedure or treatment may have committed which of the following torts?

    a. slander

    b. fraud

    c. libel

    d. assault

3. Which of the following processes grants recognition to a person who has met certain criteria established by nongovernmental association?

    a. certification

    b. accreditation

    c. licensure

    d. litigation

4. Which of the following is the *primary* reason for filling out an incident report?

    a. to document everyday occurrences

    b. to document the need for disciplinary action

    c. to improve quality of care

    d. to initiate litigation

5. The Good Samaritan Laws would protect which of the following actions performed by health practitioners?

    a. any emergency care where consent is given

    b. negligent acts performed in an emergency situation

    c. medical advice given to a neighbor regarding her child's rash

    d. emergency care for a choking victim in a restaurant

6. Protection of employees from discrimination based on race, color, religion, sex, and national origin is provided under which of the following government agencies?

    a. OSHA

    b. EEOC

    c. HUD

    d. NAACP

7. When a nurse has met all the criteria necessary for recognition by the ANA, she is said to have undergone which of the following processes?

    a. licensure

    b. accreditation

    c. certification

    d. registration

8. A nurse who comments to her co-workers at lunch that her patient with a STD (sexually transmitted disease) has been sexually active in the community, may be guilty of which of the following torts?

   a. slander

   b. libel

   c. fraud

   d. assault

9. What is the process by which an educational program is evaluated and recognized as having met certain predetermined criteria?

   a. licensure

   b. registration

   c. accreditation

   d. certification

10. Which of the following actions would be recommended for a nurse who is named as a defendant?

    a. Discuss the case with the plaintiff to ensure understanding of each other's positions.

    b. If a mistake was made on a chart, change it to read appropriately.

    c. Be prepared to tell your side to the press, if necessary.

    d. Do not volunteer any information on the witness stand.

COMPLETION

1. Give an example of how nurses could avoid the following common allegations of malpractice.

   a. Failure to ensure patient safety: _____

   _____

   _____

   b. Improper treatment or performance of treatment:

   _____

   _____

   _____

   c. Failure to monitor and report: _____

   _____

   _____

   d. Medication errors and reactions: _____

   _____

   _____

   e. Failure to follow agency procedure: _____

   _____

   _____

   f. Equipment use: _____

   _____

   _____

   g. Adverse incidents: _____

   _____

   _____

   h. Patients with HIV: _____

   _____

   _____

2. Explain the difference between voluntary standards of nursing practice and legal standards and give an example of each.

   a. Voluntary standards: _____

   _____

   _____

   Example: _____

   b. Legal standards: _____

   _____

   _____

   Example: _____

   _____

3. List four cases in which informed consent is needed from a patient.

   a. _____

   b. _____

   c. _____

   d. _____

4. Give three examples of invasion of privacy in a nurse/patient relationship.

   a. _____

   b. _____

   c. _____

5. List three strengths a nurse must possess to testify competently as an expert witness._____

   a. _____

   b. _____

   c. _____

6. What conditions are necessary for a contract to be valid? _____

   _____

   _____

   _____

   _____

7. Describe what conditions you, as a nurse, would require to accept a telephone order from a physician: _____

   _____

   _____

   _____

8. List two cases in which it would be appropriate to question a physician's order.

   a. _____

   b. _____

9. Mrs. Toole is an 85-year-old patient recovering from a hip replacement in a home-care setting. When bathing Mrs. Toole, a visiting nurse practitioner forgets to replace her bed rails, resulting in her fall from bed. Mrs. Toole is shaken up, and sore from her fall, but there appears to be no further damage to her hip.

   a. What is the nurse's liability in this situation? ____

   _____

   _____

   b. What information should be included in an incident report? _____

   _____

   _____

   c. Do you feel the patient has a case for negligence? Explain why, or why not, using the four elements of liability that must be present to prove that negligence has occurred (duty, breach of duty, causation, damages): _____

   _____

   _____

GUIDE TO CRITICAL THINKING AND DEVELOPING BLENDED SKILLS

1. Think about how you would respond in the following situation and discuss your responsibilities with your classmates. Are there ever differences between the legally prudent and morally right response?

   a. Another student tells you she inadvertently gave medications to the wrong patient. She is terrified of your nurse supervisor and has decided not to inform anyone.

   b. An elderly resident in a nursing home tells you that the evening nurses are mean and sometimes push and hit her, but she begs you not to tell anyone.

   c. You observe a surgeon contaminate a sterile field and when you inform him he tells you not to be so squeamish.

2. Watch a TV show or movie that depicts a courtroom drama involving nursing practice. Write down all the legal jargon you hear and see if you can define it. Note if the jury delivers the same verdict for the plaintiff that you would deliver. Describe your reaction to the proceedings and verdict and state how your conscience would dictate your resolution of the conflict.

3. Stage a mock jury with your peers. Have each person take a turn suggesting a legal issue. Let the jury deliberate and return a verdict in each case.

4. Interview someone in the legal department of the institution where you will be practicing. Ask them about the legal issues that face novice nurse practitioners and what the hospital does to prevent problems from arising. Discuss with this administrator what you perceive to be your legal responsibilities to patients involving patient safety, informed consent, equipment use, incident reports, and medication errors.

UNIT II

Promoting Health Across the Life Span

CHAPTER 8

Developmental Concepts

CHAPTER OVERVIEW

- Nurses provide care to all ages in the life continuum; this care involves both individuals and their families.

- Growth and developmental theories, taken together, involve all aspects of life: physiologic, cognitive, psychosocial, moral, spiritual, and family dimensions.

- Principles of growth and development state that the processes are (1) orderly and sequential, (2) continuous and complex, (3) specific for each person, (4) influenced by environmental factors, (5) directed by regular trends, and (6) quantitative and qualitative, and that they (7) become integrated, (8) have vulnerable periods, (9) have rates and patterns that can be modified, and (10) occur at different stages and different rates.

- Freud's psychosexual theory explains ego development through predictable id–superego conflicts.

- Erikson identifies personality development in a series of stages from birth to later adult years, when critical tasks must be mastered.

- Havighurst focuses on the concept of learning in order to understand growth and development.

- Piaget's theory describes cognitive development from infancy through adolescence based on assimilation, accommodation, and formation of schemata.

- Kohlberg presents a theory of moral judgment of reasoning that begins in early childhood years. Gilligan developed a theory of moral development in females that is based on caring and responsibility.

- Fowler defines faith or spirituality as comprising meaning for life, which includes values, beliefs, and, possibly, religious affiliation.

- Each developmental theory explains a portion of the process of development and provides part of the nurse's understanding of the total being and coping abilities. Such theories are limited by the specific focus and the theorist's beliefs about growth and development.

- The family plays a vital role in promoting wellness and preventing illness. Both positive and negative health practices are shared in the family and learned by younger members. Health problems affect the family unit.

■ Learning Checklist

Review the learning checklist at the end of the chapter in your textbook and be sure you can meet each objective.

■ Exercises

MATCHING

Match Erikson's stages of development listed in Part A with the appropriate example, listed in Part B. Some answers will be used more than once.

PART A

a. trust versus mistrust

b. autonomy versus shame and doubt

c. initiative versus guilt

d. industry versus inferiority

e. identity versus role confusion

f. intimacy versus isolation

g. generativity versus stagnation

h. ego integrity versus despair

PART B

1. _____ A ten-year-old child proudly displays his principal's award certificate.

2. _____ An infant believes that his parents will feed him.

3. _____ A 22-year-old woman picks a circle of friends with whom she spends her free time.

4. _____ A 13-year-old girl fights with her mother about appropriate dress.

5. _____ A nursing home resident reflects positively on her past life experiences.

6. _____ A 15-year-old boy worries about how his classmates treat him.

7. _____ A 45-year-old man meets a goal of guiding his two children into rewarding careers.

8. _____ A kindergartner learns the alphabet.

9. _____ A two-year-old boy expresses interest in dressing himself.

10. _____ A 35-year-old woman volunteers Saturday mornings to work with the homeless.

Match the stages of faith development listed in Part A, with the appropriate definition listed in Part B. Note which of the following stages you have personally experienced in your lifetime. Give an example from your past that illustrates your passage through each stage on the lines proved at the end of the definitions.

PART A

a. stage 1: intuitive–projective faith

b. stage 2: mythical–literal faith

c. stage 3: synthetic–conventional faith

d. stage 4: individuative–reflective faith

e. stage 5: conjunctive faith

f. stage 6: universalizing faith

PART B

11. _____ This stage integrates other viewpoints about faith into one's understanding of truth. One is able to see the paradoxical nature of the reality of one's own beliefs. Personal example:

_____

12. _____ This is the characteristic stage for many adolescents. An ideology has emerged, but has not been closely examined until now; attempts to stabilize own identity. Personal example:

_____

13. _____ This stage involves making tangible the values of absolute love and justice for humankind; total trust in principle of being and existence of future. Personal example:

_____

14. _____ In this stage, children imitate religious gestures and behaviors of others; they follow parental attitudes toward religious or moral beliefs without thorough understanding of them. Personal example:

_____

15. _____ This stage is critical for older adolescents and young adults because the responsibility for their commitments, beliefs, and attitudes becomes their own. Personal example:

_____

16. _____ This stage predominates in the school-age child with increased social interaction. Stories represent religious and moral beliefs, and existence of a deity is accepted. Personal example:

_____

CORRECT THE FALSE STATEMENTS

Circle the word true or false that follows the statement. If the word false has been circled, change the underlined word/words to make the statement true. Place your answer in the space provided.

1. The human processes of growth and development result from two interrelated factors: <u>heredity and environment.</u>

   True   False   _____

2. Growth and development follow <u>irregular and unpredictable</u> trends.

   True   False   _____

3. The second trend in human development is <u>proximodistal development</u>, which means that growth progresses from gross to fine motor movements.

   True   False   _____

4. Different aspects of growth and development occur at <u>the same</u> stages and rates.

   True   False   _____

5. Freud identified the underlying stimulus for human behavior as <u>faith</u>.

   True   False   _____

6. According to Freud, the <u>ego</u> is the part of the psyche concerned with self-gratification by the easiest and quickest available means.

   True   False   _____

7. In Freud's <u>phallic</u> stage, the child has increased interest in gender differences and curiosity about the genitals and masturbation increases.

   True   False   _____

8. According to Havighurst, developing a conscience, morality, and a <u>scale of values</u> should occur in middle childhood.

   True   False   _____

9. <u>Accommodation</u> is the process of integrating new experiences into existing schemata.

   True   False   _____

10. In Kohlberg's <u>preconventional level, stage 2, instrumental relativist orientation</u>, the motivation for choices of action is fear of physical consequences or authority's disapproval.

    True   False   _____

MULTIPLE CHOICE

Circle the letter that corresponds to the best answer for each question.

1. The human process of growth and development is the result of which two interrelated factors?
   a. heredity and environment
   b. heredity and religion
   c. faith and culture
   d. physical and psychosocial skills

2. Which of the following generalizations about growth and development is accurate?
   a. Growth and development do not occur in a specific order or sequence.
   b. Growth and development follow irregular and unpredictable trends.
   c. Growth and development are differentiated and integrated.
   d. Different aspects of growth and development cannot be modified.

3. Which of the following theorists listed the unconscious mind, the id, the ego, and the superego as the primary aspects of the psychoanalytic theory?
   a. Erik Erikson
   b. Robert Havighurst
   c. Jean Piaget
   d. Sigmund Freud

4. Which of Freud's stages of development marks the transition to adult sexuality during adolescence?
   a. latency stage
   b. anal stage
   c. phallic stage
   d. genital stage

5. The expansion of Freud's theory to include cultural and social influences in addition to biologic processes is credited to which of the following theorists?
   a. Erik Erikson
   b. Robert Havighurst
   c. Jean Piaget
   d. Sigmund Freud

6. Which of the following theorists believed that living and growing are based on learning, and that a person must continuously learn to adjust to changing societal conditions.
   a. Erik Erikson
   b. Robert Havighurst
   c. Jean Piaget
   d. Sigmund Freud

7. A child who learns that he must sit quietly during story hour in kindergarten, thus integrating this new experience into his existing schemata is applying the process of:
   a. accommodation
   b. dissemination
   c. assimilation
   d. orientation

8. In which stage of Piaget's Cognitive Development Theory is logical thinking developed with an understanding of reversibility, relations between numbers, and loss of egocentricity?
   a. sensorimotor stage
   b. preoperational stage
   c. concrete operational stage
   d. formal operational stage

9. According to Piaget, the use of abstract thinking and deductive reasoning occurs during which of the following stages of development?
   a. sensorimotor stage
   b. preoperational stage
   c. concrete operational stage
   d. formal operational stage

10. Which of the following theorists developed the theory that males and females have different ways of dealing with moral issues?
    a. Lawrence Kohlberg
    b. Jean Piaget
    c. James Fowler
    d. Carol Gilligan

COMPLETION

1. Complete the following chart using the first theorist (Sigmund Freud) as an example.

Complete the following table with the correct word or phrase to differentiate among the nursing roles that are listed.

Theorist and Theory	Basic Concepts of Theory	Stages of Development
EXAMPLE Sigmund Freud Psychoanalytic theory	Stressed the impact of instinctual drives on determining behavior: Unconscious mind, the id, the ego the superego, stages of development based on sexual motivation.	oral stage anal stage phallic stage latent stage genital stage
Eric Erikson		
Robert J. Havighurst		
Jean Piaget		
Lawrence Kohlberg		
Carol Gilligan		
James Fowler		

2. Describe Lawrence Kohlberg's three levels of moral development and give an example of behavior that would typify each level.

a. Preconventional level: _____

_____

_____

Example: _____

b. Conventional level: _____

_____

_____

Example: _____

c. Postconventional level:_____

_____

_____

Example: _____

3. A 6-year-old girl with leukemia is admitted to the hospital for her first session of chemotherapy. What insight into this patient's needs could be gained from the following theorists?

a. Freud: _____

_____

_____

b. Erikson: _____

_____

_____

c. Havighurst: _____

_____

_____

d. Piaget: _____

_____

_____

e. Kohlberg: _____

_____

_____

f. Gilligan: _____

_____

_____

g. Fowler: _____

_____

_____

4. Identify the stage of the theorist noted that can be used by the nurse in responding to the statement made by the patient in the following situation:

Situation: A 15-year-old boy has been admitted to the hospital following a three-wheeler accident. He has multiple fractures and several deep cuts in his face that require stitches.

a. Freud: _____ "My dad told me not to ride that thing. I should have listened to him and this never would have happened."

b. Erikson: _____ "I am going to be so ugly with these scars on my face. I won't ever be able to have a girl look at me again."

c. Piaget: _____ "Tell me the best way to be sure I don't lose strength in my muscles. If I do those exercises you taught me, I will be able to go back to school and play basketball next year."

d. Fowler:_____ "I don't believe in God. If there is a God, he never would have let this happen to me."

5. What role does the family play in health promotion and illness prevention? How has your family affected your attitudes toward health and illness?

_____

_____

_____

GUIDE TO CRITICAL THINKING AND DEVELOPING BLENDED SKILLS

1. Reflect on the nursing plan you would develop for a 3-year-old, a 10-year-old, and a 16-year-old child undergoing heart surgery. How would your plan differ to take into consideration the age differences of the patients? How would you explain the procedure to each child? Give a rationale for each nursing intervention planned. Support your rationale by using a different developmental theory for each age group's nursing plan.

2. Make a chart listing Freud's stages of psychosexual development, Piaget's psychosocial development of different ages, and Havighurst's developmental tasks. Observe children in different settings and find an example of each stage of development. Talk with classmates about how these findings would influence your nursing practice.

CHAPTER 9

Conception Through Young Adult

CHAPTER OVERVIEW

- Heredity dictates an individual child's growth potential, whereas environment and nutrition influence the degree to which that potential will be reached.

- Growth and development in childhood begin rapidly, increase at a slower, steady pace in the middle, and end rapidly.

- The development of higher levels of moral and spiritual reasoning is directly related to higher levels of cognitive ability

- The family is an integral part of a child's growth and development.

- Healthy development occurs if the tasks of each stage are completed before entering the next stage.

- The nurse's role in child healthcare is focused on preventive teaching.

- An understanding of childhood development is essential to understanding adulthood.

■ Learning Checklist

Review the learning checklist at the end of the chapter in your textbook and be sure you can meet each objective.

■ Exercises

MATCHING

Match the stage of development, listed in Part A, with the risk factor associated with that age, listed in Part B. Some risk factors will have more than one answer.

PART A

a. neonate

b. infant

c. toddler

d. preschooler

e. school-age

f. adolescent and young adult

PART B

1. _____ Hormonal changes cause physical symptoms.

2. _____ Communicable diseases and respiratory tract infections begin to develop in this stage.

3. _____ Congenital disorders, such as hypospadias, inguinal hernias, and cardiac anomalies, require surgery at this stage.

4. _____ The suicide rate is highest for this group.

5. _____ A mother who smokes cigarettes, drinks alcohol, or uses drugs may cause developmental deficits in this stage.

6. _____ Accidents, poisonings, burns, drownings, aspiration, and falls remain the major causes of death in this stage.

7. _____ Gastroenteritis, food allergies, and skin disorders are common in this stage of development.

8. _____ Scabies, impetigo, and head lice are more prevalent in this stage.

MULTIPLE CHOICE

Circle the letter that corresponds to the best answer for each question.

1. Which of the following numbers is a normal score on the Apgar rating scale for newborns taken 1 and 5 minutes after birth?
   a. 1–3
   b. 4–6
   c. 7–10
   d. 11–15

2. Which of the following statements concerning neonates is accurate?
   a. A neonate can see color and forms.
   b. A neonate cannot hear sounds.
   c. A neonate is insensitive to touch and pain.
   d. A neonate has no labile temperature control.

3. A preschooler who clings excessively to his mother and uses infantile speech patterns is exhibiting which of the following behaviors?
   a. separation anxiety
   b. regression
   c. negativism
   d. self-expression

4. In which of the following stages of puberty do ova and sperm begin to be produced by the reproductive organs?
   a. prepubescence
   b. pubescence
   c. postpubescence

5. In which of the following stages of development would a person be most likely to think in abstract and question beliefs and practices that no longer serve to stabilize identity or purpose?
   a. toddler
   b. school-age
   c. adolescent
   d. older adult

6. In which of the following stages of development of a fetus have all the basic organs been developed?
   a. preembryonic stage
   b. embryonic stage
   c. fetal stage
   d. neonatal stage

7. A child would be most likely to develop *separation anxiety* in which of the following stages of development?
   a. infant
   b. toddler
   c. preschooler
   d. school-age

8. You have been asked to implement a sex education program in the public schools. With which grade level would you begin the program?
   a. kindergarten
   b. elementary
   c. junior high
   d. high school

9. Which of the following toys would be most appropriate for the toddler?
   a. tricycle
   b. basketball
   c. building blocks
   d. stuffed animal

10. The influential group in stabilizing self-concept in the adolescent are his or her:
    a. parents
    b. siblings
    c. peers
    d. teachers

11. Which of the following cell layers of the fetus becomes the skeleton, connective tissue, cartilage, and muscles and the circulatory, lymphoid, reproductive, and urinary systems?
    a. ectoderm
    b. endoderm
    c. mesoderm

12. During which stage of development would the fetus be most susceptible to maternal use of alcohol?
    a. preembryonic stage
    b. embryonic stage
    c. fetal stage

13. When assessing the health of a neonate, the nurse should be aware of which of the following accurate statements?

    a. The neonate has not yet developed reflexes that allow sucking, swallowing, or blinking.

    b. The neonate has labile temperature control that responds slowly to environmental temperatures.

    c. The neonate is alert to the environment but cannot distinguish color and form.

    d. The neonate hears and turns toward sound and can smell and taste.

COMPLETION

1. Write down the age group in which the following physiologic characteristics and behaviors are developed. Use N for neonate, I for infant, T for toddler, P for preschooler, S for school-age, and A for adolescent/young adult.

   _____ Motor abilities include skipping, throwing and catching, copying figures, and printing letters and numbers.

   _____ Puberty begins.

   _____ Brain grows to about half the adult size.

   _____ Reflexes include sucking, swallowing, blinking, sneezing, yawning.

   _____ Temperature control responds quickly to environmental temperatures.

   _____ Walks forward and backward, runs, kicks, climbs, rides tricycle.

   _____ Drinks from a cup and uses a spoon.

   _____ Sebaceous and axillary sweat glands become active.

   _____ Height increases 2–3 inches, weight increases 3–6 lb. a year.

   _____ The feet, hands, and long bones grow rapidly, and muscle mass increases.

   _____ Alert to environment, sees color and form, hears and turns to sound.

   _____ Birth weight usually triples.

   _____ Full set of 20 deciduous teeth, baby teeth fall out and are replaced.

   _____ Body is less chubby and becomes leaner and more coordinated.

   _____ Primary and secondary development occurs with maturation of genitals.

   _____ Typically four times the birth weight and 23–37 inches in height.

   _____ Body temperature stabilizes.

   _____ Average weight is 45 pounds.

   _____ Brain reaches 90%–95% of adult size, nervous system almost mature.

   _____ Head is close to adult size.

   _____ Motor abilities develop, allowing feeding self, crawling and walking.

   _____ Can smell and taste, and is sensitive to touch and pain.

   _____ Eliminates stool and urine.

   _____ Deciduous teeth begin to erupt.

   _____ All permanent teeth present except for 2nd and 3rd molars.

   _____ Bladder control during the day and sometimes during the night.

   _____ Holds a pencil, and eventually writes in script and sentences.

   _____ Full adult size is reached.

   _____ Drinks breast milk, glucose water, and plain water.

   _____ Eyes begin to focus and fixate.

   _____ Turns pages in a book and by age 3, draws stick people.

   _____ Heart doubles in weight, heart rate slows, blood pressure rises.

   _____ Rapid brain growth; increase in length of long bones of the arms/legs.

   _____ Uses fingers to pick up small objects.

_____ Sexual organs grow but are dormant until late in this period.

2. Write down the age group in which the following psychosocial characteristics and behaviors are developed. Use N for neonate, I for infant, T for toddler, P for preschooler, S for school-age, and A for adolescent/young adult.

_____ Is in oral stage (Freud); strives for immediate gratification of needs. Strong sucking need.

_____ Developmental task of learning appropriate sex's social role.

_____ In Freud's genital stage, libido reemerges in mature form.

_____ Is in anal stage (Freud); focus on pleasure of sphincter control.

_____ Self-concept is being stabilized, with peer group as greatest influence.

_____ Develops trust (Erikson) if caregiver is dependable to meet needs.

_____ Achieving personal independence, developing conscience, morality, and scale of values.

_____ Tries out different roles, personal choices, and beliefs (identity vs. role confusion).

_____ Meets developmental tasks (Havighurst) by learning to eat/walk/talk.

_____ Develops skill in reading, writing, and calculating and concepts for everyday living.

_____ More mature relationships with both males and females of same age.

_____ Enters Erikson's stage of autonomy vs. shame and doubt.

_____ Is in Erikson's stage of initiative vs. guilt.

_____ Inner turmoil/examination of propriety of actions by rigid conscience.

_____ Getting ready to read and learning to distinguish right from wrong.

_____ One's personal appearance accepted; set of values internalized.

_____ Freud's latency stage; strong identification with own sex.

_____ Developmental tasks of learning to control elimination; begins to learn sex differences, concepts, learn language, learn right from wrong.

_____ Focus on learning useful skills; emphasis on doing, succeeding, accomplishing.

_____ Developmental tasks of describing social and physical reality through concept formation and language development.

_____ Is in phallic stage (Freud) with biologic focus on genitals.

_____ Superego and conscience begin to develop.

_____ Developmental tasks of learning sex differences and modesty.

_____ Developmental task of learning physical game skills.

_____ Is in Erikson's industry vs. inferiority stage.

3. Briefly describe the growth and development of the fetus in the following three stages of fetal growth.

a. Preembryonic stage: _____

_____

_____

b. Embryonic stage: _____

_____

_____

c. Fetal stage: _____

_____

_____

_____

4. List four critical areas of development that are assessed by using the Denver Developmental Screening test.

a. _____

b. _____

c. _____

d. _____

5. After observing infants in a neonatal unit, describe the physical symptoms of the following temperaments:

   a. "Easy" _____

   b. "Slow to warm" _____

   c. "Difficult" _____

6. Define the following infant health problems and the role of the nurse in treating/preventing them.

   a. Colic: _____

   _____

   _____

   b. Failure to thrive: _____

   _____

   _____

   c. Sudden infant death syndrome: _____

   _____

   _____

   d. Child abuse: _____

   _____

   _____

7. Describe age-appropriate methods for preparing the following age groups for eye surgery; explain why you have chosen this method.

   a. Toddler: _____

   _____

   _____

   b. Pre-schooler: _____

   _____

   _____

   c. School-age: _____

   _____

   _____

   d. Adolescent and young adult: _____

   _____

   _____

8. The nurse plays an important role in the healthcare for each stage of development. Explain how you would tailor your care plan for the various age groups listed below.

   a. Infant: _____

   _____

   _____

   b. Toddler: _____

   _____

   c. Pre-schooler: _____

   _____

   _____

   d. School-age: _____

   _____

   _____

   e. Adolescent and young adult: _____

   _____

   _____

9. Briefly describe the following stages of puberty.

   a. Prepubescence: _____

   _____

   _____

   b. Pubescence: _____

   _____

   _____

   c. Postpubescence: _____

   _____

   _____

GUIDE TO CRITICAL THINKING AND DEVELOPING BLENDED SKILLS

1. A child is admitted to the Intensive Care Unit with third degree burns. How would your nursing care plan differ for this child if he were a toddler, a pre-schooler, a school-age child, or an adolescent? Be sure to include the type of dialogue you would use to explain painful procedures to each age group.

2. No two parents are the same in their methods of raising children. Although there aren't always clear cut right or wrong ways to raise children, some parents just seem to do a better job of it than others. Interview some of your friends to find out how successful they feel their parents were when raising them. Ask them about their parents' methods of discipline, motivation, and encouragement. Compare their answers with your own thoughts about how you were raised by your parents. What is nursing's role in promoting good parenting?

CHAPTER 10

The Aging Adult

CHAPTER OVERVIEW

- Growth and development continue as a sequence of predictable patterns throughout the adult life span.

- Erikson, Levinson, and Gould have described major developmental stages and tasks for the middle adult.

- During the middle adult years, visible signs of aging and an awareness of mortality appear. Various role changes may occur, and midlife crisis may precipitate changes in lifestyle.

- Middle adults are generally healthy, but increased risk for illness results from lifestyle, developmental or situational crises, family history, and the environment.

- Nursing considerations to promote health and prevent illness in middle adulthood focus on teaching self-care activities and the importance of regular physical examinations.

- According to Erikson, the older adult continues to look forward but also reflects back on life experiences to find meaning and acceptance. Havighurst views the major tasks of older adulthood to be primarily concerned with social relationships and roles.

- In older adulthood, physiologic aging becomes more rapid, with all organ systems showing decline in efficiency. The lack of physiologic reserves places the older patient at risk for multisystem complications.

- The older adult continues to learn and problem solve; intelligence and personality remain consistent after middle age.

- Most older adults adjust well to aging and continue to live active, independent, and productive lives. Although chronic illness is common, most older adults regard themselves as healthy.

- Ageism is a form of prejudice in which the older adult is incorrectly stereotyped as being different from other members of society. Also, aging is not synonymous with disease.

- Gerontologic nursing is a specialty field in the nursing profession, with specialized knowledge of aging in both health and illness that can benefit all nurses.

- A major goal of nursing care is to help the patient regain and maintain functional health; the nurse does this by collaborating with the patient, family, and healthcare team.

■ Learning Checklist

Review the learning checklist at the end of the chapter in your textbook and be sure you can meet each objective.

■ Exercises

MATCHING

Match the term in Part A with the correct definition listed in Part B.

PART A

a. ageism

b. dementia

c. sundowning syndrome

d. Alzheimer's disease

e. reminiscence/life review

f. gerontology

g. old-old

h. functional health

i. reality orientation

j. self-transcendence

PART B

1. _____ A variety of organically caused disorders that progressively affect cognitive functioning.

2. _____ A way for older adults to relive and restructure life experiences and achieve ego integrity.

3. _____ Term used to identify people over age 85.

4. _____ Redirecting the patient's attention to what is real in the environment.

5. _____ A form of prejudice related to older adults.

6. _____ The older adult habitually becomes confused in darkness.

7. _____ The scientific and behavioral study of all aspects of aging and its consequences.

8. _____ Affects brain cells and is characterized by patchy areas of the brain that degenerate or break down.

9. _____ The ability of older adults to expand beyond personal limits to reach out to others and the environment.

MULTIPLE CHOICE

Circle the letter that corresponds to the best answer for each question.

1. Which of the following accurately describes the behavior of the middle adult?
   a. Believes in establishment of self, but fears being pulled back into the family.
   b. Usually substitutes new roles for old roles and perhaps continues formal roles in a new contest.
   c. Looks inward, accepts life span as having definite boundaries and has special interest in spouse, friends, and community.
   d. Looks forward, but also looks back and begins to reflect on his/her life.

2. Which of the following aging theories assumes that healthy aging is related to the ability of the older adult to continue similar patterns of behavior that existed in young to middle adulthood?
   a. identity-continuity theory
   b. disengagement theory
   c. activity theory

3. After what age is one considered an older adult?
   a. 45
   b. 55
   c. 65
   d. 75

4. Based on an understanding of the cognitive changes that normally occur with aging, what would you expect a newly hospitalized older adult to do?
   a. talk rapidly, but be confused
   b. withdraw from strangers
   c. interrupt with frequent questions
   d. take longer to respond and react

5. Which of the following nursing actions would help maintain safety in the older adult?
   a. Treat each patient as a unique individual.
   b. Orient the patient to new surroundings.
   c. Encourage independence.
   d. Provide planned rest and activity times.

6. As defined by Erikson, in what stage of human development is the older adult?
   a. intimacy versus isolation
   b. identity versus role diffusion
   c. ego-integrity versus despair
   d. generativity versus stagnation

7. According to Havighurst, which of the following is a developmental task of older adulthood?
   a. adjusting to declining physical strength and health
   b. moving from one's own home to the home of others
   c. learning to live by oneself after losing a spouse
   d. establishing oneself in the community

8. Which of the following adult developmental theorists viewed the middle years as a time when adults increase their feelings of self-satisfaction, value spouse as a companion, and become more concerned with health?
   a. Erikson
   b. Levinson
   c. Piaget
   d. Gould

9. Which of the following is a developmental task of the middle adult?

   a. selecting a life partner

   b. establishing and guiding the next generation

   c. establishing a social network

   d. forming a personal philosophical and ethical structure

10. Which of the following statements about the older adult is accurate?

    a. Old age begins at age 65.

    b. Personality is not changed by chronologic aging.

    c. Most older adults are ill and institutionalized.

    d. Intelligence declines with age.

COMPLETION

1. Briefly describe the following characteristics of middle and older adulthood.

   a. Middle adulthood: _____

   _____

   Physiologic development: _____

   _____

   _____

   Psychosocial development: _____

   _____

   _____

   Cognitive, moral, spiritual development: _____

   _____

   _____

   b. Older adulthood: _____

   _____

   Physiologic development: _____

   _____

   _____

   Psychosocial development: _____

   _____

   _____

   Cognitive, moral, spiritual development: _____

   _____

   _____

2. Explain the concept "generation sandwich."

   _____

   _____

   _____

   _____

3. List five health promotion activities recommended for all middle adults.

   a. _____

   b. _____

   c. _____

   d. _____

   e. _____

4. Briefly describe the following theories on aging.

   a. Genetic theory: _____

   _____

   _____

   b. Immunity theory: _____

   _____

   _____

   c. Cross linkage theory: _____

   _____

   _____

   d. Free radical theory: _____

   _____

   _____

5. You are a visiting nurse for a patient with Alzheimer's disease. Describe what physical and psychologic changes you would expect to occur in this patient over time: _____

   _____

   _____

   _____

6. Briefly describe the following aging theories.

a. Disengagement theory: _____

_____

_____

b. Activity theory: _____

_____

_____

c. Identity-continuity theory: _____

_____

_____

_____

7. Give an example of how older adulthood may affect the following body organs:

a. Integumentary: _____

b. Musculoskeletal: _____

c. Neurologic: _____

d. Cardiopulmonary: _____

e. Gastrointestinal: _____

f. Genitourinary: _____

GUIDE TO CRITICAL THINKING AND DEVELOPING BLENDED SKILLS

1. Due to the advancement of modern medical technology and the focused awareness of the necessity of eating right and exercising, there is a dramatic increase in the number of active older adults. Although this age group on the whole is healthier than the generations that preceded them, they still have specific health risks and needs that must be identified by the nursing process. Consider the older adults you know personally and identify nursing strategies that would enhance their cognitive development and overall functioning (physiologic, social, emotional, and spiritual).

2. Examine your family and friends to identify healthy middle age adults and older adults. Interview them to learn about their physical, emotional, and spiritual selves. Compare their long-range and short-range goals, life stressors, physical ability, and emotional stability. How have age factors affected their life experiences? What can you learn from this healthy group to help others?

3. Take a look at the way older adults are portrayed on TV dramas. Are these dramas a realistic representation of this age group? Identify several health risks for older adults and preventive methods to promote health and safety.

UNIT III

Community-Based Settings for Patient Care

CHAPTER 11

Community-Based Healthcare

CHAPTER OVERVIEW

- Healthcare policy and reform issues are creating changes in healthcare that provide nurses with opportunities to shape healthcare for the future.

- Community-based healthcare is care that is provided in all types of healthcare settings, is provided to people who live in a defined geographic area with common needs, is holistic, and is designed to meet the needs of people as they move between and among healthcare settings.

- Community-based healthcare is provided in homes, hospitals, primary care centers, ambulatory care centers, specialized care centers, rehabilitation centers, long-term care facilities, hospices, and agencies. Nurses care for patients in all these settings and more.

- Healthcare services provided to patients in the home include skilled nursing assessment, teaching and support of patients and family members, and direct care.

- Hospitals provide a wide variety of inpatient and outpatient services and are classified as either private or public, for-profit or not-for-profit. Care in the hospital setting is focused on the acute care needs of patients.

- Primary healthcare services are provided in offices by physicians and nurse practitioners.

- Ambulatory care centers are often located in convenient areas, may offer walk-in services, and are open for a longer period than offices. Urgent-care centers provide emergency care services, and ambulatory surgical centers are sites for surgical procedures and care.

- Specialized care centers provide services for a specific population or group; they include day-care centers, mental health centers, rural health centers, schools, industry, and homeless shelters.

- Long-term care centers provide care and support for physically and mentally challenged people of any age. Care, which may range from only a few days to years, includes transitional subacute care, intermediate and long-term care, and skilled care. Settings for long-term care include hospitals, nursing homes, retirement centers, and residential institutions.

- Hospices provide special services for terminally ill patients and their families.

- Agencies that provide community-based healthcare services include voluntary agencies, religious agencies, and government agencies. Veterans hospitals, the Public Health Service, and public health agencies are also agencies that provide care and services to patients.

- Methods of ensuring continuity of care and cost-effective care include managed care systems, case-management, and primary healthcare.

- Members of the healthcare team collaborate to promote patient wellness and to restore health to patients who require healthcare services.

- Healthcare costs are financed through federally funded programs, group plans, and private healthcare insurance.

- Medicare is a federal health insurance program in the United States for people aged 65 years or older, people with permanent kidney failure, and certain physically challenged individuals. Medicaid is a federally funded health insurance program for people with low income.

- The National Medical Care insurance program provides hospital care to all citizens of Canada.

- Current societal issues influencing healthcare delivery focus on wellness promotion, changes in patient care needs, cost containment, and consumer rights. Patients are better educated about health matters, prefer more control and more participation in decision making about personal health, and are becoming active participants in planning and implementing healthcare.

■ Learning Checklist

Review the learning checklist at the end of the chapter in your textbook and be sure you can meet each objective.

■ Exercises

MATCHING

Match the type of healthcare provided, listed in Part A, with its definition, listed in Part B.

PART A

a. respite care
b. hospice services
c. mental health centers
d. voluntary agencies
e. rehabilitation centers
f. day-care centers
g. parish nursing centers
h. ambulatory care centers
i. homeless shelters
j. public health agencies
k. long-term care facilities
l. rural health centers
m. hospitals
n. schools
o. home care
p. industry
q. primary care centers

PART B

1. ___F___ Care for infants and children whose parents work, elderly who cannot be home alone, and patients with special needs who do not need to be in a healthcare institution.

2. ___D___ Not-for-profit community agencies financed by private donations, grants, or fund-raisers.

3. ___G___ Community health nursing practice that emphasizes holistic healthcare, health promotion and disease prevention, hopefully reaching people before they are sick; often volunteer and church oriented.

4. ___B___ Special services available to terminally ill individuals and their families, providing inpatient and home care committed to maintaining quality of life and dignity in the dying person.

5. ___E___ Provides services for patients requiring psychologic or emotional rehabilitation and for treatment of chemical dependency.

6. ___J___ Those local, state, or federal agencies that provide public health services to communities of various sizes.

7. ___H___ Urgent care center that provides walk-in emergency care services.

8. ___L___ Often located in geographically remote areas with few healthcare providers. Many of these centers are run by nurse practitioners.

9. ___C___ Provide 24-hour services and hot lines for people who are suicidal, who are abusing drugs or alcohol, and who require psychologic or psychiatric counseling.

10. ___I___ Living units that provide housing for people who do not have regular shelter.

11. ___M___ The traditional acute care provided for people who were too ill to care for themselves at home, who were severely injured, required surgery or complicated treatments, or were having babies.

12. ___Q___ Healthcare services are provided by physicians and advanced practice nurses in offices and clinics offering the diagnosis and treatment of minor illnesses, minor surgical procedures, obstetric care, well-child care, counseling, and referrals.

13. ___A___ The type of care provided to home-bound ill, disabled, or elderly patients to enable the primary caregiver some time away from the responsibilities of day-to-day care.

14. ___N___ Nurses in this setting are often the major source of health assessment, health education, and emergency care for the nation's children.

15. ___P___ Occupational health nurses practicing in these settings focus on preventing work-related illnesses and injuries by conducting health assessments, teaching health promotion, and caring for minor injuries and illnesses.

Match the team member in Part A with the role they play in the healthcare system, listed in Part B.

PART A

a. physician

b. physician's assistant

c. physical therapist

d. respiratory therapist

e. occupational therapist

f. speech therapist

g. dietitian

h. pharmacist

i. social worker

j. unlicensed assistive personnel

k. chaplain

PART B

16. __H__ Licensed to formulate and dispense medications.

17. __F__ Trained to help hearing-impaired patients speak more clearly.

18. __A__ Responsible for the diagnosis of illness and medical or surgical treatment of that illness.

19. __J__ Help nurses provide direct care to patients; titles include nursing assistants, orderlies, attendants, or technicians.

20. __G__ Responsible for managing and planning for dietary needs of patients.

21. __e__ Licensed to assist the physically challenged patient to adapt to limitations.

22. __b__ Has completed a specific course of study and a licensing examination in preparation for providing support to the physician.

23. __c__ Seeks to restore function or prevent further disability in a patient after an injury or illness.

24. __i__ Counsels patients and family members and informs them of and refers them to various community resources.

25. __D__ Has been trained in techniques that improve pulmonary function and oxygenation.

MULTIPLE CHOICE

1. In which of the following healthcare insurance plans is the patient most limited in choice of healthcare provider?

   a. HMO

   b. PPO

   c. POS

   d. LTC

2. Which of the following types of health-care plans allows a third party payor to contract with a group of healthcare providers to provide services at a lower fee in return for prompt payment and volume guarantee?

   a. HMO

   b. PPO

   c. POS

   d. LTC

3. In which of the following types of care can patients move to a living space, such as an apartment, while they are still physically able to care for themselves, and then have access to progressively more healthcare services, as needed, as long as they live?

   a. aging in place

   b. rest homes

   c. nursing homes

   d. aging gracefully

4. Diagnosis-related groups were implemented by the federal government to meet what healthcare problem?

   a. increasing numbers of ill elderly

   b. increasing fragmentation of care

   c. increasing consumer complaints

   d. increasing healthcare costs

5. Which of the following abilities would be most important for a nurse who works in a crisis intervention center?

   a. well-developed technical skills

   b. low tolerance for frustration

   c. strong communication and counseling skills

   d. ability to relate to co-workers on a professional level

6. Which of the following programs illustrates a focus on health in our society?

   a. research on the treatment of AIDS

   b. incarceration of drug addicts

   c. anti-smoking ads on television

   d. aggressive therapy for cancer

7. What does the term *fragmentation of care* mean?

   a. Care is provided only on certain days, such as Monday through Friday.

   b. Care is provided only to those with the resources to pay for it.

   c. The healthcare provider performs total care.

   d. Care is given by many different providers.

8. Which of the following nursing functions would most likely be found in an ambulatory care facility?

   a. serving as an administrator or manager

   b. providing direct patient care

   c. educating individuals or groups

   d. assessing the home environment

9. Which of the following patients would be covered by Medicare?

   a. people who have kidney failure

   b. infants of low-income families needing immunizations

   c. all people with disabilities

   d. dependents of people who are 65 years or older

10. Which of the following statements is a characteristic of case management?

    a. The primary objective is to identify specific protocols and timetables for care and treatment.

    b. In many of these cases, the cost of services has skyrocketed.

    c. Nurses who are case managers give direct care to the patients.

    d. Continuity of care is sacrificed under the case management system.

COMPLETION

1. List four factors that have influenced the need for increased home healthcare.

   a. _____

   b. _____

   c. _____

   d. _____

2. Describe the role of the nurse in the following healthcare centers:

   a. Primary care offices: _____

   _____

   _____

   b. Ambulatory care centers and clinics: _____

   _____

   _____

   c. Mental health centers: _____

   _____

   _____

   d. Rehabilitation centers: _____

   _____

   _____

   e. Long-term care centers: _____

   _____

   _____

3. How have recent changes in the healthcare system affected the role of the hospital as a provider of healthcare services? _____

   _____

   _____

4. List five services that can be performed during outpatient care.

   a. _____

   b. _____

   c. _____

   d. _____

   e. _____

5. Explain the term DRG and how it is implemented in hospitals: _____

_____

_____

_____

7. Define the term "fragmentation of care" and its effect on the healthcare system: _____

_____

_____

_____

6. Complete the following chart describing healthcare payment plans and their advantages and disadvantages if any.

Plan	Description	Advantages	Disadvantages
a. HMO			
b. PPO			
c. PPA			
d. Private			
e. LTC			
f. Medicare			
g. Medicaid			

GUIDE TO CRITICAL THINKING AND DEVELOPING BLENDED SKILLS

1. Think about a group of individuals in your community that is underserved and lacks access to nursing resources. How might the needs of this group be better addressed?

2. Visit a local healthcare clinic in your community. Find out what type of services are performed and the backgrounds of the patients seeking these services. Check out how the clinic is funded and how the staff is reimbursed for its services. Would you feel comfortable being cared for in this clinic?

3. Look at the promotional materials for a local healthcare plan and interview people on the plan. Which features of the plan are most important for the insured? What does the plan lack? Is the insured party free to choose his/her own doctors or treatment plans?

4. Compare the roles and responsibilities of a physical therapist vs. an occupational therapist, a physician vs. a physician's assistant, and a social worker vs. a chaplain. Write down the responsibilities of each professional, where they overlap to provide continuity of care for the patient, and where they diverge to meet the specific needs of each patient. How will this information help you as a nurse to coordinate the efforts of the interdisciplinary team?

CHAPTER **12**

Continuity of Care

CHAPTER OVERVIEW

- The nurse is the primary person responsible for ensuring continuity of care as patients move from one type of health care setting to another.

- Continuity of care is the coordination of services provided to patients. It ensures a smooth transition between ambulatory or hospital care and home care or other types of community-based care.

- Continuity of care is provided by including discharge planning as part of the care plan from admission, collaborating with other members of the healthcare team, and involving the patient and family in planning.

- Anxiety about the unknown can be reduced by establishing a therapeutic nurse–patient relationship on admission to a setting that provides healthcare.

- Although admission and dismissal from ambulatory and hospital settings differ, the focus is on meeting patient needs and providing individualized care. The nurse is responsible for assessments, teaching, and developing a care plan with the patient and family.

- Transfer of a patient from one level of care to another is common. The nurse provides care to meet comfort, safety, and knowledge needs of the patient and family, ensuring continuity of care.

- Discharge planning is a systematic process of preparing a patient to leave a healthcare agency and for maintaining continuity of care. This process is coordinated and multidisciplinary and is carried out with consideration of each patient's needs when moving to a different level of care. Information about medications, diet, procedures and treatments, referrals, and health promotion activities may be included in the teaching plan for discharge.

■ Learning Checklist

Review the learning checklist at the end of the chapter in your textbook and be sure you can meet each objective.

■ Exercises

CORRECT THE FALSE STATEMENT

Circle the word true *or* false *that follows the statement. If the word* false *has been circled, change the underlined word/words to make the statement true. Place your answer in the space provided.*

1. The <u>physician</u> is the person who most often is responsible for helping the patient make a smooth transition from one type of care setting to another.

   True   False   _____

2. <u>Discharge planning</u> is the coordination of services provided to patients before they enter a healthcare setting, during the time they are in the setting, and after they leave the setting.

   True   False   _____

3. People who enter a healthcare setting must take on the role of <u>patient</u>.

   True   False   _____

4. <u>Ambulatory facilities</u> are those in which the patient receives healthcare services but does not remain overnight.

   True   False   _____

5. The <u>admitting diagnosis</u> is generally included on the identification bracelet that is placed on the patient's wrist during treatment at a health facility.

   True   False   _____

6. Hospital admissions and lengths of hospital stay are <u>increasing</u>.

   True   False   _____

7. Discharge planning <u>is not</u> indicated when a patient is to be placed in a nursing home or other continued care setting.

   True   False   _____

8. When <u>goals</u> are established with the patient, compliance with the treatment regimen is more likely.

   True   False   _____

9. When transferring a patient to a long-term facility for care, the original chart is <u>sent with the patient</u>.

   True   False   _____

10. Your patient says, "I'm going home today!" You verify this by checking the <u>nursing care plan</u>.

    True   False   _____

MULTIPLE CHOICE

Circle the letter that corresponds to the best answer for each question.

1. Mrs. Rogers is in acute respiratory distress from pneumonia, but refuses to stay for treatment. It is the nurse's responsibility to do which of the following?

   a. Restrain the patient until a social worker can talk to her about the results of her actions.

   b. Call for psychologic counseling to see is she is mentally stable.

   c. Notify physician; discuss the outcomes of the patient's decision and have her sign a release form.

   d. Call the patient's family and have them discharge her.

2. Which of the following actions must be performed by the nurse upon discharging a patient from a healthcare agency?

   a. coordinating future care for the patient

   b. write a discharge order for the patient

   c. write any orders for future home visits that may be necessary for the patient

   d. send the patient's records to the attending physician

3. When patients are transferred within or among health-care settings, which of the following is *most* essential in ensuring continuity of care?

   a. notification of all departments of room change

   b. careful moving of all personal items

   c. asking family members to take home patient's jewelry, money, or other valuables

   d. accurate and complete communication

4. Which of the following health-care providers is responsible for the comfort and well-being of the patient on arrival to the unit?

   a. nurse

   b. physician

   c. nurse's aide

   d. admitting office clerk

5. Which of the following statements best describes the use of the word *ambulatory* in ambulatory healthcare facilities?

   a. The patient must be able to walk upright.

   b. The patient does not remain overnight.

   c. The patient does not have surgery.

   d. The patient remains overnight, but is not bedfast.

6. Which of the following *cognitive skills* would a nurse need to ensure continuity of care for a patient?

   a. The ability to provide the technical nursing assistance to meet the needs of patients and their families.

   b. The ability to establish trusting professional relationships with patients, family caregivers, and healthcare professionals in different practice settings.

   c. The knowledge of how to effectively communicate patient priorities and the related plan of care as a patient is transferred between different settings.

   d. Commitment to securing the best setting for care to be provided for patients and the best coordination of resources to support the level of care needed.

COMPLETION

1. Describe how a nurse could help reduce anxiety for a patient who expresses the following concerns upon being admitted to a healthcare facility.

   a. Who will take care of my children when I'm in here?

   _____

   _____

b. Will the procedure the doctor ordered be painful?

_____

_____

_____

c. Will I be able to afford to be hospitalized?

_____

_____

_____

d. Who will take care of me after my surgery?

_____

_____

_____

2. Briefly describe how a nurse should instruct a patient in the following areas of care prior to discharge.

a. Medications: _____

_____

_____

b. Procedures and treatments: _____

_____

_____

c. Diet: _____

_____

_____

d. Referrals: _____

_____

_____

e. Health promotion: _____

_____

_____

3. Describe how the following methods help provide continuity of care for patients:

a. Discharge planning: _____

_____

_____

b. Collaboration with other members of healthcare team: _____

_____

_____

c. Involving patient and family in planning:

_____

_____

_____

4. List five guidelines that should be followed when admitting and discharging a patient from a hospital according to the standards established by the Joint Commission on Accreditation of Healthcare Organizations.

a. _____

b. _____

c. _____

d. _____

e. _____

5. List four factors the nurse should assess prior to discharge planning for the following patient: A 38-year-old woman hospitalized for a miscarriage in her second month, who has been trying to conceive a child for 2 years, is being discharged:

a. _____

b. _____

c. _____

d. _____

6. Describe the appropriate nursing actions that would be performed during the following patient transfers:

a. Transfer within the hospital setting: _____

_____

_____

b. Transfer to a long-term facility: _____

_____

_____

c. Discharge from a healthcare setting: _____

_____

_____

_____

7. What is the proper procedure for discharging a patient AMA (against medical advice)?

_____

_____

_____

8. Describe how you would prepare a hospital room for a patient who is arriving on a stretcher and is receiving oxygen.

_____

_____

GUIDE TO CRITICAL THINKING AND DEVELOPING BLENDED SKILLS

1. More and more hospital services are being performed on an outpatient basis. While this practice is cost efficient, in many cases patients are being sent home without the fundamental knowledge to care for their conditions. Think about what can be done to bridge the gap between hospital and home healthcare. How would you use this knowledge to discharge a 59-year-old woman who lives alone and is recovering from back surgery?

2. Imagine that your elderly mother is being discharged from the hospital with a stroke that left her partially paralyzed and she is no longer able to live alone. Community living options include a life care community, live-in companion, living with you, or living in a nursing home. Think about the information and support you would need to make this decision. How might this knowledge influence your nursing practice?

CHAPTER 13

Home Healthcare

CHAPTER OVERVIEW

- Home healthcare is a rapidly expanding component of the healthcare system.

- Home healthcare is provided in the patient's home, encompassing the care of patients of all ages and with both chronic and acute healthcare needs.

- Home healthcare began in England, emerged in the United States in the 1880s, and expanded to the older population in the 1960s.

- Nurses who provide home healthcare are increasingly specializing to implement technology and meet patient needs.

- Home healthcare nurses provide care that adapts to the patient's environment. They must have knowledge and skill, be independent, and be accountable.

- Home health nurses are providers of care, and are a patient advocate, coordinator of services, and educator.

- The home visit has two phases: pre-entry and entry. During pre-entry, the nurse collects patient information, gathers supplies, and ensures personal safety. During entry, the nurse develops rapport with the patient and family, mutually determines outcomes, makes assessments, implements care, and provides teaching.

- Caregiver needs are also an important consideration in home healthcare.

- Hospice nursing (care for the dying patient) is often provided in the home, with a focus on improving quality of life and preserving dignity in death.

■ Learning Checklist

Review the learning checklist at the end of the chapter in your textbook and be sure you can meet each objective.

■ Exercises

MATCHING

Match the role of the home healthcare nurse in Part B with the appropriate example of that role in Part B. Answers may be used more than once.

PART A

a. patient advocate

b. coordinator of services

c. patient/family educator

PART B

1. _____ The nurse convinces her patient's insurance carrier that there is a need for continued home health services.

2. _____ The nurse provides information on wound care to a patient's family member.

3. _____ The nurse designs a diet for her patient and explains it to the household cook.

4. _____ The nurse arranges for a physical therapist to visit her patient recovering from a broken hip.

5. _____ The nurse calls in a mental health worker to assess the ability of her patient's husband to provide adequate care.

6. _____ The nurse reports the condition of her patient to his physician.

CORRECT THE FALSE STATEMENT

Circle the word true *or* false *that follows the statement. If the word* false *has been circled, change the* underlined *word/words to make the statement true. Place your answer in the space provided.*

1. One of the changes in the healthcare industry in the past 5 years has been a shift from <u>community-based care to hospital-based care</u>.

   True   False   _____

2. The focus of hospice care is on <u>improving quality of life</u> as opposed to prolonging the length of life.

   True   False   _____

3. The focus of home healthcare is on patients of all ages with <u>acute</u> healthcare needs.

   True   False   _____

4. Once the nurse crosses the threshold of the patient's home, <u>the patient must adapt to the plan of care dictated by the nurse</u>.

   True   False   _____

5. Lillian Wald and <u>William Rathbone</u> opened the Henry Street Settlement House in New York City in 1893.

   True   False   _____

6. The introduction of DRGs in the hospital setting created an <u>earlier</u> discharge from the hospital than patients previously experienced.

   True   False   _____

7. Prior to the late 1980s, home care nurses were considered <u>specialists</u>.

   True   False   _____

8. Nurses providing care in the home <u>are not responsible</u> for independent decision making.

   True   False   _____

9. The <u>home care nurse</u> is responsible for coordinating community resources needed by the patient.

   True   False   _____

10. During the <u>entry phase</u> of the home visit, the nurse develops rapport with the patient and family, mutually determines desired outcomes, makes assessments, plans and implements prescribed care, and provides teaching.

    True   False   _____

11. Home care is meant to be <u>long term</u>.

    True   False   _____

12. <u>Hospice care</u> provides terminally ill patients a humane option of dying with dignity.

    True   False   _____

13. Home nursing agencies emerged in major cities in the <u>late 1800s</u> to meet the needs of the large influx of a growing population due to an influx of immigrants.

    True   False   _____

MULTIPLE CHOICE

1. Which of the following statements concerning the characteristics of a home care nurse is accurate?

   a. Clinical skills are less important in a home care setting than in a hospital setting.

   b. The nurse should not make independent decisions about patient care.

   c. Increased autonomy of the nurse reduces the nurse's legal risks.

   d. Physical assessment, nursing diagnoses, and infection control are all part of the nurse's role.

2. Which of the following statements concerning the unique role of the home care nurse is accurate?

   a. Home care is provided to the patient in a setting that is controlled by the nurse.

   b. The nurse should not feel that she is only a "guest" in the patient's home.

   c. The nurse must adapt to the patient's environment instead of the patient adapting to a strange environment.

   d. Home care nurses do not need the patient's permission to adjust furniture or patient belongings to provide a safe environment.

3. Which of the following activities would be performed by a home care nurse in the pre-entry phase of the home visit?

   a. The nurse gathers supplies that may be needed for the patient.

   b. The nurse develops rapport with the patient and family.

   c. The nurse determines desired outcomes, makes assessments, and plans and implements care.

   d. The nurse provides teaching to promote independence in self-care.

4. The 1990s were a time of transition for the home care industry. Which of the following statements accurately describes a probable trend for future home care?

a. Acuity levels of patients will be lower due to increased care in the hospital setting.

b. More complex services will be provided in the home setting.

c. Families will have less responsibility in caring for loved ones at home.

d. Nursing services will be more generalized to meet the greater demand for home nurses.

COMPLETION

1. Complete the following chart describing the history of home care nursing from the 1800s to the present:

Date	Home Health Care Provider/Location	Type of Care
1893	Henry Street Settlement House NYC	
Prior to WWII	Physician	
During and Post WWII	Nurses	
Mid 1960s	1965 Social Security Act	
Post 1980	Home care specialists	
2000s	Nurses and families	

3. Give a brief definition and example of the following roles of the home health nurse.

a. Patient advocate: _____

_____

_____

b. Coordinator of services: _____

_____

_____

c. Educator: _____

_____

_____

2. Give an example of how you personally have used or witnessed the following characteristics of a home care nurse in your practice.

a. Knowledge and skills: _____

_____

_____

b. Independence: _____

_____

c. Accountability: _____

_____

_____

4. List the four basic premises behind the bag technique:

a. _____

b. _____

c. _____

d. _____

5. Describe how teaching is designed and implemented in the home care situation: _____

_____

_____

6. Explain why the family is so important to the patient's recovery as healthcare continues to shift from the hospital setting to community based care:

_____

_____

7. What type of care and skills would a hospice nurse employ in caring for a 35-year-old mother, dying of AIDS, who is living at home with her husband and two children, 13 and 6? _____

_____

_____

GUIDE TO CRITICAL THINKING AND DEVELOPING BLENDED SKILLS

1. Identify care priorities for the patients listed below who are being transferred to a home healthcare setting. Be sure to include physical, psychologic, socioeconomic, environmental, spiritual, and cultural assessments for each patient. Think about nursing's role in making necessary resources available to the patient and family.

   a. A 76-year-old male patient with advanced cancer is being sent home with a catheter and a patient-controlled analgesic pump. He lives alone, but his son lives 45 minutes away and has promised to check on him once a day. Members of his church have offered to visit him and bring him a meal once a day.

   b. A 32-year-old male with advanced AIDS is being sent home to spend his remaining days with his parents. His life partner died of AIDS the previous year, and he is angry about his situation. His parents do not accept his condition and lifestyle, but offer to take care of his healthcare needs.

   c. A young single mother who lives with her boyfriend is released from the hospital with an infant who has Down syndrome. Both the mother and her boyfriend work and need two incomes to maintain the household. The mother has expressed concerns about being able to take care of her infant and give him the proper treatment and attention.

2. Volunteer to help a home healthcare nurse who is practicing in the field. See how this professional bridges the gap between hospital and long-term facility care. Interview some of the patients and ask them if they feel their healthcare needs are being met by home healthcare agencies. Ask the home healthcare nurse if she feels the system is working and, if appropriate, what could be done to provide a higher quality of care for these patients.

The Nursing Process

CHAPTER 14

Blended Skills and Critical Thinking Throughout the Nursing Process

CHAPTER OVERVIEW

- The nursing process is a systematic method that directs the nurse and patient as they together determine the need for nursing care (assessing and diagnosing) and then plan, implement, and evaluate care.

- The primary purpose of the nursing process is to help the nurse manage each patient's nursing care scientifically, holistically, and creatively.

- In each step of the nursing process, the nurse and patient work together as partners. The patient's health state and resources influence his or her level of participation.

- Assessment is the systematic and continuous collection, validation, and communication of patient data.

- Diagnosing is the analysis of patient data to identify (1) data clusters that indicate actual or potential problems in the way the patient is responding to the illness, (2) factors that contribute to or cause these problems, and (3) coping patterns or other strengths the patient can draw on to prevent or resolve the problem.

- During the planning step of the nursing process, the nurse, working with the patient, (1) develops patient goals/expected outcomes that, if achieved, prevent, reduce, or eliminate the problems specified in the nursing diagnoses, and (2) identifies the nursing interventions most likely to achieve these goals/outcomes.

- Implementation is simply the carrying out of the plan of nursing care. It includes all the actions performed by the nurse to promote wellness, prevent disease and illness, restore health, and facilitate coping with altered functioning.

- During evaluation, the nurse and patient measure how well the patient has achieved the goals/outcomes specified in the plan of care and identify factors that positively or negatively influenced goal achievement. Patient responses to the plan of care determine if nursing care is to be continued without change, modified, or terminated.

- Underlying the science and art of nursing is a successful blend of the scientific problem-solving method and the intuitive method.

- The nursing process is systematic, each step depending on the accuracy of the previous step and influencing the steps that follow. The steps of the nursing process are interrelated; each step is fluid and moves into the rest.

- The nursing process is an interpersonal process that is always patient-centered rather than task-centered. As nurses help patients to use their strengths to meet all their human needs, nurses themselves grow personally and professionally.

- A goal-oriented process, the nursing process offers a means for nurses and patients to work together to identify the specific health goals that are most important to the patient and to match these with the appropriate nursing interventions.

- The unique challenges now confronting nurses demand that nurses be proficient in cognitive, technical, interpersonal, and ethical/legal competencies.

- Cognitive competencies enable nurses to "make sense" of their world and to grasp conceptually what is necessary to achieve valued goals. It is impossible to practice nursing successfully without using critical thinking skills.

- Nurses wishing to develop critical thinking skills will find it helpful to work through five sets of considerations when posed with a thinking challenge: (1) purpose of thinking, (2) adequacy of knowledge, (3) potential problems, (4) helpful resources, and (5) critique of judgment/decision.

- Technical competencies enable nurses to use equipment and procedures with sufficient competence and ease to achieve goals with minimal distress to the involved participants.

- Interpersonal competencies enable nurses to establish and maintain caring relationships that facilitate the achievement of valued goals while affirming the worth of participants in the relationship.

- Ethical and legal competencies enable nurses to conduct their lives in a manner that is consistent with their personal moral code and professional role responsibilities.

- Professional codes of ethics obligate nurses to report professional conduct that is incompetent, unethical, or illegal.

■ Learning Checklist

Review the learning checklist at the end of the chapter in your textbook and be sure you can meet each objective.

■ Exercises

MATCHING

Match the step of the nursing process, listed in Part A, with the related task listed in Part B. Answers will be used more than once.

PART A

a. assessing

b. diagnosing

c. planning

d. implementing

e. evaluating

PART B

1. __a__ A nurse performs an initial patient interview.

2. __d__ A home care nurse helps the physical therapist exercise his patient's limbs.

3. __e__ A nurse sits down with the healthcare team halfway through treatment of a patient to see how effective the treatment has been.

4. __b__ A nurse analyzes data to determine what health problems might exist.

5. __c__ A nurse sets a goal for an obese teenager to lose 2 pounds a week.

6. __a__ A nurse consults with a patient's support people and other healthcare professionals to learn more about a patient problem.

7. __e__ A nurse decides whether to continue, modify or terminate the healthcare plan.

8. __b__ A nurse identifies the strengths a patient with cancer possesses.

9. __c__ A home care nurse determines how much nursing care is needed by an elderly stroke patient living with her daughter.

10. __e__ A nurse weighs a patient after 3 weeks to determine if his new diet has been effective.

11. __d__ A nurse documents respiratory care performed on a patient.

12. __a__ A nurse reviews a patient's past medical records.

Match the competencies listed in Part A with the appropriate example of competencies listed in Part B. Answers will be used more than once.

PART A

a. cognitive competencies

b. technical competencies

c. interpersonal competencies

d. ethical/legal competencies

PART B

13. __c__ A nurse skillfully conducts a patient interview in which her patient relaxes and "opens up" to her.

14. __b__ A nurse skillfully attaches a heart monitor to a patient.

15. __d__ A nurse carefully fills out an incident report, documenting a fall.

16. __a__ A nurse understands the need for palpating the lungs of a patient with pneumonia.

17. __d__ A nurse checks the side rails on a bed of an elderly patient with a history of falls.

18. __b__ A nurse successfully performs a catheterization of a patient.

19. __a__ A nurse is familiar with the various types of medications for high blood pressure and their side effects.

20. __c__ A nurse calms the mother of an infant brought to the ER with a high fever.

21. __b__ A nurse competently starts an IV drip on a patient.

22. __d__ A nurse checks a patient's bracelet before administering medications.

MULTIPLE CHOICE

1. Which of the following statements concerning the nursing process is accurate?

   a. The nursing process is nurse-oriented.

   b. The steps of the nursing process are separate entities.

   c. The nursing process is nursing practice in action.

   d. The nursing process comprises four steps to promote patient well-being.

2. Which of the following groups legitimized the steps of the nursing process in 1973, by developing standards of practice to guide nursing practice?

   a. American Nurses Association Congress for Nursing Practice

   b. Joint Commission on Accreditation of Health Care Organizations

   c. The National League of Nursing

   d. American Association of Critical Care Nursing

3. Which of the following characteristics of the nursing process could be defined as an overlapping and great interaction among the five steps with each step being fluid and flowing into the next step?

   a. interpersonal

   b. dynamic

   c. systematic

   e. universally applicable

4. Which of the following statements accurately depicts a step in the critical thinking process?

   a. The first step when thinking critically is to gather as much data related to the question as possible.

   b. Nurses who think critically allow emotions to direct their thinking.

   c. Nurses who use the critical thinking process ultimately must identify alternative decisions and reach a conclusion.

   d. The critical thinking process is based on intuition and excludes the use of outside resources.

5. In which of the following cases is the nursing process applicable?

   a. When nurses work with patients who are able to participate in their care

   b. When families are clearly supportive and wish to participate in care

   c. When patients are totally dependent on the nurse for care

   d. In all the nursing situations listed above

6. Which of the following interpersonal skills is displayed by a nurse who is attentive and responsive to the healthcare needs of individual patients and ensures the continuity of care when leaving the patient?

   a. establishing caring relationships

   b. enjoying the rewards of mutual interchange

   c. developing accountability

   d. developing ethical/legal skills

7. Which of the following traits helps nurses develop the attitudes and dispositions to think critically?

   a. thinking independently

   b. being intellectually humble

   c. being curious and persevering

   d. all of the above

8. A nurse who is responsible for "whistle-blowing" has acted in which of the following manners?

   a. The nurse has conferred with a physician suspected of malpractice.

   b. The nurse has investigated a charge of nurse incompetence.

   c. The nurse has complained about insurance fraud.

   d. The nurse has reported employer violation of law.

COMPLETION

1. List three patient and three nursing benefits of using the nursing process correctly.

   Patient:

   a. _____

   b. _____

   c. _____

Nursing:

a. _____

b. _____

c. _____

2. Describe how the nurse and patient work together to accomplish the following tasks of the nursing process.

a. Determining the need for nursing care: _____

_____

_____

b. Planning and implementing the care: _____

_____

_____

c. Evaluating the results of the nursing care: _____

_____

_____

3. Define the nursing process: _____

_____

_____

_____

What are the primary goals of the nursing process? _____

_____

_____

What skills are necessary to use the nursing process successfully? _____

_____

_____

Which of these skills do you personally possess and which do you need to develop in your practice? _____

_____

_____

4. Describe what the following words mean to you and how they apply to your use of the nursing process:

a. Systematic: _____

_____

_____

b. Dynamic: _____

_____

_____

c. Interpersonal: _____

_____

_____

d. Goal-oriented: _____

_____

_____

e. Universally applicable: _____

_____

_____

5. Briefly explain how the following considerations are relevant to the successful use of critical thinking competencies.

a. Purpose of thinking: _____

_____

_____

b. Adequacy of knowledge: _____

_____

_____

c. Potential problems: _____

_____

_____

d. Helpful resources: _____

_____

_____

e. Critique of judgment/decision: _____

_____

_____

6. List four good habits nurses should develop to help them master the manual competencies essential to quality nursing process.

a. _____

b. _____

c. _____

d. _____

7. Think of three people you know personally, preferably of different ages/professions/cultures. What about each of these individuals causes you to respect their human dignity? Are some people more deserving of respect than others? How do you show respect for them in your daily contact with them?

_____

_____

_____

8. Follow three different nurses around on their daily rounds of patients, noticing how they relate to their patients. Does their attitude say "drop dead," "you mean nothing to me," or "I care about you"? Note what each nurse said or did to display this attitude.

a. Nurse one: _____

_____

_____

b. Nurse two: _____

_____

_____

c. Nurse three: _____

_____

_____

9. Nurses skilled in developing caring relationships often need to direct the conversations with their patients. Develop four opening statements/questions designed to elicit information from a patient that you could use in your own practice.

a. _____

_____

_____

b. _____

_____

_____

c. _____

_____

_____

d. _____

_____

_____

10. List four areas a nurse should consider when seeking to develop a sense of legal and ethical accountability to a patient.

a. _____

_____

_____

b. _____

_____

_____

c. _____

_____

_____

d. _____

_____

_____

GUIDE TO CRITICAL THINKING AND DEVELOPING BLENDED SKILLS

1. Assess your personal blend of the skills nurses need: cognitive, technical, interpersonal, ethical/legal. Would you want *you* to be your nurse? What skills do you need to develop to better meet the needs of those entrusted to your care?

2. Think about major health problems on campus. How might the school of nursing use the nursing process to address one or more of these problems? Do you as a nursing student have an obligation to address the health problem you encounter widely?

3. Think about a stressful situation you had to deal with in your past, such as changing a course of study, accepting a job in another city, dealing with a sick relative, deciding on a life partner, and so on. What methods did you use to weigh all your options in making a life decision? Where did you turn for information or assistance? How did you come to your final decision? Relate the method you used in your personal life to the models of problem solving listed in this chapter. Which process most accurately describes your personal process of problem solving? Compare this process to the nursing process.

4. Write down all the qualities you admire in your friends. What is it about them that makes you respect them? What attributes of their personality don't you like? How might this knowledge help you to understand your responses to patients with different personality traits? Are some patients more worthy of your respect than others? Do you feel your attitude toward a patient affects the outcome of their treatment?

CHAPTER 15

Assessing

CHAPTER OVERVIEW

- Assessing is the systematic and continuous collection, validation, and communication of patient data. A database is all the pertinent patient information collected by the nurse and other healthcare professionals that enables a comprehensive and effective plan of care to be designed and implemented for the patient.

- Ongoing nursing assessment alerts the nurse to changes in the patient's responses to health and illness and suggests necessary changes in the plan of care.

- Unlike medical assessments, whose primary purpose is to define the existence of medical problems and identify the underlying pathology, nursing assessments are focused primarily on patient responses to health problems.

- Objective data are perceptible to the senses and verifiable by another person observing the same data. Subjective data can be perceived only by the affected person and cannot be perceived or verified experientially by another.

- Common methods used for collecting data in nursing are observation, interview, and physical assessment. Observation is the conscious and deliberate use of the five senses to gather data. Skilled nurses observe patients for significant data during each nurse–patient interaction.

- Strong interviewing skills are needed by the nurse to obtain a comprehensive nursing history that captures the unique qualities and characteristics of the patient in a way that makes individualized care planning possible.

- During the nursing physical assessment, the nurse assesses the patient for objective data to better define the patient's condition and help the nurse in planning care. The nursing examination focuses primarily on the patient's functional abilities.

- The primary source of patient data is the patient. Unless otherwise specified, it is assumed that the data recorded in the nursing history are from the patient. Other important sources of patient data are the patient's support people, the patient record, other healthcare professionals, and the nursing and related healthcare literature.

- A database nursing assessment is done during the nurse's initial contact with the patient, and involves collecting data about all aspects of the patient's health. A focused assessment may be done during any nurse–patient interaction. Its purpose is to gather data about a specific problem.

- Before beginning to collect data, the nurse should have a good sense of the type of data needed to develop a satisfactory plan of care. Assessment priorities are influenced by the patient's health orientation, developmental stage, and need for nursing.

- Using systematic assessment guidelines specifically developed for a nursing assessment ensures that comprehensive, holistic data are collected for each patient and that those data easily lead to the formulation of nursing diagnoses.

- Problems related to data collection include inappropriate organization of database, omission of pertinent data, irrelevant or duplicate data, erroneous or misinterpreted data, too little data acquired from the patient, recording of interpretation of data rather than observed behavior, and failure to update database.

- Validation is the act of confirming or verifying. The purpose of validation is to keep data as free from error, bias, and misinterpretation as possible. Data need to be verified when they contain discrepancies and lack objectivity.

- Patient data collected by the nurse, both initially and as patient contact continues, are of no benefit to the patient and the nursing and healthcare teams unless they are appropriately communicated. It is important to learn when significant data need to be communicated verbally immediately and how to document data.

- Patient data should be summarized and written so that they communicate a unique sense of the patient and are comprehensive, concise, and easily retrievable.

■ Learning Checklist

Review the learning checklist at the end of the chapter in your textbook and be sure you can meet each objective.

■ Exercises

MATCHING

Match the term in Part A with the definition in Part B.

PART A

a. database

b. focused assessment

c. nursing interview

d. health assessment

e. nursing history

f. objective data

g. physical assessment

h. subjective data

i. validation

j. observation

k. time-lapsed assessments

PART B

1. _____ Observable and measurable information that can be seen, heard, or felt by someone other than the person experiencing them.

2. _____ The conscious and deliberate use of the five physical senses to gather information

3. _____ Clearly identifies patient strengths and weaknesses, health risks, and potential and existing health problems.

4. _____ A planned communication to obtain patient data.

5. _____ The examination of a patient for objective data that may better define the patient's condition and help the nurse in planning care.

6. _____ The act of confirming or verifying data.

7. _____ Compares a patient's current status to baseline data obtained earlier.

8. _____ Includes all the pertinent patient information collected by the nurse and other healthcare professionals, enabling a comprehensive and effective plan of care to be designed and implemented for the patient.

9. _____ The gathering of data about a specific problem that has already been identified.

10. _____ May be used by nurses to help patients identify potential and actual health risks and to explore their habits, behaviors, beliefs, attitudes, and values that influence their health.

Match the examples of data in Part B with the type of data in Part A. Answers may be used more than once.

PART A

a. objective data

b. subjective data

PART B

11. _____ Redness and swelling are noticed at the site of an incision.

12. _____ A patient complains of pain in his left arm.

13. _____ A patient has a violent spell of coughing.

14. _____ A patient recovering from knee surgery favors his impaired leg when walking.

15. _____ A patient is nauseated at the sight of food.

16. _____ A patient worries about her children during her hospital stay.

MULTIPLE CHOICE

Circle the letter that corresponds to the best answer for each question.

1. Which of the following statements concerning nursing assessments is accurate?

   a. Nursing assessments duplicate medical assessments.

   b. Nursing assessments target data pointing to pathology.

   c. Nursing assessments focus on patient responses to health problems.

   d. Nursing assessments focus on the identification of a medical diagnosis.

2. Data that can be observed by one person and verified by another person observing the same patient are known as

   a. subjective data

   b. covert data

   c. symptomatic data

   d. objective data

3. During which of the following phases of the nurse–patient interview does the nurse gather all the information needed to form the subjective database?

   a. preparatory phase

   b. introduction

   c. working phase

   d. termination

4. Which of the following nurse/patient positions facilitates an easy exchange of information?

   a. If the patient is in bed, the nurse stands at the foot of the bed.

   b. When seated, the nurse/patient's chairs should be placed at right angles to each other, 1 foot apart.

   c. If the patient is in bed, a chair should be placed at a 45-degree angle to the bed.

   d. If the patient is in bed, the nurse stands at the side of the bed.

5. Which of the following sources of patient data is usually the primary and best source?

   a. patient

   b. support people

   c. patient records

   d. reports of diagnostic studies

6. Mrs. Smith is admitted to the hospital with c/o left-sided weakness and difficulty speaking. Which of the following assessments contains the data that best represent a nursing assessment?

   a. Neurologic exam reveals partial paralysis and aphasic speech.

   b. Brain scan shows evidence of a clot in the middle cerebral artery.

   c. Unable to communicate basic needs and perform hygiene measures with left hand.

   d. Left-sided weakness and speech deficit indicate probable stroke.

7. Mr. Martin is an energetic 80-year-old man, admitted to the hospital with c/o difficulty urinating, bloody urine, and burning on urination. In assessing Mr. Martin, which of the following data collection priorities should be included?

   a. Assessing only the urinary system

   b. Focusing on altered patterns of elimination common in the elderly

   c. Obtaining a detailed assessment of the patient's sexual history

   d. Conducting a thorough systems review to validate data on the patient's record

8. During the nursing examination, Mrs. Jones becomes very tired. There are still questions the nurse practitioner would have liked to address in order to have data for planning care. Which of the following actions would be most appropriate in this situation?

   a. Ask Mrs. Jones to wake up and try to answer your questions.

   b. Ask Mrs. Jones's husband to come in and answer your questions.

   c. Wait until the next day to obtain the answers to your questions.

   d. Ask Mrs. Jones if she objects to your interviewing her husband to obtain the needed data.

9. Mrs. Anderson is a 50-year-old woman admitted to your unit with the diagnosis of scleroderma. You are unfamiliar with this condition. Which of the following would be your best source of information?

   a. Consult with the patient.

   b. Consult with the patient's doctor.

   c. Read the patient's chart.

   d. Consult nursing and medical literature.

COMPLETION

1. List the five functions of the initial comprehensive nursing assessment.

   a. _____

   b. _____

   c. _____

   d. _____

   e. _____

2. Identify eight sources of patient data and give an example of each.

   a. _____

   b. _____

   c. _____

   d. _____

   e. _____

   f. _____

   g. _____

   h. _____

3. Briefly describe why the following characteristics of data are important when collecting and recording patient data:

   a. Complete: _____

   b. Factual and accurate: _____

   c. Relevant: _____

4. Give an example of three observations nurses should make each time they encounter a patient.

   a. _____

   b. _____

   c. _____

5. List three patient goals that should be accomplished by the end of the introduction phase of the patient interview.

   a. _____

   b. _____

   c. _____

6. Give two examples of closed questions, open-ended questions, and reflective questions that could be employed to elicit information from the following patient:

   A 42-year-old mother of three young children, who was recently diagnosed with diabetes, is admitted to the hospital overnight for observation.

   a. Closed questions: _____

   _____

   _____

   b. Open-ended questions: _____

   _____

   _____

   c. Reflective questions: _____

   _____

   _____

7. Explain how the following factors affect assessment priorities when collecting patient data.

   a. Patient's health orientation: _____

   _____

   _____

b. Patient's developmental stage: _____

   _____

   _____

c. Patient's need for nursing: _____

   _____

   _____

8. Give two examples of when data need to be validated.

   a. _____

   b. _____

9. Explain when the immediate communication of data is indicated.

   _____

   _____

   _____

GUIDE TO CRITICAL THINKING AND DEVELOPING BLENDED SKILLS

1. Roleplay the following nursing interviews with your classmates:

   a. A 50-year-old woman with diabetes and diabetic foot ulcers is admitted to the ER for observation after she experienced a blackout.

   b. An 85-year-old African American man is admitted to the ICU after experiencing a possible stroke.

   c. A teenage boy is admitted to the hospital with severe stomach pains and possible ruptured appendix.

   Talk about which approaches and types of questions (closed, open-ended, reflective, direct) resulted in the best interviews.

2. Recall the last time you went to a doctor's office for a check-up or medical problem. How were you treated by the doctor's staff? Did they do anything to make you feel comfortable/uncomfortable? What did they do to include you in the process? How did it feel to be a patient at the mercy of others? What would you do to incorporate this learning into your own nursing practice?

CHAPTER 16

Diagnosing

CHAPTER OVERVIEW

- The purpose of diagnosing is the identification of (1) problems in the way the patient is responding to health or illness, (2) factors that contribute to or cause these problems (etiologies), and (3) strengths the patient can draw on to prevent or resolve the problems.

- Actual or potential health problems that independent nursing intervention can prevent or resolve are termed nursing diagnoses.

- Once significant patient data are detected, the nurse looks for data clusters that signal a patient strength or problem, and checks out these findings with the patient.

- The interpretation and analysis of patient data may lead to the identification of nursing diagnoses or collaborative problems (best treated by nurses working together with other healthcare professionals) or, when shared with a physician, may contribute to medical diagnoses.

- Most nursing diagnoses are written as either two-part statements that contain the patient problem and its etiology connected by the words *related to*, or as three-part statements that include the problem's defining characteristics.

- A wellness diagnosis is a one-part statement that contains the label *Potential for Enhanced* followed by the desired higher-level wellness.

- The problem component of the nursing diagnosis identifies what is unhealthy about the patient, indicating the need for change. It suggests the patient goals. The etiology identifies the factors that are maintaining the unhealthy state or response and suggests the appropriate nursing intervention. The defining characteristics are the subjective and objective data that initially signaled the existence of the problem. They suggest evaluative criteria.

- Although nursing care may be related to the following, they are not nursing diagnoses and should not appear in the diagnostic statement: medical diagnosis, medical pathology, diagnostic tests, treatments, equipment, therapeutic patient needs,

therapeutic patient goals, a single sign or symptom, and *unvalidated* nursing inferences.

- Other sources of error when writing nursing diagnoses include making legally inadvisable statements, reversing the clauses, identifying environmental factors rather than patient factors as the problem, identifying as a patient response what is not necessarily unhealthful, having both clauses say the same thing, and identifying as a patient problem what cannot be changed.

■ Learning Checklist

Review the learning checklist at the end of the chapter in your textbook and be sure you can meet each objective.

■ Exercises

MATCHING

Match the examples listed in Part B with the four steps involved in the interpretation and analysis of data listed in Part A. Answers will be used more than once.

PART A

a. recognizing significant data

b. recognizing patterns or clusters

c. identifying strengths and problems

d. reaching conclusions

PART B

1. _____ A nurse notes that a patient's refusal to stop smoking will adversely affect his recovery from cardiac surgery.

2. _____ A nurse compares a 15-month-old child's motor abilities with the norms for that age group.

3. _____ A nurse recognizes an unhealthy situation developing around a woman recovering from a mastectomy who cries at night, refuses to eat meals, and sleeps all day.

4. _____ A nurse decides no further nursing response is indicated for a woman who recovered from gallbladder surgery according to schedule.

5. _____ A maternity nurse notices a newborn's skin tone is markedly different than that of the other babies and checks for jaundice.

6. _____ A nurse determines that a man with a history of diabetes is highly motivated to develop a healthy pattern of nutrition in response to his problem.

7. _____ A nurse notices that a patient with AIDS has an adverse reaction to a drug and consults the prescribing physician.

CORRECT THE FALSE STATEMENTS

Circle the word true or false that follows the statement. If the word false has been circled, change the underlined word/words to make the statement true. Place your answers in the space provided.

1. Actual or potential health problems that can be prevented or resolved by independent nursing intervention are termed underline{collaborative problems}.

   True   False   _____

2. underline{Medical diagnoses} represent situations that are the primary responsibility of nurses.

   True   False   _____

3. A underline{cue} is a generally accepted rule, measure, pattern, or model that can be used to compare data in the same class or category.

   True   False   _____

4. A underline{data cluster} is a grouping of patient data or cues that points to the existence of a patient health problem.

   True   False   _____

5. Nursing diagnoses should be derived from underline{a single cue}.

   True   False   _____

6. underline{The NANDA list} is a beginning list of suggested terms for health problems that may be identified and treated by nurses.

   True   False   _____

7. The underline{problem statement} of a nursing diagnosis identifies the physiologic, psychologic, sociologic, spiritual, and environmental factors believed to be related to the problem as either a cause or a contributing factor.

   True   False   _____

8. The underline{etiology} of nursing diagnoses directs nursing intervention.

   True   False   _____

9. A underline{possible} nursing diagnosis is written when the health problem is likely to occur unless the nurse intervenes.

   True   False   _____

10. A underline{possible} nursing diagnosis is written when the nurse suspects that a health problem exists, but needs to gather more data to confirm the diagnosis.

    True   False   _____

11. A underline{wellness diagnosis} is a clinical judgment about an individual, family, or community in transition from a specific level of wellness to a higher level of wellness.

    True   False   _____

12. In the diagnosing step, the nurse underline{collects patient data}.

    True   False   _____

13. A underline{possible nursing diagnosis} is a clinical judgment that an individual, family, or community is more vulnerable to develop the problem than others in the same or similar situation.

    True   False   _____

MULTIPLE CHOICE

Circle the letter that corresponds to the best answer for each question.

1. Which of the following statements regarding nursing diagnoses is accurate?
   a. Nursing diagnoses remain the same for as long as the disease is present.
   b. Nursing diagnoses are written to identify diseases.
   c. Nursing diagnoses are written to describe patient problems that nurses can treat.
   d. Nursing diagnoses focus on identifying healthy responses to health and illness.

2. Which of the following is an actual or potential health problem that can be prevented or resolved by independent nursing intervention?

    a. Nursing diagnoses

    b. Nursing assessments

    c. Medical diagnoses

    d. Collaborative problems

3. Which of the following would be an appropriate nursing diagnosis for a toddler who has been treated on two different occasions for lacerations and contusions due to parental negligence in providing a safe environment for their child.

    a. High risk/injury related to abusive parents

    b. Injury, high risk for, related to impaired home management

    c. Child abuse related to unsafe home environment

    d. High risk for injury related to unsafe home environment

4. Which of the following nursing diagnoses would be written when the nurse suspects that a health problem exists, but needs to gather more data to confirm the diagnosis?

    a. Actual

    b. Potential

    c. Possible

    d. Apparent

5. Which of the following is an example of a properly written wellness diagnosis?

    a. Potential for enhanced self-esteem

    b. Possible enhanced self-esteem

    c. Enhanced self-esteem potential

    d. Potential for enhanced self-esteem related to nutrition education

6. Which of the following guidelines for writing a nursing diagnosis is accurate?

    a. Phrase the nursing diagnosis as a patient *need* as opposed to a patient *problem*.

    b. Check to make sure the etiology precedes the patient problem and that the two are linked by the words "related to."

    c. Make sure any included defining characteristics follow the etiology and are linked by the phrase "as manifested by" or "as evidenced by."

    d. Use defining characteristics and medical diagnoses to support the problem statement.

COMPLETION

1. Place a check next to the nursing diagnoses that are written correctly and identify the errors in the incorrect diagnoses on the lines that follow.

    a. _____ High risk for injury related to absence of restraints and side rails.

    _____

    b. _____ Impaired skin integrity related to mobility deficit.

    _____

    c. _____ Grieving related to loss of breast.

    _____

    d. _____ Self-care deficit: bathing related to immobility.

    _____

    e. _____ Sleep pattern disturbance related to insomnia.

    _____

    f. _____ Nutrition, alteration in: less than body requirements; related to loss of appetite.

    _____

    g. _____ Powerlessness related to poor family support system.

    _____

    h. _____ Anxiety: mild, related to changing life style/diet.

    _____

    i. _____ Ineffective airway clearance related to 20-year smoking habit.

    _____

    j. _____ Alteration in bowel elimination: constipation related to cancer of bowel.

    _____

    k. _____ Nausea and vomiting related to medication side effects.

    _____

    l. _____ Knowledge deficit related to noncompliance with diet.

    _____

    m. _____ Alteration in parenting related to knowledge deficit: child growth and development, discipline.

    _____

n. _____ Pain related to discomfort in abdomen.

_____

o. _____ Impaired physical mobility: amputation of left leg related to gangrene.

_____

p. _____ Alteration in nutrition: more than body requirements related to obesity.

_____

q. _____ Noncompliance related to unresolved hostility.

_____

r. _____ Needs assistance walking to bathroom:

related to immobility.

_____

2. What questions would you ask a patient to validate the following nursing diagnoses?

a. Altered urinary elimination: _____

_____

_____

b. Impaired social interaction: _____

_____

_____

c. Ineffective individual coping: _____

_____

_____

d. Sleep pattern disturbance: _____

_____

_____

3. Describe the appropriate nursing response to each of the following basic conclusions after interpreting and analyzing patient data.

a. No problem: _____

_____

_____

b. Possible problem: _____

_____

_____

c. Actual or potential nursing diagnosis: _____

_____

_____

d. Clinical problem other than nursing diagnosis:

_____

_____

4. Give three examples of how standards may be used to identify significant cues.

a. _____

_____

_____

b. _____

_____

_____

c. _____

_____

_____

Read the three mini-cases that follow and in each, underline the cues that form a data cluster indicating a nursing diagnosis, and write the appropriate nursing diagnosis as a three-part statement.

5. Mr. Klinetob, age 86, has been seriously depressed since the death 6 months ago of his wife of 52 years. Although he suffers from degenerative joint disease and has talked for years about having "just a touch of arthritis," this never kept him from being up and about. Recently, however, he spends all day sitting in a chair and seems to have no desire to engage in self-care activities. He tells the visiting nurse that he doesn't get washed up anymore because he's "too stiff" in the morning to bathe and "just doesn't seem to have the energy." The visiting nurse notices that his hair is matted and uncombed, his face has traces of previous meals, and he has a strong body odor. His children have complained that their normally fastidious father seems not to care about personal hygiene any longer.

Nursing Diagnosis: _____

_____

_____

_____

_____

6. Miss Ebenezer sustained a right-sided cerebral infarct that resulted in left hemiparesis (paralysis on the left side of the body) and left "neglect." She ignores the left side of her body and actually denies its existence. When asked about her left leg, she stated that it belonged to the woman in the next bed—this while she was in a private room. This patient was previously quite active; she walked for 45–60 minutes four or five times a week, and was an avid swimmer. At present, she cannot move either her left arm or leg.

Nursing Diagnosis: _____

_____

_____

_____

_____

7. Ted and Rosemary Hines tried to conceive a child, unsuccessfully, for 11 years. At this time, they sought the assistance of a fertility specialist who was highly recommended by a friend. It was determined that Ted's sperm was inadequate, and Rosemary was inseminated with sperm from an anonymous donor. The Hines were told that the donor was healthy and that he was selected because he resembled Ted. Rosemary became pregnant after the second in vitro fertilization attempt and delivered a healthy baby girl named Sarah.

At the time they present for counseling, their child is 7 years old, and Ted and Rosemary have learned from blood tests that their fertility specialist is the biologic father of their child. It seems that he lied to some couples about using sperm from anonymous donors, and deceived others into thinking the wives had become pregnant when he had simply injected them with hormones. Ted and Rosemary have joined other couples in pressing charges against this physician.

Rosemary informs the nurse in her pediatrician's office that she is concerned about how all this is affecting her family. "Ted and I both love Sarah and would do nothing to hurt her, but I am so angry about this whole situation that I am afraid I may be taking it out on her." Questioning reveals that Rosemary has found herself yelling at Sarah for minor disobedience and spanking her, something she rarely did before. Both Ted and Rosemary had commented before about Sarah's striking physical resemblance to the fertility specialist, but attributed this to coincidence. "Whenever I see her now I can't help but see Dr. Clowser and everything inside me

clenches up and I want to scream." Both Ted and Rosemary express great remorse that Sarah, who is innocent, is bearing the brunt of something that is in no way her fault.

Nursing Diagnosis: _____

_____

_____

_____

_____

GUIDE TO CRITICAL THINKING AND DEVELOPING BLENDED SKILLS

1. With a partner or several classmates, write appropriate nursing diagnoses for the following patient. Be sure to include actual, potential, and possible diagnoses. Compare your diagnoses with your partner's and note similarities and differences. Decide which diagnoses best suit the patient's situation.

   a. A 35-year-old woman presents with chills, fever, and severe vaginal bleeding. She tells you she's 2 months pregnant and has had a miscarriage two previous times. She is overwrought and says she feels God is punishing her for an abortion she had when she was in college. Although she and her husband have been trying to have children for years, they haven't been successful and were counting on this pregnancy to come to term.

2. Interview members of your family or several close friends. Identify wellness diagnoses for each person. What factors contributed to these diagnoses?

CHAPTER 17

Planning

CHAPTER OVERVIEW

- During planning, the nurse works with the patient and family to (1) develop patient goals/outcomes that, if achieved, prevent, reduce, or eliminate the problems specified in the nursing diagnoses; and (2) identify the nursing interventions most likely to help the patient achieve these goals.

- Conscious, deliberate planning individualizes care, helps communication among nurses, identifies priorities of care, promotes continuity of care, coordinates care, facilitates evaluation of the patient's responses to care, and promotes the nurse's professional development.

- The three types of planning essential to comprehensive nursing care are initial, ongoing problem-oriented, and discharge.

- When planning care, the nurse reviews the prioritized list of nursing diagnoses to see that diagnoses are ranked according to the level of threat they present to patient well-being. Any changes in the patient's health status or in the way the patient is responding to health and illness or the treatment plan may signal the need to reestablish patient priorities.

- A patient goal/outcome describes an expected patient behavior. Patient goals are derived from the problem statement of the nursing diagnosis, and once achieved, they contribute to the prevention or resolution of this problem.

- Each patient goal/outcome must have a subject (the patient), a verb (which clearly indicates the action the patient is expected to perform), and criteria that describe in observable, measurable terms the expected patient behavior.

- Patient goals/outcomes should be valued by the patient, be supportive of the total treatment plan, be brief, be specific, and be stated positively.

- Nursing interventions are derived from the etiology of the nursing diagnosis. The effective nurse chooses from various possible nursing interventions those that specifically address factors that cause or contribute to the patient's problems.

- Effective nursing interventions are consistent with standards of care; realistic in terms of the abilities, time, and resources available to the nurse and patient; compatible with the patient's values, beliefs, and psychosocial background; valued by the patient; and compatible with other planned therapies.

- Nursing orders clearly and concisely describe the nursing intervention to be performed; are signed by the nurse prescribing the order, and dated; use acceptable abbreviations, symbols, and key phrases; and refer nurses to procedure manuals for the steps of lengthy, routine procedures.

- Comprehensive nursing orders specify what observations need to be made and how often; what nursing interventions need to be done, how they are to be done, and when; and the teaching, counseling, and advocacy needs of patients and families.

- The plan of nursing care is the written guide that directs the efforts of the nursing team as they work with patients to meet health goals. Primarily, nursing care plans ensure that nursing care is goal-oriented, efficient, effective, and individualized.

- The nurse who best knows the patient develops the plan of care in a reasonable time frame, dictated by the patient's condition. The plan is written in ink (part of the patient's permanent record) and signed and dated by the nurse who develops the plan. Alternatively, the plan of care is entered into the computer as dictated by agency policy.

- Many institutions use a Kardex system of care planning, which specifies nursing care related to basic human needs, prioritized nursing diagnoses, and the medical plan of care. Each patient's 6 × 11–inch Kardex care plan is placed in a central Kardex file.

- Standardized plans are prepared plans of care that specify care guidelines and outcomes for groups of patients with common care needs. These plans may be computerized. Interdisciplinary critical pathways are an example of one type of standardized plan.

- Most student care plans are designed to help students systematically proceed through each of the five steps of the nursing process. The assessment data establishing and validating nursing diagnoses often are recorded on the plan, scientific rationales and references may be requested for the nursing order chosen, and evaluative statements are documented.

- Some of the common problems encountered while developing plans of nursing care are insufficient data collection, nursing diagnoses developed from inaccurate or insufficient data, stating goals/outcomes too broadly, developing goals/outcomes from poorly developed nursing diagnoses, failure to write nursing orders clearly, writing nursing orders that do not adequately resolve the problem, failure to involve the patient in the planning process, and failure to update the plan of care.

■ Learning Checklist

Review the learning checklist at the end of the chapter in your textbook and be sure you can meet each objective.

■ Exercises

MATCHING

Match the definition in Part B with the type of care plan listed in Part A. Answers may be used more than once.

PART A

a. initial care plan

b. ongoing, problem-solving care plan

c. discharge care plan

d. standardized care plan

e. Kardex care plan

f. computerized care plan

g. case management care plan

h. critical care plan

PART B

1. _____ A care plan developed by the nurse who performs the admission nursing history and physical assessment.

2. _____ A care plan which is concisely recorded on a 6 × 11–inch card and filed in a central file.

3. _____ Benefits of this type of care plan include ready access to expanded knowledge base, improved record keeping and documentation, and decreased paperwork.

4. _____ The chief purpose of this type of planning is to keep the plan up to date.

5. _____ Prepared plans of care that identify the nursing diagnoses.

6. _____ This type of plan for leaving the institution is best prepared by the nurse who has worked most closely with the patient in conjunction with a social worker familiar with the patient's community.

7. _____ The emphasis on this care plan is to clearly state expected patient outcomes and the specific times in which it is reasonable to achieve these outcomes.

8. _____ The emphasis of this type of care plan is to individualize the plan to meet unique patient needs.

Match the patient goals in Part B with the type of goal listed in Part A. Answers may be used more than once.

PART A

a. cognitive goals

b. psychomotor goals

c. affective goals

PART B

9. _____ By 3/30/02, patient will successfully navigate length of hallway with walker.

10. _____ By 3/30/02, patient will list five low-fat snacks to replace high-fat foods.

11. _____ By 3/30/02, patient will bathe infant on her own.

12. _____ By 3/30/02, patient will value her health sufficiently to stop smoking.

13. _____ By 3/30/02, patient will list three reasons to continue taking blood pressure medication.

14. _____ By 3/30/02, patient will show concern for his well-being and participate in AA meetings.

Match the descriptions in Part B, with the type of planning being performed, listed in Part A. Answers may be used more than once.

PART A

a. initial planning

b. ongoing planning

c. discharge planning

PART B

15. _____ Used to keep the nursing plan up-to-date.

16. _____ Addresses each problem listed in the prioritized nursing diagnoses and identifies appropriate patient goals and related nursing care.

17. _____ States nursing diagnoses more clearly and develops new diagnoses.

18. _____ Should be carried out by the nurse who has worked most closely with the patient and family.

19. _____ Involves teaching and counseling skills to effectively help the patient and family carry out self care behaviors at home.

20. _____ Standardized care plans provide an excellent basis for this type of planning if the nurse individualizes them.

MULTIPLE CHOICE

Circle the letter that corresponds to the best answer for each question.

1. Which of the following actions would be performed during the planning step of the nursing process?

   a. Interpreting and analyzing patient data

   b. Establishing the data base

   c. Identifying factors contributing to patient's success or failure

   d. Selecting nursing measure

2. Which of the following is a correctly written goal for a patient who is scheduled to ambulate following hip surgery?

   a. Over the next 24-hour period, the patient will walk the length of the hallway assisted by the nurse.

   b. The nurse will help the patient ambulate the length of the hallway once a day.

   c. Offer to help the patient walk the length of the hallway each day.

   d. Patient will become mobile within a 24-hour period.

3. Mr. Conner is a 48-year-old patient, post-colostomy. Which of the following patient goals for Mr. Conner is written correctly?

   a. Explain to Mr. Conner the proper care of the stoma by 3/29/02.

   b. Mr. Conner will know how to care for his stoma by 3/29/02.

   c. Mr. Conner will demonstrate proper care of stoma by 3/29/02.

   d. Mr. Conner will be able to care for stoma and cope with psychologic loss by 3/29/02.

4. The etiology of the nursing diagnosis contains which of the following factors?

   a. Identification of the unhealthy response preventing desired change

   b. Identification of factors causing undesirable response and preventing desired change

   c. Suggestion of patient goals to promote desired change

   d. Identification of patient strengths

5. Mr. Rose is an overweight, highly stressed 50-year-old executive, being discharged from the hospital post-coronary bypass surgery. Which of the following demonstrates an affective goal for this patient?

   a. By 6/30/02, the patient will list three benefits of daily exercise.

   b. By 6/30/02, the patient will correctly demonstrate breathing techniques to reduce stress.

   c. By 6/30/02, the patient will value his health sufficiently to reduce the cholesterol in his diet.

   d. By 6/30/02, the patient will be able to plan healthy weekly menus.

6. Which of the following statements concerning nursing orders is accurate?

   a. Nursing orders are a separate entity from the original goal/outcome.

   b. Nursing orders are dated when written and when the plan of care is reviewed.

   c. Nursing orders are signed by the attending physician.

   d. Nursing orders do not describe the nursing action to be performed.

7. According to Maslow's hierarchy of human needs, which of the following examples would be the highest priority for a patient?

   a. self-actualization needs

   b. love and belonging needs

   c. physiologic needs

   d. safety needs

COMPLETION

1. Give an example of an appropriate nursing order for the following patients:

   a. A child with asthma who must be taught to use an inhaler:

   _____

   _____

   b. An elderly woman recovering from hip surgery who must learn to ambulate with a walker:

   _____

   _____

   c. An obese teenager who needs weight counseling:

   _____

   _____

   d. A new mother who must ambulate post C-section:

   _____

   _____

2. Briefly define the following elements of planning. Explain why they are necessary to the planning step of the nursing process.

   a. Establishing priorities

   _____

   _____

   b. Writing goals/outcomes that determine the evaluative strategy:

   _____

   _____

   c. Selecting appropriate nursing interventions: _____

   _____

   _____

d. Communicating the plan of nursing care:

   _____

   _____

3. List two examples of informal planning.

   _____

   _____

4. Explain how a formal plan of care benefits the nurse and patient.

   _____

   _____

5. Individualize the following standard plans to meet the patient's specific goals.

   a. Manage pain for a terminally ill patient:

   _____

   _____

   b. Explore support people for patient with AIDS:

   _____

   _____

   c. Provide sensory stimulation for an elderly man in a nursing home:

   _____

   _____

   d. Teach self-help to stroke patient in home care setting:

   _____

   _____

6. Describe the following types of nursing care and give an example of each type.

   a. Nursing care related to basic human needs:

   _____

   _____

   Example: _____

   b. Nursing care related to nursing diagnoses:

   _____

   _____

   Example: _____

   _____

c. Nursing care related to the medical plan of care:

_____

_____

Example: _____

_____

7. List four considerations a nurse should employ when planning nursing care for each day.

a. _____

b. _____

c. _____

d. _____

8. Place a check mark next to the patient goals that are written correctly, and on the line below rewrite those that are written incorrectly.

a. _____ Teach Mrs. Myer one lesson per day on the nutritional value of foods.

_____

b. _____ Mrs. Gray will know the dangers of smoking after viewing a film on smoking.

_____

c. _____ By end of shift, patient ambulates in hallway using crutches.

_____

d. _____ By 2/7, patient correctly demonstrates sub Q injections using normal saline.

_____

e.. _____ By next visit, the patient will understand the benefits of psychotherapy.

_____

f. _____ By 6/12, patient correctly demonstrates application of wet to dry dressing on leg ulcer.

_____

9. Identify a patient goal that shows a direct resolution of the health problem expressed in the nursing diagnoses below.

a. Nursing diagnosis: Fluid Volume Deficit—related to decreased fluid intake during fever.

Patient goal: _____

_____

b. Nursing diagnosis: Altered Sexual Patterns—Loss of desire related to change in body image and feelings of unattractiveness following mastectomy.

Patient goal: _____

_____

c. Nursing diagnosis: Stress Incontinence—related to age-related degenerative changes and weak pelvic muscles and structural supports.

Patient goal: _____

_____

d. Nursing Diagnosis: Activity Intolerance—related to decreased amount of oxygenated blood available to tissues.

Patient goal: _____

_____

e. Nursing Diagnosis: Acute Postoperative Pain—related to fear of taking prescribed analgesics.

Patient goal: _____

_____

GUIDE TO CRITICAL THINKING AND DEVELOPING BLENDED SKILLS

1. Think about what type of goals would be appropriate in each of the three stages of planning—initial planning, on-going planning, and discharge planning—using the following patient data:

a. A mother brings her 5-year-old son to the ER. She says he has been running a low fever and complaining of abdominal pain and headache. You notice his skin is pale and there are several bruises on his arms and legs. On examination, you notice the spleen is enlarged and the abdominal area is tender. A medical diagnosis confirms the child has acute leukemia.

b. A 45-year-old man presents with low fever, weight loss, chronic fatigue, and heavy sweating at night. He has a productive cough with yellowish mucus and chest pain. A TB skin test comes back positive.

c. A 12-year-old girl presents with fatigue, weight loss, excessive thirst, and frequent urination. Laboratory tests confirm a diagnosis of diabetes mellitus.

Why is the identification of goals in each stage necessary for optimal care and outcomes?

2. Some nurses may tell you that care plans are a waste of time. Think about what knowledge and experience you need to respond to this comment. If possible, interview nurses or search through literature to discover how plans can make a difference.

CHAPTER 18

Implementing

CHAPTER OVERVIEW

- Implementing, the fourth step of the nursing process, is the carrying out of the plan of care. Its purpose is to assist patients to achieve desired health goals—to promote wellness, prevent disease and illness, restore health, and facilitate coping with altered functioning.

- The plan of care is best implemented when patients who are able and willing to participate have maximal opportunity to do so.

- Whereas other healthcare professionals focus on select aspects of the patient's treatment regimen, nursing is concerned with how the *person* is responding in general to the plan of care.

- Nurses implement nurse-initiated or independent nursing actions, physician-initiated, or interdependent nursing actions, and collaborative interventions, or interdependent nursing actions.

- A taxonomy of nursing interventions now exists, which offers a means of standardizing nomenclature, expanding nursing knowledge, developing information systems, teaching decision making, costing out nursing, allocating nursing resources, communicating nursing to non-nurses, and linking nursing content.

- While carrying out the plan of care, nurses use cognitive, interpersonal, technical, and ethical and legal skills. Nursing's first challenge is the determination of how much nursing assistance the patient needs to reach desired goals/outcomes.

- The nurse's teaching, counseling, and advocacy skills are used to assist patients to develop the self-care behaviors that enable them to direct and manage their own care.

- Nothing about the care plan or the way it is implemented is fixed. Patient and nurse variables, as well as available resources, current standards of care, research findings, and ethical and legal guides to practice, may influence the plan's implementation.

- Ongoing data collection directs the revision of the plan of care.

- Improved personal health enables nurses to practice more effectively and to be a health model for patients and their families.

■ Learning Checklist

Review the learning checklist at the end of the chapter in your textbook and be sure you can meet each objective.

■ Exercises

Matching

Match the examples in Part B with the types of nursing interventions listed in Part A. Answers may be used more than once.

PART A

a. nurse-initiated independent intervention

b. physician-initiated dependent intervention

c. collaborative interdependent intervention

PART B

1. _____ A nurse notices her patient is extremely anxious prior to surgery and recommends psychiatric evaluation by the psychiatric nurse specialist.

2. _____ A nurse administers the prescribed dosage of pain medication for his patient recovering from knee surgery.

3. _____ A nurse teaches the daughter of a patient with leg ulcers how to apply the dressings.

4. _____ A nurse meets with a patient's physician to describe what she feels is the patient's lack of response to prescribed therapy.

5. _____ A nurse prepares a patient for surgery by performing a bowel cleansing.

6. _____ A nurse meets in conference with a patient's physician, social worker, and psychiatrist to discuss the patient's failure to progress.

Correct the False Statements

Circle the word true or false that follows the statement. If the word false has been circled, change the underlined word/words to make the statement true. Place your answer in the space provided.

1. The <u>physician</u> is legally responsible for the assessments nurses make and for their nursing responses.

   True   False   _____

2. <u>Nurse-initiated interventions</u> involve carrying out nurse-prescribed orders written on the nursing plan of care.

   True   False   _____

3. In 1992, McCloskey and Bulechek published <u>Nursing Interventions Classification</u>, a report of research to construct a taxonomy of nursing interventions.

   True   False   _____

4. <u>Standing orders</u> are written plans that detail the nursing activities to be executed in specific situations.

   True   False   _____

5. The <u>physician</u> plays the role of coordinator within the healthcare team.

   True   False   _____

6. The <u>nursing team</u> carries out the nursing orders detailed in the nursing plan of care.

   True   False   _____

7. When working with patients to achieve the goals/outcomes specified in the plan of care, it is important to remember that <u>everything about the plan of care is fixed</u>.

   True   False   _____

8. When choosing nursing interventions, it is important to consider the <u>patient's</u> background.

   True   False   _____

9. Sincere motivation to benefit the patient and conscientious attempt to implement nursing orders <u>is sufficient</u> to protect a nurse from legal action due to negligence.

   True   False   _____

10. When a patient fails to follow the plan of care in spite of the nurse's best efforts, it is time to <u>change the patient's</u> attitude toward his care.

    True   False   _____

11. If a plan of care is well written, <u>carrying out its orders</u> is the nurse's most important task and should receive top priority.

    True   False   _____

12. <u>All nursing actions for implementing the plan of care</u> must be consistent with standards for practice.

    True   False   _____

13. It is <u>the medical profession</u> that determines the scope of nursing practice.

    True   False   _____

Multiple Choice

Circle the letter that corresponds to the best answer for each question.

1. Which of the following phrases best describes the unique focus of nursing implementation?
   a. The selected aspects of the patient's treatment regimen
   b. The response of the patient to the plan of care in general
   c. The response of the patient to his illness
   d. The patient's ability to work with support people to promote wellness

2. Which of the following nursing actions is considered an independent (nurse-initiated) action?
   a. Executing physician orders for a catheter
   b. Meeting with other healthcare professionals to discuss a patient
   c. Helping to allay a patient's fears pending surgery
   d. Administering medication to a patient

3. Which of the following terms denotes a nurse's authority to initiate actions that normally require the order or supervision of a physician?

   a. protocols

   b. nursing interventions

   c. collaborative orders

   d. standing orders

4. As the nurse bathes a patient, she notes his skin color and integrity, his ability to respond to simple directions, and his muscle tone. Which of the following statements best explains why such continuing data collection is so important?

   a. It is difficult to collect complete data in the initial assessment.

   b. It is the most efficient use of the nurse's time.

   c. It enables the nurse to revise the care plan appropriately.

   d. It meets current standards of care.

5. Your patient, who presented with high blood pressure, is put on a low-salt diet and instructed to quit smoking. You find him in the cafeteria eating a cheeseburger and French fries. He also tells you there is no way he can quit smoking. What is your *first* objective when implementing care for this patient?

   a. Explain to the patient the effects of a high-salt diet and smoking on blood pressure.

   b. Identify why the patient is not following the therapy.

   c. Collaborate with other healthcare professionals about the patient's treatment.

   e. Change the nursing care plan.

Completion

1. List three duties nurses perform when acting as coordinator for the healthcare team.

   a. _____

   b. _____

   c. _____

2. Give an example of a nurse variable, a patient variable, and a healthcare variable that might influence the implementation of the plan of care:

   a. Nurse variable: _____

   b. Patient variable: _____

   c. Healthcare variable: _____

3. Explain why the following nursing actions are important to the continuity of nursing care.

   a. Promoting self-care: teaching, counseling, and advocacy: _____

   _____

   _____

   b. Assisting patients to meet health goals:

   _____

   _____

   _____

4. Mr. Franks is a new resident in a nursing home and recovering from minor surgery. He shows no interest in his condition and refuses to participate in self-care. You suspect an underlying problem of loneliness and boredom stemming from his admittance to the home, which was not mentioned in his original plan of care. How would you reevaluate the nursing care plan and incorporate self-care for Mr. Franks, taking into consideration his mental state?

   _____

   _____

   _____

5. Your patient is a pregnant woman, living in a subsidized housing development, whom you feel is not receiving proper nutrition for her condition. She has two other children and complains that there is not enough money to put three square meals a day on the table. When evaluating her plan of care, you notice that there is no mention of providing counseling in this area. How would you reevaluate the nursing care plan for this patient to include options for proper nutrition?

   _____

   _____

   _____

6. List seven factors a nurse should consider before delegating a nursing intervention.

   a. _____

   b. _____

   c. _____

   d. _____

   e. _____

   f. _____

   g. _____

7. Explain why the following *rights* of delegation are important when deciding whether or not to delegate a nursing intervention.

   a. The *right* task _____

   b. The *right* person _____

   c. The *right* communication _____

   d. The *right* feedback _____

   e. The *right* time _____

GUIDE TO CRITICAL THINKING AND DEVELOPING BLENDED SKILLS

1. Work with your classmates to list all the factors (nurse, healthcare team, patient/family, healthcare setting, resources, and so on) that might interfere with the nurse's ability to successfully implement a plan of care for the following patients. Then identify facilitating factors. Think about how you can use this knowledge.

   a. A 5-year-old girl with cystic fibrosis is being discharged into the care of her family. Her family consists of a single working mother and two older brothers.

   b. A 17-year-old single mother who is living with her parents is being sent home with her newborn son. She is trying to nurse the baby, but is having difficulty. The baby is being treated for jaundice.

2. Spend some time observing nurses as they care for patients. Make a list of all the nursing actions you observe. Determine whether these actions involved the use of the nurse's cognitive skills, interpersonal skills, technical skills, or ethical/legal skills, or a blend of these skills. Rate your own skills in these areas and note in which areas you feel confident and in which areas you need improvement. Write a plan of action to help you improve these skills.

CHAPTER 19

Evaluating

CHAPTER OVERVIEW

- During evaluation, the nurse and patient measure how well the patient has achieved the goals/outcomes specified in the plan of care. Factors that have positively or negatively influenced goal/outcome achievement are identified, and a decision is made to terminate, continue, or modify care.

- When evaluation points to the need to modify nursing care, each preceding step in the nursing process is reviewed for accuracy.

- The type of evaluative data collected to support the decision regarding goal/outcome achievement (goal met, partially met, or not met) is determined by the nature of the goal/outcome. Goals/outcomes may be cognitive, psychomotor, or affective, or they may describe physical changes in the patient.

- It is important for nurses to evaluate patient goal/outcome achievement as early as possible. Achievement, when celebrated with the patient, encourages further goal achievement. Failure directs necessary revisions in the plan of care. Waiting until a patient is about to be discharged to evaluate goals/outcomes is the most common mistake nurses make in evaluation.

- Evaluative statements recorded on the plan of care alert the entire nursing staff to the patient's level of goal/outcome achievement. Each evaluative statement includes a decision about how well the goal/outcome was achieved and the patient data or behavior that supports the decision. The statement is dated and signed.

- Sensitivity to the patient, nurse, and healthcare system variables that influence goal/outcome achievement enables the nurse to manipulate factors that will help the patient reach desired goals.

- Common problems encountered during evaluation that may require a revision of the plan of care include inaccurate or incomplete database, vague or missing nursing diagnoses, standardized plan of care, improperly developed nursing goals, superficial nursing orders, plan that is not kept up-to-date, failure to use evaluation to improve quality of nursing care, and insufficient communication among nurses.

- Historically, nursing has been a strong advocate for quality healthcare. The current availability of fewer resources to treat patients in hospitals and the unavailability of sufficient alternative treatment settings pose a serious challenge to nursing.

- Quality assurance programs are evaluative programs designed to secure and implement excellence in nursing and healthcare. These programs may include process, structure, or outcome standards and have as their focus the patient, the nurse, the institution, or the healthcare system.

- Quality assurance/quality improvement programs enable nursing to be accountable to society for the quality of its service. They also are a response to the public mandate for professional accountability and the mandate of professional nursing law. They ensure professional survival, encourage nursing's fidelity to its moral and ethical responsibilities, and assist nursing to comply with other external pressures.

- Self-evaluation skills promote professional development, enhance self-esteem, and develop self-awareness.

■ Learning Checklist

Review the learning checklist at the end of the chapter in your textbook and be sure you can meet each objective.

■ Exercises

MATCHING

Match the term in Part A with the correct definition listed in Part B.

PART A

a. concurrent evaluation

b. retrospective evaluation

c. outcome evaluation

d. process evaluation

e. structure evaluation

f. introspective evaluation

PART B

1. _____ An evaluation that focuses on the environment in which care is provided.

2. _____ An evaluation that focuses on measurable changes in the health status of the patient.

3. _____ An evaluation of nursing care and patient goals while the patient is receiving the care.

4. _____ An evaluation that focuses on the nature and sequence of activities carried out by the nurse implementing the nursing process.

5. _____ An evaluation to collect data post-discharge.

Match the measurement tool in Part A with its appropriate example listed in Part B. Answers may be used more than once.

PART A

a. criteria

b. standard

PART B

6. _____ Patient will be able to walk length of hall by 5/15/02.

7. _____ The admission database will be completed on all patients within 24 hours of admission to the unit.

8. _____ All patients in active labor will have continuous external fetal heart monitoring.

9. _____ Upon completion of an ECG course, the nurse will be able to recognize common arrhythmias when they appear on a heart monitor.

10. _____ The student will be able to name and describe steps of nursing procedure by end of semester.

MULTIPLE CHOICE

Circle the letter that corresponds to the best answer for each question.

1. Which of the following actions is the most important act of evaluation performed by the nurse?

   a. Evaluating patient's goal/outcome achievement.

   b. Evaluating the plan of care.

   c. Evaluating the competence of nurse practitioners.

   d. Evaluating the types of healthcare services available to the patient.

2. The nurse collects data in the evaluation step to determine which of the following?

   a. patient health problems

   b. assessment of patient's underlying health problems

   c. solution for health problems through goal achievement

   d. effect of medical diagnosis

3. Which of the following patient goals would be considered a psychomotor goal?

   a. By 8/18/02, patient will value his health sufficiently to quit smoking.

   b. By 8/18/02, patient will have full motion in left arm.

   c. By 8/18/02, patient will list three foods that are low in salt.

   d. By 8/18/02, patient will learn three exercises designed to strengthen leg muscles.

4. Which of the following statements concerning quality improvement is accurate?

   a. Quality improvement is externally driven.

   b. Quality improvement follows organizational structure rather than patient care.

   c. Quality improvement focuses on individuals rather than processes.

   d. Quality improvement has no endpoints.

5. Which of the following actions should the nurse take when patient data indicate that the stated goals have not been achieved?

    a. Collect more data for the database.

    b. Review each preceding step of the nursing process.

    c. Implement a standardized plan of care.

    d. Change the nursing orders.

6. For a patient with self-care deficit, the long-term goal is that the patient will be able to dress himself by the end of the 6-week therapy. For best results, the nurse should evaluate the patient's progress toward this goal at which of the following times?

    a. When the patient is discharged

    b. At the end of the 6-week therapy

    c. Only when the patient shows some progress

    d. As soon as possible

7. The quality assurance model of the ANA identifies three essential components of quality care. Which one of these components does the nurse use when determining whether or not a patient has met the goals stated on the care plan?

    a. structure

    b. process

    c. retrospective

    d. outcome

8. Which of the following actions would be an appropriate nursing action when evaluating a patient's responses to a plan of care?

    a. Terminate the plan of care when each expected outcome is achieved.

    b. Modify the plan if there are difficulties achieving the goals/outcomes.

    c. Continue the plan of care if more time is needed to achieve the goals/outcomes.

    d. All of the above

COMPLETION

1. Explain how you would evaluate whether or not a patient has achieved the following goals:

    a. Cognitive goals: _____

    b. Psychomotor goals: _____

    c. Affective goals: _____

2. Explain how the following elements of evaluation help to determine whether goals/outcomes have been met.

    a. Identifying evaluative criteria: _____

    _____

    _____

    b. Determining if these criteria and standards are met: _____

    _____

    _____

    d. Terminating, continuing, or modifying the plan: _____

    _____

    _____

3. Give an example of a variable that may influence goal/outcome achievement in the following areas:

    a. Patient: _____

    b. Nurse: _____

    c. Healthcare system: _____

4. Mr. Bogash is a 28-year-old man recovering from leukemia. He recently had a bone marrow transplant. His medical condition has improved, but he is unable to meet his goal of being up and alert during the daytime hours. What would be the appropriate step to take after evaluating Mr. Bogash? How would you document Mr. Bogash's failure to progress? How would you revise his plan of care?

    _____

    _____

    _____

5. Explain the following three essential components of quality care and how nursing care is evaluated in each area.

    a. Structure:

    _____

    _____

    b. Process:

    _____

    _____

c. Outcome: _____

_____

_____

7. Explain why the following revisions may be made to a plan of care.

a. Delete or modify the nursing diagnosis: _____

_____

_____

b. Make the goal statement more realistic: _____

_____

_____

c. Adjust time criteria in goal statement: _____

_____

_____

d. Change nursing interventions: _____

_____

_____

8. Would you rather work in an environment that ensures the quality of the profession by quality by inspection or quality as opportunity? Explain your answer: _____

_____

_____

GUIDE TO CRITICAL THINKING AND DEVELOPING BLENDED SKILLS

1. Interview friends and family members who have experienced a stay in the hospital. Ask them if they were aware of specific nursing plans geared to their recovery. See if they were given goals and taught behaviors to accomplish them. Was goal attainment evaluated before they were discharged? Were further goals incorporated into their discharge plan? What do they feel could have been done to help them attain their health goals? How can you use this knowledge to help you develop the blended skills necessary to help patients achieve goals?

2. Reflect on the role that evaluation plays in promoting your scholastic achievement. Has it been positive or negative? Think of specific ways nurses can use evaluation to motive patients to achieve healthy goals.

CHAPTER 20

Documenting, Reporting, and Conferring

CHAPTER OVERVIEW

- Nurses are responsible for documenting each step of the nursing process in the patient record. Most health-care institutions and professional and regulatory agencies have standards for documentation that detail the nurse's responsibilities.

- The patient record is the only legal document that provides a comprehensive picture of the nursing care given to the patient.

- Patient-specific data and information are used to facilitate patient care, serve as a financial and legal record, help in clinical research, and support decision analysis.

- Documentation should be consistent with professional and agency standards; complete, accurate, relevant, factual, and timely; orderly and sequential; legally prudent; and confidential.

- Each healthcare group keeps data on its own separate form in the source-oriented patient record. In the problem-oriented record, recording is organized around the patient's problems rather than around sources of information.

- The case management model of documentation uses a critical or collaborative pathway tool for groups of patients with the same diagnosis. The pathway includes expected outcomes and lists the interventions needed to secure these outcomes and the timing and sequence of these interventions.

- Computer records have simplified nursing documentation in many ways. Use of computer terminals at the patient's bedside enables nurses to document care immediately.

- There are distinct advantages and disadvantages linked to common formats used by nurses to document patient progress toward expected outcomes and related nursing care. Examples of these formats include narrative notes, SOAP notes, PIE charting, focus charting, charting by exception, and flow sheets.

- One out of four malpractice suits is decided from the patient's record. No nurse can afford to be ignorant of or careless with respect to agency policies and professional standards for documentation.

- Reporting is the oral, written, or computer-based communication of patient data with the purpose of informing others. Common methods for reporting among health practitioners, other than the patient record, include face-to-face meetings, the telephone, a messenger, the written message, the audiotaped message, and the computer message.

- To confer is to consult with someone to exchange ideas or to seek information, advice, or instructions. When nurses detect problems they are unable to solve because they lie outside the scope of independent nursing practice or outside the scope of their expertise, they make referrals to other professionals. The process of sending or guiding someone to another source for assistance is called a referral.

■ Learning Checklist

Review the learning checklist at the end of the chapter in your textbook and be sure you can meet each objective.

■ Exercises

MATCHING

Match the formats of nursing documentation listed in Part A with their appropriate example listed in Part B.

PART A

a. initial nursing assessment

b. plan of nursing care

c. critical/collaborative pathways

d. progress notes

e. graphic record

f. 24-hour fluid balance record

g. medication record

h. 24-hour nursing care record

i. discharge and transfer summary

j. home care documentation

k. long-term care documentation

PART B

1. _____ The nurse documents the case management plan for a patient population with a designated diagnosis which includes expected outcomes, interventions to be performed, and the sequence and timing of these interventions.

2. _____ The nurse documents her diabetic patient's intake and output of fluids.

3. _____ The nurse summarizes her patient's reason for treatment, significant findings, procedures performed and treatment rendered, and any specific instructions for the patient/family.

4. _____ The nurse uses this form to record his patient's pulse, respiratory rate, blood pressure, body temperature, weight, and bowel movements.

5. _____ The nurse documents patient's routine aspects of care that promote goal achievement, safety, and well-being.

6. _____ The nurse records the database obtained from the nursing history and physical assessment.

7. _____ The nurse documents the administration of Cipro IV, 400 mg every 12 hours.

8. _____ The nurse documents her patient's diagnosis of AIDS, expected outcomes, and specific nursing interventions.

9. _____ A nurse documents that her patient is homebound and still needs nursing care.

10. _____ A nurse uses RAI to document care.

MULTIPLE CHOICE

Circle the letter that corresponds to the best answer for each question.

1. Which of the following is a nurse's best defense against allegations of negligence by a patient or patient's surrogate?
   a. Nursing team
   b. Flow sheet
   c. Medication record
   d. Patient record

2. Which of the following statements regarding the patient record is accurate?
   a. A patient's chart may be shared only with close family members.
   b. Student nurses are not granted access to patient records.
   c. The patient record is generally the responsibility of one caregiver.
   d. Most patient records are microfilmed and stored in computers.

3. In which of the following systems would a nurse organize data according to the SOAP format?
   a. Source-oriented method
   b. PIE-charting method
   c. Problem-oriented method
   d. Focus charting method

4. Abnormal status can be seen immediately with narrative easily retrieved in which of the following documentation formats?
   a. Charting by exception
   b. PIE
   c. Narrative notes
   d. SOAP notes

5. Which of the following is a key component to facilitate data and outcome comparisons by using uniform definitions to create a common language among multiple healthcare data users?
   a. Kardex care plan
   b. minimum data sets
   c. computer-based records
   d. critical/collaborative pathways

6. You are finding it difficult to plan and implement care for Mr. Rivers, and decide to have a nursing care conference. Which of the following best defines this action?
   a. You consult with someone in order to exchange ideas or seek information, advice, or instructions.
   b. You meet with nurses or other health professionals to discuss some aspect of patient care.
   c. You and other nurses visit similar patients individually at each patient's bedside in order to plan nursing care.
   d. You send or direct someone for action in a specific nursing care problem.

7. Which of the following is an accurately written documentation of the effectiveness of a patient's pain management?

   a. Mr. Gray is receiving sufficient relief from pain medication.

   b. Mr. Gray appears comfortable and is resting adequately.

   c. Mr. Gray reports that on a scale of 1–10, the pain he is experiencing would be a 3.

   d. Mr. Gray appears to have a low tolerance for pain and complains frequently about the intensity of his pain.

8. Which of the following guidelines for charting patient information is accurate?

   a. Nursing interventions should be charted chronologically on consecutive lines.

   b. If a mistake is made on a chart, correcting fluid should be used to change the mistake.

   c. Charting should be done in pencil to facilitate correction of mistakes.

   d. If a procedure is repeated frequently, it is proper to use dittos to decrease recording time.

9. Which of the following is a form used to record specific patient variables such as pulse, respiratory rate, blood pressure readings, body temperature?

   a. progress notes

   b. flow sheets

   c. graphic sheets

   d. medical records

COMPLETION

1. List four areas of nursing care data that, according to JCAHO, must be permanently integrated into the patient record.

   a. _____

   b. _____

   c. _____

   d. _____

2. Briefly describe the following methods of reporting patient data.

   a. Change-of-shift reports: _____

   _____

   _____

   b. Telephone reports: _____

   _____

   _____

   c. Telephone orders: _____

   _____

   _____

   d. Transfer and discharge reports: _____

   _____

   _____

   e. Reports to family members and significant others: _____

   _____

   f. Incident reports: _____

   _____

   _____

   g. Conferring about care: _____

   _____

   h. Consultations and referrals: _____

   _____

   i. Nursing care conference: _____

   _____

   j. Nursing care rounds: _____

   _____

3. Briefly explain the following purposes of the patient record.

   a. Communication: _____

   _____

   _____

   b. Care planning: _____

   _____

   _____

   c. Quality review: _____

   _____

   _____

   d. Research: _____

   _____

   _____

e. Decision analysis: _____

_____

f. Education: _____

_____

g. Legal documentation: _____

_____

_____

h. Reimbursement: _____

_____

_____

i. Historical document: _____

_____

_____

4. List five guidelines nurses should follow when reporting a significant change in a patient's condition to other healthcare professionals by telephone.

a. _____

b. _____

c. _____

d. _____

e. _____

5. Complete the following chart listing the purpose, advantages, and disadvantages of the following methods of documentation.

Documentation Method	Description/Advantages/Disadvantages
SOURCE-ORIENTED RECORD	Advantages: Disadvantages:
PROBLEM-ORIENTED MEDICAL RECORDS	Advantages: Disadvantages:
PIE–PROBLEM, INTERVENTION, EVALUATION	Advantages: Disadvantages:
FOCUS CHARTING	Advantages: Disadvantages:
CHARTING BY EXCEPTION	Advantages: Disadvantages:
CASE MANAGEMENT MODEL	Advantages: Disadvantages:

(continues)

Documentation Method	Description/Advantages/Disadvantages
VARIANCE CHARTING	Advantages: Disadvantages:
COMPUTERIZED RECORDS	Advantages: Disadvantages:

GUIDE TO CRITICAL THINKING AND DEVELOPING BLENDED SKILLS

1. Consider the following case:

A 79-year-old woman with Alzheimer's disease is admitted to a long-term care unit. She has a history of falls and has fractured her left hip in the past. She no longer recognizes her daughter, who was taking care of her. The daughter states she can no longer handle her mother's condition. The daughter insists that the nurses restrain her mother physically to prevent falls.

Think about the information the team will need to provide safe, quality care for this patient. What types of data should the admitting nurse record, and what system of documentation is most likely to bring the information to the attention of everyone who needs it?

2. How would you go about scheduling a consultation for a male amputee who needs physical therapy? Write a brief summary of the patient's condition and how you would present his case to the referred agency.

3. Make an appointment to interview the risk manager of a healthcare system. Find out how important the documentation of patient care is to the patient, nurse, and health agency when legal questions arise. How can this knowledge help to safeguard your practice?

UNIT V

Roles Basic to Nursing Care

CHAPTER 21

Communicator

CHAPTER OVERVIEW

- Nurses communicate thoughts, ideas, experiences, and facts to other nurses, patients, physicians, other healthcare workers, and families as part of their promotion of wellness and prevention of illness.

- The communication process can be defined in two ways: (1) the process of sharing information and (2) the process of generating and transmitting meanings. Communication, as a foundation of life, is a reciprocal process with simultaneous participation.

- People communicate one to one or in small or large groups by verbal and nonverbal means.

- Nonverbal communication includes touch, eye contact, facial expressions, posture, gait, gestures, physical appearance, modes of dress and grooming, sounds, and silence.

- Factors that can influence the process of communication include development, gender, sociocultural differences, roles and responsibilities, space and territoriality, physical and mental/emotional state, values, and environment.

- The ability of the nurse to communicate with others is essential to effective use of the nursing process.

- The three phases in the helping relationship are (1) orientation phase, (2) working phase, and (3) termination phase. A helping relationship is dynamic, purposeful, and time limited, and involves one person in a dominant role.

- Factors that benefit the helping relationship by promoting effective communication include having specific objectives, a comfortable environment, privacy, confidentiality, and patient focus, as well as using nursing observations, allowing optimal pacing, and providing personal space.

- Effective communication techniques are conversational skills, listening skills, use of silence and touch, and interviewing techniques. The interview is a major tool for data collection in the assessment step of the nursing process.

- Interpersonal skills such as warmth and friendliness, openness, empathy, competence, and consideration of patient variables are essential to a therapeutic nurse–patient relationship.

- Assertive skills enable nurses to communicate with patients, nurses, and other members of the healthcare team in a direct, honest fashion that is respectful of the rights of all parties in the communication.

- The nurse must develop communication skills for special circumstances, especially when the patient is visually impaired, hearing impaired, unconscious, cognitively impaired, has a physical barrier such as a laryngectomy or endotracheal tube, or speaks a foreign language.

- In functional groups members communicate with one another for the purpose of achieving a goal. Group members may serve task, maintenance, or self-serving roles. When groups are studied to determine their effectiveness or ineffectiveness, the study is called group dynamics.

■ Learning Checklist

Review the learning checklist at the end of the chapter in your textbook and be sure you can meet each objective.

■ Exercises

MATCHING

Match the elements of the communication process in Part A with the appropriate definition in Part B.

PART A

a. source

b. message

c. channel

d. receiver

e. noise

f. communication

g. feedback

PART B

1. _____ The actual product of the encoder.

2. _____ He/she must translate and make a decision about the product.

3. _____ Verbal and nonverbal evidence that patient received and understood the product.

4. _____ He/she prepares and sends the product.

5. _____ The medium selected to convey the product.

6. _____ Factors that distort the quality of the product.

Match the examples of patient goals in Part B with the appropriate phase in which they should occur, listed in Part A. Answers may be used more than once.

PART A

a. orientation phase

b. working phase

c. termination

PART B

7. _____ The patient will demonstrate ability to maneuver on crutches.

8. _____ The patient will acknowledge goals he has accomplished in physical therapy.

9. _____ The patient will learn the name of the physical therapist and address him by his name.

10. _____ An anorexic patient will establish an agreement with her healthcare professional to gradually return to a normal eating pattern.

11. _____ The patient will express his desire to go home despite the excellent care he received at the agency.

12. _____ The patient will attend a counseling session dealing with smoking.

13. _____ The patient will verbalize the goals set forth in his transition to a home healthcare setting.

14. _____ The patient will establish an agreement with the home healthcare worker about the frequency and length of contacts.

15. _____ The patient will express his concerns about pending surgery to the nurse.

Match the interviewing questions in Part B with the interviewing techniques useful in nurse–patient interactions, listed in Part A.

PART A

a. validating question/comment

b. clarifying question/comment

c. reflective question/comment

d. sequencing question/comment

e. directing question/comment

PART B

16. _____ "You say you've always been healthy and active; is this the first time you've been hospitalized?"

17. _____ "You expressed concern about your children at home…"

18. _____ "At home you've been treating your ulcer with antacid. Did you take any today?"

19. _____ You've been on your present medication for 3 years. Did you experience any side-effects?"

20. _____ "Your chest pain began after exercising on a lifecycle?"

21. _____ "You've been upset about taking medication…"

MULTIPLE CHOICE

Circle the letter that corresponds to the best answer for each question.

1. Which of the following statements about the communication process is accurate?

   a. Communication is a reciprocal process in which both the sender and receiver of messages take turns participating.

   b. One-to-one communication occurs when three or more people are involved in the communication process.

   c. Nursing instructors and students seldom experience the communication process in large groups.

   d. Communicating people receive and send messages through verbal and nonverbal means, which occur simultaneously.

2. In which of the following phases of the helping relationship is an agreement or contract about the relationship established?

    a. orientation phase

    b. working phase

    c. termination phase

    d. all of the above

3. An active listener in a group is performing which of the following group roles?

    a. task roles

    b. maintenance roles

    c. self-serving roles

    d. administrative roles

4. A group member who delegates responsibilities to other members is performing which of the following group roles?

    a. task roles

    b. maintenance roles

    c. self-serving roles

    d. administrative roles

5. In a helping relationship, the nurse would most likely perform which of the following activities?

    a. Encourage the patient to independently explore goals that allow his/her human needs to be satisfied.

    b. Set up a reciprocal relationship in which patient and nurse are both helper and person being helped.

    c. Establish communication that is continuous and reciprocal.

    d. Establish goals for the patient that are not set in a specific time frame.

6. Which of the following is a characteristic of a helping relationship?

    a. There is an equal sharing of information.

    b. The relationship is dynamic.

    c. Nonspecific goals are set within a certain time frame.

    d. The relationship is spontaneous.

7. Which of the following techniques would a nurse employ when using listening skills appropriately?

    a. The nurse would try to avoid body gestures when listening to the patient.

    b. The nurse would not allow conversation to lapse into periods of silence.

    c. The nurse would listen to the themes in the patient's comments.

    d. The nurse would stand close to the patient when communicating with him and maintain eye contact.

8. Which of the following senses is most highly developed at birth?

    a. hearing

    b. taste

    c. sight

    d. touch

9. When a nurse unblocks and redirects congested areas of energy in a patient's body, she is applying the phenomenon known as:

    a. "unruffling" touch

    b. interpersonal touch

    c. tactile manipulation

    d. therapeutic touch

10. When communicating with an unconscious patient, which of the following facts should be considered?

    a. Hearing is the first sense to be lost; therefore, it is most likely that the patient cannot hear the nurse.

    b. An unconscious patient needs to be spoken to in a clear, louder-than-normal voice.

    c. Environmental noise should be controlled to allow the patient to focus on the communicator.

    d. An unconscious patient should not be subjected to the use of touch because it is ineffective and may be detrimental to the patient.

11. A 36-year-old patient who is 4 days post hysterectomy says to the nurse, "I wonder if after all this surgery, I will still feel like a woman." Which of the following responses would most likely encourage the patient to expand on this and express her concerns in more specific terms?

    a. "When did you begin to wonder about this?"

    b. "Do you want more children?"

    c. "Feel like a woman..."

    d. Remaining silent

12. When a nurse attends a staff meeting, he/she is participating in which of the following types of communication?

    a. intrapersonal communication

    b. interpersonal communication

    c. small group communication

    d. organizational communication

COMPLETION

1. Give an example of the following nonverbal forms of communication and explain how they can provide clues to the patient's health status.

    a. Touch: _____

    _____

    _____

    b. Eye contact: _____

    _____

    _____

    c. Facial expressions: _____

    _____

    _____

    d. Posture: _____

    _____

    _____

    e. Gait: _____

    _____

    f. Gestures: _____

    _____

    _____

    g. General physical appearance: _____

    _____

    _____

    h. Mode of dress and grooming: _____

    _____

    _____

    i. Sounds: _____

    _____

    _____

    j. Silence: _____

    _____

    _____

2. Briefly describe how you would alter your explanation of a surgical procedure to take into account the developmental considerations of the following patients:

    a. An 8-year-old boy: _____

    _____

    b. A 16-year-old girl: _____

    _____

    c. A 65-year-old male with a hearing impairment: _____

    _____

3. What clues to a person's identity can sometimes be determined by knowing that person's occupation? _____

    _____

    _____

4. Briefly explain the role communication plays in the following steps of the nursing process.

    a. Assessing: _____

    _____

    b. Diagnosing: _____

    _____

    _____

c. Planning: _____

_____

_____

d. Implementing: _____

_____

_____

e. Evaluating: _____

_____

_____

f. Documenting: _____

_____

_____

5. Explain why the following variables must be considered when establishing rapport between a nurse and patient.

a. Having specific objectives: _____

_____

_____

b. Providing a comfortable environment: _____

_____

_____

c. Providing privacy: _____

_____

_____

d. Maintaining confidentiality: _____

_____

e. Maintaining patient focus: _____

_____

_____

f. Using nursing observations: _____

_____

_____

g. Using optimal pacing: _____

_____

_____

h. Providing personal space: _____

_____

_____

i. Developing therapeutic communication skills: _____

_____

_____

j. Developing listening skills: _____

_____

_____

k. Using silence as a tool: _____

_____

_____

6. Rewrite the following questions/statements in order to promote more effective communication with the patient.

a. Did you have a good night? _____

_____

_____

b. Are you ready to try walking on that foot?

_____

_____

c. I can't believe you stopped taking your insulin:

_____

_____

d. You aren't afraid of taking that test, are you?

_____

_____

e. No one should be afraid of that procedure; it's been done a million times: _____

_____

_____

f. Don't worry; everything will be all right:

_____

_____

7. Underline the nonverbal communication in the following paragraph.

   Mrs. Clarke is a 42-year-old woman post mastectomy. She has a husband and two children, ages 10 and 5. When the nurse enters Mrs. Clarke's room, she finds her patient's eyes are teary and a worried expression on her face. When asked how she is feeling, Mrs. Clarke replies "fine," although her face is rigid and mouth drawn in a firm line. She is moving her foot back and forth under the covers. Upon further investigation, the nurse finds out Mrs. Clarke is worried about her children and her own ability to be a healthy, functioning wife and mother again. After prompting, Mrs. Clarke states, "I don't know if my husband will still love me like this." She sighs and falls silent, reflecting upon her recovery. The nurse tries to make Mrs. Clarke comfortable and puts her hand over Mrs. Clarke's hand. She establishes eye contact with Mrs. Clarke and reassures her that things have a way of working out and to give her situation some time.

8. Mr. Uhl is a 72-year-old man with early signs of Alzheimer's disease. He is living with his daughter and son-in-law in a large city, where he is functioning well under supervision. His doctor suggests a day care center to fill in the gaps when the daughter is away at her part-time job. Nurse Parish, employed by the day care center, enters into a helping relationship with Mr. Uhl, even though she knows she will be starting a new job at the end of the month which will force them to terminate their relationship. Write two patient goals the nurse may prepare for Mr. Uhl in the following phases of their short helping relationship.

   a. Orientation phase:

      1. _____

      2. _____

   b. Working phase: _____

      1. _____

      2. _____

   c. Termination phase:

      1. _____

      2. _____

9. Give an example of the following interpersonal skills necessary for the promotion of a healthy nurse–patient relationship. Rate your own skills in these areas on a scale of 1–10.

   a. Warmth and friendliness: _____

   b. Openness: _____

   c. Empathy: _____

   d. Competence: _____

   e. Consideration of patient's variables: _____

   _____

10. Mr. Johnson is a 69-year-old patient diagnosed with prostate cancer. He is despondent and refuses to participate in his own care. Give an example of a nurse's dialogue with Mr. Johnson in each component of the assertive response:

    a. Empathic component: _____

    _____

    b. Description: _____

    _____

    c. Expectation: _____

    _____

    d. Consequence: _____

    _____

    _____

11. List five common blocks to communication and describe nursing's role in overcoming these obstacles.

    a. _____

    b. _____

    c. _____

    d. _____

    e. _____

GUIDE TO CRITICAL THINKING AND DEVELOPING BLENDED SKILLS

1. Write down a general script for communicating with patients beginning with "Hello, my name is..." to the end of the conversation. Make your script specific to the needs of the following patients:

   a. A 4-year-old boy is admitted to the hospital with multiple fractures following a car accident.

   b. A teen-age girl is admitted to the burn unit with third degree burns following a fire in her home.

   c. A 29-year-old rape victim is brought to the ER for treatment and testing.

   d. A 60-year-old man with a history of strokes is brought to the ER with left side paralysis.

How competent and comfortable are you in each situation? What skills do you need to develop?

2. Pick a partner and try to communicate the following messages using only nonverbal communication:

   a. I'm thirsty.

   b. I have a pain in my stomach.

   c. It's too hot in here.

   d. I'd like you to read me a story.

   e. I'd like to go home now.

   f. Where is the bathroom?

   g. Can I have another pain reliever?

   h. I'd like to go to sleep now.

   i. It's too noisy in here.

   j. I can't fall asleep.

Reflect on the importance of nonverbal communication.

3. Observe and interpret a patient's nonverbal communication, and then ask the patient if your interpretation was correct, for example, "You seem to be in a lot of pain, is that correct?"

4. Ask a friend who has been a close confidant of yours to rate you on the following attributes that stimulate a healthy nurse–patient relationship: warmth and friendliness, openness, empathy, competence, consideration of variables. See if this evaluation is consistent with your own feelings when practicing patient care. Work on the areas that rated a lower score the next time you are with patients.

CHAPTER 22

Teacher and Counselor

CHAPTER OVERVIEW

- Nurses use communication skills in their roles as teachers and counselors.

- The nursing roles of teacher and counselor require the use of the nursing process; the teaching–learning process follows the steps of the nursing process.

- With the trend toward shorter hospital stays, patients and families need more extensive instruction for home care. However, as the importance of teaching increases, the hospital time for teaching decreases. Consequently, the quality of teaching must improve.

- The outcomes of effective teaching and counseling include high-level wellness and related self-care practices; disease prevention or early detection; quick recovery from illness with minimal to no sequelae; enhanced ability to adjust to developmental life changes and acute, chronic, and terminal illness; and family acceptance of the lifestyle changes necessitated by the illness or disability of a family member.

- Learning can be divided into the following three domains: (1) cognitive learning, which involves the storing and recalling of new knowledge and information in the brain; (2) psychomotor learning, which indicates that a physical skill has been learned; and (3) affective learning, which involves changes in attitudes, values, and feelings.

- Assessment of learning needs focuses on the knowledge, attitude, and skills the patient needs to independently manage healthcare; learning readiness; the physical ability to learn; and patient strengths. Factors affecting each are explored, often in consultation with the family and significant others.

- Nursing diagnoses are developed that identify health problems related to patient deficits in knowledge, attitudes, or skills.

- Teaching plans specify measurable learning objectives, related content, and specific teaching strategies and learning activities. A contractual agreement may facilitate learning.

- Implementing the teaching plan requires use of interpersonal skills as well as effective communication techniques. Teaching is part of the working phase of the helping relationship.

- The evaluation of learning provides the information needed for revisions and for documenting that learning has occurred. Positive reinforcement affirms and encourages learning.

- Counseling involves the nurse in teaching and assisting the patient to learn problem-solving techniques.

- The three types of counseling are (1) short-term counseling, which focuses on an immediate problem; (2) long-term counseling, which extends over a prolonged period; and (3) motivational counseling, which involves discussing feelings and incentives with the patient.

- Counseling may be needed for assisting the patient through crises or for motivating the patient to work toward health promotion.

■ Learning Checklist

Review the learning checklist at the end of the chapter in your textbook and be sure you can meet each objective.

■ Exercises

MATCHING

Match the examples in Part B with the appropriate teaching strategy listed in Part A. Answers may be used more than once.

PART A

a. role modeling
b. lecture
c. discussion
d. demonstration
e. discovery
f. role-playing
g. AV materials
h. printed material
i. computer-assisted instruction programs

PART B

1. _____ A nurse speaks to a group of patients about the dangers of smoking.

2. _____ A nurse chooses a low-calorie meal for herself when having lunch with an obese patient.

3. _____ A nurse performs a bath procedure on a newborn infant in front of several new mothers.

4. _____ A nurse obtains pamphlets for a 16-year-old that describe how STDs are transmitted.

5. _____ One student pretends to be a patient while another student conducts a nursing interview.

6. _____ A nurse uses a videotape to teach a patient about heart disease.

7. _____ A nurse describes the symptoms of an anxiety attack to a patient with panic disorder and lets him choose measures to take during and after the attack.

8. _____ A nurse shows a film on relaxation techniques to a cardiac patient.

9. _____ A nurse shows a diabetic patient how to give herself insulin by injecting an orange.

10. _____ A nurse exchanges information with a patient about the patient's feelings of powerlessness following a TIA.

Match the examples of teaching strategies in Part B with the aims of nursing listed in Part A. Some answers may be used more than once.

PART A

a. promoting wellness
b. preventing illness
c. restoring health
d. facilitating coping

PART B

11. _____ A nurse demonstrates to a postoperative patient the proper way to bandage his incision.

12. _____ A nurse explains to a new mother the importance and availability of immunizations for her baby.

13. _____ A nurse counsels a woman in her first trimester on proper nutrition.

14. _____ A nurse refers a recovering alcoholic to a local group meeting.

15. _____ A nurse presents a lecture on baby-proofing a home to a group of parents.

16. _____ A nurse teaches a young athlete stretching exercises to be used before running track.

17. _____ A nurse refers the daughter of a terminally ill patient to a counseling session on coping with death and dying.

18. _____ A nurse introduces a patient recovering from a broken hip to the physical therapy staff.

19. _____ A nurse refers a 42-year-old woman to a clinic providing free mammograms.

20. _____ A nurse teaches relaxation techniques to a patient recovering from coronary bypass surgery.

Match the learning domain listed in Part A with the example of the domain listed in Part B. Answers may be used more than once.

PART A

a. cognitive learning
b. psychomotor learning
c. affective learning

PART B

21. _____ A patient learns how to care for his surgical wound.

22. _____ A patient explains how eating a proper diet will lower his cholesterol.

23. _____ A patient learns how to use range-of-motion exercises post surgery.

24. _____ A patient expresses renewed self-confidence following successful completion of a class to stop smoking.

25. _____ A patient decides to get dressed in the morning following treatment for depression.

26. _____ A patient reiterates the need for prenatal and infant care to her social worker.

MULTIPLE CHOICE

Circle the letter that corresponds to the best answer for each question.

1. Which of the following developmental considerations is the nurse assessing when he determines that an 8-year-old boy is not equipped to understand the scientific explanation of his disease?
   a. intellectual development
   b. motor development
   c. emotional maturity
   d. psychosocial development

2. Which of the following is the best source of assessment information for the nurse?
   a. nursing plan of care
   b. physician
   c. patient
   d. family/friends

3. Which of the following diagnoses would best describe a situation in which a patient has a knowledge deficit concerning child safety for her toddler, who is currently being treated for burns and was previously treated for a fracture from a fall?
   a. Knowledge Deficit: Child Safety, related to inexperience with the active developmental stage of a toddler.
   b. Toddler at High Risk for Injury, related to mother's lack of knowledge about child safety.
   c. Potential for Enhanced Parenting, related to child safety knowledge deficit.
   d. Knowledge Deficit: Child Safety, related to mother's lack of experience and socioeconomic level.

4. When writing learner objectives for a patient, the nurse should consider which of the following statements?
   a. It is better to use one or two broad objectives than several specific objectives.
   b. The objectives written in the Learner Objectives column of the sample teaching plan are general statements that could be accomplished in any amount of time.
   c. Planning of learner objectives should be done by the nurse or other healthcare professionals before obtaining input from the patient/family.
   d. One long-term objective could be stated for each diagnosis followed by several specific objectives.

5. When deciding what information the patient needs to meet learner objectives successfully, the nurse is planning which part of the teaching plan?
   a. content
   b. teaching strategies
   c. learning activities
   d. learning domains

6. A nurse could attempt to help a patient solve a situational crisis during which of the following types of counseling sessions?
   a. long-term counseling
   b. motivational counseling
   c. short-term counseling
   d. professional counseling

7. When a patient says: "I don't care if I get better; I have nothing to live for, anyway," which type of counseling would be appropriate?

   a. long-term counseling

   b. motivational counseling

   c. short-term counseling

   d. professional counseling

8. When teaching an adult patient how to control stress through relaxation techniques, the nurse should consider which of the following assumptions concerning adult learners?

   a. As an adult matures, his/her self-concept becomes more dependent; therefore, this patient must be made aware of the importance of reducing stress.

   b. The adult learner is not as concerned with the immediate usefulness of the material being taught as he is with the quality of the material.

   c. As patients, adults are the least likely to resist learning because of preconceived ideas about the teaching/learning process.

   d. The nurse should be able to draw from the previous experience of the patient to elaborate the importance of stress reduction.

9. Which of the following principles of teaching–learning is an accurate guideline for the nurse/teacher?

   a. Patient teaching should occur independent of the nursing process.

   b. Past life experience should not be a factor when helping patients assimilate new knowledge.

   c. The teaching–learning process can be facilitated by the existence of a helping relationship.

   d. Planning learner objectives should be done by the teacher alone.

10. When planning for learning, who must decide who should be included in the learning sessions?

    a. the healthcare team

    b. the doctor and nurse

    c. the nurse and the patient

    d. the patient and the patient's family

COMPLETION

1. Briefly explain how teaching and counseling patients can facilitate the following nursing aims.

   a. Promoting wellness: _____

   _____

   _____

   b. Preventing illness: _____

   _____

   _____

   c. Restoring health: _____

   _____

   _____

   d. Facilitating coping: _____

   _____

   _____

2. How would you modify your teaching plan to motivate the following patients to learn a new skill?

   a. An adult who has a fear of failure: _____

   _____

   _____

   b. An adult who resists learning because of preconceived ideas about the process and your expectations of him/her: _____

   _____

   _____

   _____

   c. An older adult who is afraid to learn something new: _____

   _____

   _____

3. Mr. Lang is a 75-year-old man recovering from a stroke in a home care setting. He has partial paralysis of his left side and must be taught exercises for rehabilitation. List three teaching strategies you would use in treating this patient, and give an example of each.

   a. _____

   _____

   _____

   b. _____

   _____

   _____

   c. _____

   _____

   _____

4. List two solutions to the problem time constraints place on the nurse when planning patient learning.

   a. _____

   b. _____

5. Briefly describe the following types of teaching, and give an example of each:

   a. Formal: _____

   _____

   b. Informal: _____

   _____

6. Give an example of a method that could be used to evaluate the following types of learning:

   a. Cognitive domain: _____

   b. Affective domain: _____

   c. Psychomotor domain: _____

7. How would you document successfully teaching a new mother how to bathe her infant?

   _____

   _____

   _____

8. Define the following types of counseling, and give an example of a case in which each type would be used by the nurse.

   a. Short-term counseling: _____

   _____

   _____

   _____

   b. Long-term counseling: _____

   _____

   _____

   c. Motivational counseling: _____

   _____

   _____

9. List four elements that should be considered in each assessment of patient learning needs.

   a. _____

   b. _____

   c. _____

   d. _____

10. Give an example of the following teaching strategies that you have experienced in your personal/student life. Which of these strategies do you feel were most effective for you?

    a. Role modeling: _____

    b. Lecture: _____

    c. Discussion: _____

    d. Panel discussion: _____

    e. Demonstration: _____

    f. Discovery: _____

    g. Role playing: _____

    h. AV materials: _____

    i. Programmed instruction: _____

    j. Computer-assisted instruction: _____

GUIDE TO CRITICAL THINKING AND DEVELOPING BLENDED SKILLS

1. As a child, you learned many things from your parents. Consider the types of teaching that you experienced and think about how you could use both formal and informal teaching to help children accomplish the following goals.

    a. Avoiding drugs and alcohol

    b. Learning how to cook a healthy meal

    c. Dealing with peer pressure

2. Observe nurses teaching and counseling patients and family members to promote health, prevent illness, restore health, or facilitate coping. What methods did the nurse use to identify each patient's learning needs? Was the nurse successful in teaching this patient? How would you have handled the teaching process differently? Assess each patient's knowledge, attitude, and skills needed to independently manage their own healthcare.

3. Devise a plan to teach a woman how to lose weight by reducing the fat content in her diet and developing an exercise routine using the following methods:

    a. Lecture

    b. Discussion

    c. Demonstration

    d. Role playing

    What was the advantage/disadvantage of each method?

CHAPTER 23

Leader, Researcher, and Advocate

CHAPTER OVERVIEW

- Nurses have the basic qualities and skills for leadership; they need to work toward developing these qualities and skills.

- Nurses choose leadership styles according to their own personality traits, the objectives to be achieved, and the characteristics of the followers.

- Nurse leaders are responsible for effecting positive changes, managing patient and staff activities, and using administrative knowledge appropriately.

- Nursing leadership is involved in working for the benefit of the patient, the nursing team, the nursing profession, and society.

- Research provides an important step toward expanding the professional role of nursing, acquiring new knowledge to improve patient care, and remaining competitive in the healthcare marketplace.

- Beginning nurses can use research findings to improve their care; identify researchable problems; and protect the rights of research subjects to informed consent, confidentiality, and freedom from harm.

- Making choices about health is a fundamental human right that promotes patient dignity and well-being.

- As an advocate, the nurse informs the patient of rights and supports patient decisions concerning rights and healthcare choices.

- Assertiveness is a necessary tool for the nurse to use in both advocacy and leadership roles. Nurses may also need to teach assertiveness techniques to patients and families.

- Educating the public about the benefits of advance directives is an important nursing advocacy role.

■ Learning Checklist

Review the learning checklist at the end of the chapter in your textbook and be sure you can meet each objective.

■ Exercises

MATCHING

Match the examples of leadership in Part B with the types of leadership they imply, listed in Part A. Some answers may be used more than once.

PART A

a. autocratic leadership

b. democratic leadership

c. laissez-faire leadership

d. transformational leadership

e. situational leadership

PART B

1. _____ A nurse unites with other nurses to create a shelter for battered women in their neighborhood.

2. _____ A nurse opens a discussion among healthcare team members to determine the best care plan for a patient.

3. _____ A nurse takes control during a "code blue" and directs all activities to resuscitate the patient.

4. _____ A nurse leads other nurses in developing a schedule to cook meals for the homeless.

5. _____ A nurse manager adjusts the work schedule of her unit each week to accommodate the current caseload.

6. _____ A nurse in charge of scheduling suggests that the nurses meet and work out the schedule on their own.

7. _____ A nurse seeks input from her co-workers to solve a problem of understaffing.

8. _____ A head nurse makes schedules of meetings of the ANA available to any staff members who are interested.

9. _____ A head nurse directs the triage unit after several earthquake victims arrive at the emergency room.

10. _____ A head nurse issues a memo describing step-by-step documentation procedures that she wants initiated in the ER.

CORRECT THE FALSE STATEMENTS

Circle the word true or false that follows the statement. If the word false has been circled, change the underlined word/words to make the statement true. Place your answer in the space provided.

1. Planned change is a purposeful, systematic effort to alter or bring about change through the intervention of a change agent.

   True   False   _____

2. Preceptorship is a relationship in which an experienced individual advises and assists a less experienced individual.

   True   False   _____

3. Nursing research is fundamental to the recognition of nursing as an occupation.

   True   False   _____

4. Scientific knowledge comes from an expert and is accepted as truth based on a perceived level of expertise.

   True   False   _____

5. Independent variables are the factors the researcher introduces into the study and can control.

   True   False   _____

6. Informed consent is the patient's right to knowledgeably participate in a study without coercion, or to refuse to participate without jeopardizing the care he/she will receive.

   True   False   _____

7. Assertiveness involves combining the three roles of teacher, counselor, and leader to form a new role through which the nurse protects and supports the patient's rights.

   True   False   _____

8. Advocacy is necessary only for those patients who are unable to defend themselves.

   True   False   _____

9. A Patient's Bill of Rights includes the rights and responsibilities of the patient while receiving care in the hospital.

   True   False   _____

10. Nurses as advocates make ethical decisions for their patients.

    True   False   _____

11. Leadership, advocacy, and research are separate and distinct entities.

    True   False   _____

12. Implied power is the power a person has by virtue of his/her position.

    True   False   _____

13. A decentralized management system invites greater accountability and responsibility among employees.

    True   False   _____

MULTIPLE CHOICE

Circle the letter that corresponds to the best answer for each question.

1. Which of the following is an essential element that differentiates an occupation from a profession?
   a. working conditions
   b. employee responsibility
   c. knowledge base
   d. research facilities

2. The most important goal of clinical nursing research is to do which of the following?
   a. Increase the knowledge base.
   b. Improve the quality of patient care.
   c. Increase the professionalism of the nurses.
   d. Test new nursing theories.

3. Which of the following statements concerning advocacy is accurate?

    a. Nurses who are advocates make decisions for their patients.

    b. Advocacy is necessary only for those who cannot defend themselves.

    c. Nurses have always been advocates for their patients' rights.

    d. Patients who participate in scientific studies give up their patient rights.

4. In which of the following styles of leadership are group satisfaction and motivation primary benefits?

    a. democratic

    b. autocratic

    c. laissez-faire

    d. transformational

5. Which of the following styles of leadership is rarely used in a hospital setting because of the difficulty of task achievement by independent nurses?

    a. democratic

    b. autocratic

    c. laissez-faire

    d. transformational

6. When a nurse arranges all the resources available to teach a juvenile how to manage her asthma, he is performing which of the following roles of a nurse manager?

    a. planning role

    b. organizing role

    c. directing role

    d. controlling role

7. In which of the following examples is a nurse accurately performing her role as an advocate for her patient?

    a. A nurse makes decisions about treatment for a patient with Alzheimer's disease.

    b. A nurse practices advocacy only on patients who cannot defend themselves.

    c. A nurse withholds information from an emotionally distraught patient to protect her mental stability.

    d. A nurse interprets the rights of a patient who is HIV positive.

8. The Freedom of Information Act of 1967 and the Privacy Act of 1974 were enacted to accomplish which of the following?

    a. Opening all medical records to patients described in them

    b. Sealing all medical records from patients in federally funded institutions

    c. Opening personal government records to patients described in them

    d. Guaranteeing patients rights in the new climate of managed care

COMPLETION

1. Describe what the following leadership qualities mean to you, and how they would help motivate patients in your practice to achieve their goals.

    Leaders should:

    a. Be dynamic: _____

    _____

    _____

    b. Be enthusiastic: _____

    _____

    c. Be self-directed: _____

    _____

    _____

    d. Have a positive self-image: _____

    _____

    _____

    e. Be role models: _____

    _____

    _____

    f. Have vision: _____

    _____

    _____

2. Mr. Eng is a 75-year-old man dying of lung cancer in a hospice. Give an example of how a nurse may use each of the following leadership skills to help relieve his suffering.

   a. Communication skills: _____

   _____

   _____

   b. Problem-solving skills: _____

   _____

   _____

   c. Management skills: _____

   _____

   _____

   d. Self-evaluation skills: _____

   _____

   _____

3. List the steps you would employ to change a nursing unit from paper records to a computerized method of record-keeping. How would you handle people who resist the change?

   _____

   _____

   _____

4. Briefly describe the following reasons why people resist change, and state how you would confront the problem in your own practice:

   a. Threat to self: _____

   _____

   _____

   b. Lack of understanding: _____

   _____

   _____

   c. Limited tolerance to change: _____

   _____

   _____

   d. Disagreements about the benefits of change:

   _____

   _____

   e. Fear of increased responsibility: _____

   _____

   _____

5. List four ways nurses can contribute to nursing research:

   a. _____

   b. _____

   c. _____

   d. _____

6. Explain how you, as a nurse practitioner, can help change the negative portrayals of nursing in the media.

   _____

   _____

   _____

7. Explain how informed consent protects the rights of individuals who are research subjects:

   _____

   _____

   _____

8. Describe the role you would assume as an advocate for the following patients.

   a. A 37-year-old woman, recently arrived in the United States from Guatemala and diagnosed with ovarian cancer, who does not speak English: _____

   _____

   _____

   b. An 88-year-old patient, post stroke, who refuses surgical repair of hernia: _____

   _____

   _____

9. Describe how you would use the following management functions to organize fellow students to form a group to help control binge drinking on campus.

   a. Planning: _____

   b. Organizing: _____

   c. Motivating: _____

   d. Controlling: _____

10. Give an example from your present situation (home, school, work), where you feel that you may have the power to influence change. Explain what steps you would take to overcome resistance to this change: _____

_____

_____

11. List four contributions nurses can make to nursing research.

    a. _____

    b. _____

    c. _____

    d. _____

GUIDE TO CRITICAL THINKING AND DEVELOPING BLENDED SKILLS

1. Explain why the following patients need a nurse advocate and what you would do to facilitate their needs.

    a. A 10-year-old child is admitted to the ER for contusions that you feel could have been caused by the mother.

    b. A 15-year-old boy with end stage cancer wants his parents to honor his right to die a dignified death by signing a DNR order.

    c. A 60-year-old homeless, alcoholic patient who has shown periods of violence on the ward spends most of her day in restraints.

2. Advance directives enable people to specify their preferences and end-of-life care. See if you can help family members and friends complete an advanced directive. How will this experience help you to be a better patient advocate?

3. Review the leadership styles of the people who have been authority figures in your life. What makes them effective or ineffective leaders? Which leadership styles have you tried? Which do you feel will be most helpful to you as you try to help patients/family and health teams achieve health goals?

4. Think about all the formal and informal research you have used to make life choices and its relationship to the outcome of your choices. How might these experiences influence your approach to nursing research?

UNIT VI

Actions Basic to Nursing Care

CHAPTER 24

Vital Signs

CHAPTER OVERVIEW

- Assessing vital signs, a traditional nursing responsibility, involves obtaining temperature, pulse, respiration, and blood pressure as part of the baseline data from which a plan of care is developed.

- The frequency of assessing vital signs is governed by the healthcare agency's policies and the patient's health status.

- Humans are warm blooded and maintain body temperature independently of their environment. The hypothalamus in the central nervous system maintains body temperature of the well human within a fairly constant range, called a set point.

- Pyrexia, or fever, an elevation of normal body temperature, is a common symptom of disease. Most fevers are self-limiting. On the other hand, hypothermia is a temperature below the lower limit of normal. Both may be means by which the body fights disease.

- Temperature may be assessed by glass clinical thermometer, electronic thermometer, disposable single-use thermometer, temperature-sensitive patch or tape, or automated monitoring device. Although most agencies measure temperature by the oral route, rectal and axillary routes are alternative sites.

- When the left ventricle of the heart contracts to eject blood into the filled aorta, arterial walls expand or distend; this expansion can be felt as a wave and is called the pulse. Pulse rate is the number of pulsations felt in a minute; pulse rhythm is the pattern of the pulsations and the pauses between them; and pulse amplitude describes the quality of the pulse.

- Arteries most commonly used for assessment are peripheral pulses or those close to the skin surface (i.e., temporal, carotid, brachial, radial, femoral, popliteal, posterior tibial, and dorsalis pedis). The radial pulse at the wrist is most commonly used.

- Respiration is the act of breathing and includes the body's use of oxygen and elimination of carbon dioxide. Inspiration or inhalation is the act of breathing in. Expiration or exhalation is the act of breathing out.

- Healthy adults breathe about 16 to 20 times per minute with a fairly consistent relationship of pulse rate to respiratory rate of one respiration to about four heartbeats.

- Apnea refers to periods in which there is no breathing; dyspnea is difficult or labored breathing, demonstrated by rapid and shallow breathing. Dyspneic patients often are able to breathe easier in an upright position. Being able to breathe easier in this manner is known as orthopnea.

- Blood pressure refers to the force of blood against arterial walls. The highest pressure, exerted when the left ventricle of the heart pushes blood through the aortic valve into the aorta during systole, is called systolic pressure. When the heart rests between beats (diastole), the pressure drops; the lowest pressure is called diastolic pressure. Blood pressure, measured in millimeters of mercury (mm Hg), is recorded as a fraction. The numerator is the systolic pressure; the denominator is the diastolic pressure (e.g., 120/80).

- Deviations from normal blood pressure are likely due to alterations in any one or more of these functions: peripheral resistance, heart's pumping action, blood volume, blood viscosity, and elasticity of vessel walls.

- Blood pressure can be within a wide range and still be normal. Many factors influence a normal, healthy adult's blood pressure.

- Hypertension is a state in which a person's blood pressure is above normal. Primary or essential hypertension has an unknown cause, whereas secondary hypertension is due to known pathologic factors. Blood pressure below normal is called hypotension. Orthostatic or postural hypotension is associated with weakness or fainting when rising to an erect position.

- A sphygmomanometer, consisting of a cuff and manometer, and a stethoscope are necessary for obtaining an indirect measurement of blood pressure. The series of sounds heard in this measurement are called Korotkoff sounds. They are written as fractions (e.g., 120/80).

- Blood pressure also can be assessed using palpation, electronic indirect blood pressure meters, or direct electronic measurements.
- Patients providing self-care at home need to know how to take their own temperature, pulse, and blood pressure.

▪ Learning Checklist

Review the learning checklist at the end of the chapter in your textbook and be sure you can meet each objective.

▪ Exercises

MATCHING

Match the following definitions related to pulse in Part B with the appropriate term listed in Part A.

PART A

a. pulse

b. pulse rate

c. tachycardia

d. palpitation

e. bradycardia

f. pulse rhythm

g. pulse amplitude

h. arrhythmia

i. stroke volume

j. cardiac output

k. ventricular contraction

l. pulse deficit

PART B

1. _____ Number of pulsations felt in a minute.

2. _____ Quantity of blood forced out of left ventricle with each contraction.

3. _____ Person is aware of own heartbeat without having to feel for it.

4. _____ Quality of the pulse in terms of fullness; reflects strength of left ventricular contraction.

5. _____ Light tap caused by expansion of aorta sending a wave through walls of the arterial system.

6. _____ Irregular pattern of heartbeats.

7. _____ Heart rate 60 beats/minute in an adult.

8. _____ The amount of blood pumped/minute.

9. _____ A rapid heart rate.

10. _____ The pattern of pulsations and pauses between them.

11. _____ The difference between the apical and radial pulse rates.

Match the term in Part A with the correct definition in Part B.

PART A

a. inspiration

b. expiration

c. apnea

d. dyspnea

e. orthopnea

f. internal respiration

g. external respiration

h. eupnea

i. tachypnea

j. pulmonary ventilation

k. bradypnea

PART B

12. _____ A fast respiratory rate.

13. _____ The exchange of oxygen and carbon dioxide between the alveoli of the lungs and the circulating blood.

14. _____ Difficult or labored breathing.

15. _____ The act of breathing in.

16. _____ The exchange of oxygen and carbon dioxide between the circulating blood and tissue cells .

17. _____ Movement of air in and out of the lungs.

18. _____ Normal respirations with equal rate and depth.

19. _____ Being able to breathe more easily in an upright position.

20. _____ Periods during which there is no breathing.

21. _____ Slow breathing.

Match the definitions of body temperatures and variations in Part B with the appropriate term listed in Part A.

PART A

a. pyrexia

b. febrile

c. afebrile

d. hyperpyrexia

e. hypothermia

f. hyperthermia

g. ineffective thermoregulation

PART B

22. _____ Body temperature below limit of normal.

23. _____ State in which temperature fluctuates between above and below normal ranges.

24. _____ Body temperature is elevated above normal range.

25. _____ Body temperature above normal.

26. _____ Person with normal body temperature.

27. _____ High fever, usually above 105.8°F.

Draw lines from the pulse assessment sites listed in Part A to their appropriate location depicted in Part B.

PART A

a. temporal

b. carotid

c. brachial

d. femoral

e. posterior tibial

f. popliteal

g. radial

h. dorsalis pedis

PART B

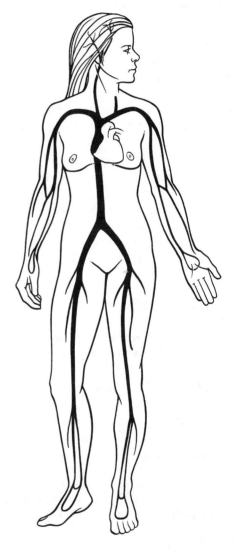

MULTIPLE CHOICE

Circle the letter that corresponds to the best answer for each question.

1. Which of the following is the primary source of heat in the human body?

   a. metabolism

   b. hormones

   c. sympathetic neurotransmitters

   d. hypothalamus

2. Which of the following is the primary mechanism or site of heat loss?

   a. contraction of pilomotor muscles of the skin

   b. warming and humidifying of inspired air

   c. skin surface

   d. urine and feces

3. What would be the cardiac output of an adult with a stroke volume of 75 mL and a pulse of 78 beats/minute?

   a. 5000 mL

   b. 5550 mL

   c. 5850 mL

   d. 6000 mL

5. Which of the following conditions occurs when an adult has a pulse rate of 100–180 beats/minute?

   a. bradycardia

   b. arrhythmia

   c. pulse amplitude

   d. tachycardia

5. Which of the following statements concerning respiratory rates is accurate?

   a. Infants and young children have a lower respiratory rate than adults.

   b. Healthy adults breathe about 16–20 times per minute.

   c. The respiratory rate decreases in response to the increased metabolic rate during pyrexia.

   d. An increase in intracranial pressures stimulates the respiratory center and increases the respiration rate.

6. Which of the following statistics regarding blood pressure is accurate?

   a. Blood pressure tends to be lower in a prone or supine position than in a seated or standing position.

   b. Men usually have a lower blood pressure than women of the same age.

   c. Blood pressure decreases after eating.

   d. Blood pressure is usually highest on arising in the morning.

7. Which of the following blood pressure measurement devices would be most appropriate for a patient to use in his own home?

   a. sphygmomanometer

   b. electronic indirect blood pressure meter

   c. Doppler ultrasound

   d. direct electronic measurement

8. The average normal temperature in degrees Fahrenheit for well adults in the rectal site is which of the following?

   a. 94.0

   b. 97.6

   c. 98.6

   d. 99.5

9. Which of the following conditions tends to lower blood pressure?

   a. high viscosity of the blood

   b. low blood volume

   c. decreased elasticity of walls of arterioles

   d. strong pumping action of blood into the arteries

10. After taking vital signs, you write down your findings as: T = 98.6, P = 66, R = 18, BP = 124/82. Which of the numbers above is the systolic blood pressure?

    a. 98.6

    b. 124

    c. 82

    d. 66

COMPLETION

1. Briefly describe how the following factors affect body temperature.

   a. Circadian rhythms: _____

   _____

   _____

   b. Age: _____

   _____

   _____

   c. Gender: _____

   _____

   _____

   d. Stress: _____

   _____

   _____

   e. Environmental temperatures: _____

   _____

   _____

2. Complete the following chart describing the types
   of thermometers used to assess temperature.

Type of Thermometer	Brief Description	Contraindication	Normal Reading
A. GLASS oral rectal			
B. ELECTRONIC			
C. TYMPANIC MEMBRANE			
D. TEMPERATURE SENSITIVE PATCH			
E. AUTOMATED MONITORING DEVICE			

3. List three methods that can be used to assess the
   pulse by palpating or auscultating.

   a. _____

   _____

   _____

   b. _____

   _____

   _____

   c. _____

   _____

   _____

4. Briefly describe how the following variables may
   affect a patient's blood pressure.

   a. Pumping action of the heart: _____

   _____

   _____

b. Blood volume: _____

   _____

   _____

c. Viscosity of blood: _____

   _____

   _____

d. Elasticity of vessel walls: _____

   _____

   _____

5. List four parts in blood pressure measurement
   equipment that should be checked to make sure
   they are functioning properly.

   a. _____

   b. _____

   c. _____

   d. _____

6. Briefly define the following NANDA nursing diagnoses for altered respirations.

   a. Impaired gas exchange: _____

   _____

   _____

   b. Ineffective airway clearance: _____

   _____

   _____

   c. Ineffective breathing pattern: _____

   _____

   _____

   d. Inability to sustain spontaneous ventilation: ____

   _____

   _____

7. Briefly define the following NANDA nursing diagnoses for alterations in pulse and blood pressure.

   a. Altered tissue perfusion: _____

   _____

   _____

   b. Risk for fluid volume imbalance: _____

   _____

   _____

   c. Fluid volume excess: _____

   _____

   _____

   d. Fluid volume deficit: _____

   _____

   _____

   e. Decreased cardiac output: _____

   _____

   _____

8. Describe the use of the following equipment used to assess the pulse and blood pressure.

   a. Stethoscope: _____

   _____

   _____

   b. Sphygmomanometer: _____

   _____

   _____

GUIDE TO CRITICAL THINKING AND DEVELOPING BLENDED SKILLS

1. Using a partner, locate the nine sites for pulse assessment. Practice the technique for obtaining radial and apical pulses. Then practice the technique for measuring respirations and assessing blood pressure. Why is it important to be proficient in assessing and reporting vital sign measurements? If you were unsure of one of your vital sign assessments, what would you do?

2. An obese woman in the clinic needs a large blood pressure cuff and one is not available. The resident tell you just to use the cuff you have. What do you do and why?

3. Using a mannequin in your nursing laboratory, practice the method of taking oral, rectal, and axillary temperatures. Research any new devices used for taking temperature and familiarize yourself with their use. Why do nurses need to be competent using different methods and devices?

CHAPTER 25

Health Assessment

CHAPTER OVERVIEW

- Data collection during a health assessment includes a health history and a physical assessment. Data from nursing assessments are used to formulate nursing diagnoses.

- Four techniques are used in performing a health assessment: inspection, palpation, percussion, and auscultation.

- The nurse should plan the health assessment at a time that is appropriate for both the patient and the nurse. The nurse should prepare the room, gather instruments and equipment, ensure privacy, and meet the patient's physical and psychologic needs.

- Various positions are used during the health assessment. The patient's privacy and comfort should be considered in each position.

- Each body system is assessed for normal and abnormal findings; included are the integument, the head and neck, the thorax and lungs, the breasts and axillae, the abdomen, the male and female genitalia, the rectum and anus, the musculoskeletal system, and the neurologic system. The techniques of assessment are used to assess the health status of the patient systematically.

- The nurse carefully documents normal and abnormal findings.

- Diagnostic tests provide valuable information about a patient's health status. Nursing responsibilities associated with diagnostic tests may include witnessing a patient's consent, scheduling the test, physical and emotional preparation of the patient, nursing care after the test, disposal of equipment, and proper care of any specimen.

■ Learning Checklist

Review the learning checklist at the end of the chapter in your textbook and be sure you can meet each objective.

■ Exercises

MATCHING

Match the organs listed in Part B with their proper location listed in Part A. Answers may be used more than once.

PART A

a. right upper quadrant

b. left upper quadrant

c. right lower quadrant

d. left lower quadrant

e. midline

PART B

1. _____ Liver

2. _____ Stomach

3. _____ Gallbladder

4. _____ Sigmoid colon

5. _____ Cecum

6. _____ Spleen

7. _____ Urinary bladder

8. _____ Left ureter and lower kidney pole

9. _____ Appendix

10. _____ Right kidney and adrenal gland

11. _____ Body of pancreas

12. _____ Left ovary and fallopian tube

Match the terms in Part A with the correct definitions for findings during skin assessment listed in Part B.

PART A

a. flushing

b. cyanosis

c. jaundice

d. pallor

e. ecchymosis

f. petechiae

g. lesion

h. turgor

i. bruits

PART B

13. _____ Yellow color

14. _____ Redness

15. _____ Dusky, blue color

16. _____ Purplish discoloration

17. _____ Diseased or injured tissue

18. _____ Paleness

19. _____ Elasticity of the skin

20. _____ Very small hemorrhagic spots

Match each nerve listed in Part A with its function listed in Part B.

PART A

a. olfactory (I) nerve

b. optic (II) nerve

c. oculomotor (III), trochlear (IV), and abducens (VI) nerves

d. trigeminal (V) nerve

e. facial (VII) nerve

f. acoustic (VIII) nerve

g. glossopharyngeal (IX) nerve

h. vagus (X) nerve

i. accessory (XI) nerve

j. hypoglossal (XII) nerve

PART B

21. _____ A sensory nerve that is tested by assessing hearing ability.

22. _____ A sensory nerve whose function is vision. Vision is tested for acuity and visual fields.

23. _____ A sensorimotor nerve that is assessed by observing the facial muscles for deviation of the jaw to one side and by palpating facial muscles for tone while patient clenches jaw.

24. _____ A motor nerve that affects the movement and strength of the tongue.

25. _____ A sensory nerve whose function is the sense of smell.

26. _____ Motor nerves that control the movement of the eyes through the cardinal fields of gaze; pupil size, shape, response to light, and accommodation; and opening of the upper eyelids.

27. _____ A sensorimotor nerve that innervates the muscles of the face and functions to provide the taste sensation of the anterior two thirds of the tongue.

28. _____ A motor nerve that is assessed by asking the patient to open the mouth and say "Ah" as the upward movement of the soft palate is observed.

29. _____ A motor nerve that controls the movement of the heard and shoulders.

Match the positions listed in Part A with their description and function listed in Part B.

PART A

a. sitting position

b. supine position

c. dorsal recumbent position

d. Sims' position

e. prone position

f. lithotomy position

g. knee–chest position

h. standing position

PART B

30. _____ The patient kneels, using the knees and chest to bear the weight of the body. The position is used to assess the rectal area.

31. _____ The patient lies on the left or right side with lower arm behind the body and upper arm bent at the shoulder and elbow. The knees are both bent, with the uppermost leg at a more acute angle. The position is used to assess the rectum or vagina.

32. _____ The patient is in the dorsal recumbent position with the buttocks at the edge of the

examining table and feet supported in stirrups. This position is used to assess female rectum and genitalia.

33. _____ The patient may sit upright in a chair or on the side of examining table or bed. This position allows visualization of the upper body and facilitates lung expansion. It is used to take vital signs and assess head, neck, posterior and anterior thorax and lungs, breasts, heart, and upper extremities.

34. _____ The patient lies on the back with legs separated, knees bent, and soles of the feet flat on the bed. This position is used to assess head and neck, anterior thorax and lungs, breasts, heart, extremities, and peripheral pulses.

35. _____ The patient lies flat on the back with legs together but extended and slightly bent at the knees. This position is used to assess the head and neck, anterior thorax and lungs, breasts, heart, abdomen, extremities, and peripheral pulses.

36. _____ The patient lies on the abdomen, flat on the bed, with the head turned to one side. This position is used to assess the hip joint and posterior thorax.

Match the structures of the thorax listed in Part A with the location on the illustration depicted in Part B.

PART A

a. arch of aorta

b. left lung

c. parietal pleura

d. right lung

e. right bronchus

f. parietal pericardium

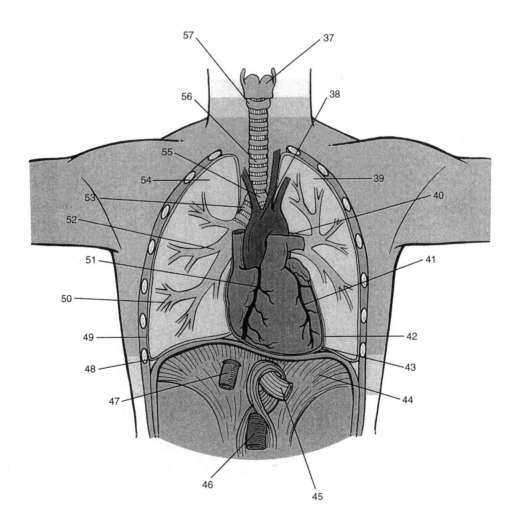

g. thyroid cartilage

h. terminal bronchiole

i. hepatic vein

j. visceral pericardium

k. abdominal aorta

l. diaphragm

m. esophagus

n. left coronary artery and vein

o. visceral pleura

p. right coronary artery and vein

q. bronchiole

r. hilum

s. left bronchus

t. trachea

u. cricoid cartilage

PART B

MULTIPLE CHOICE

Circle the letter that corresponds to the best answer for each question.

1. Which of the following describes a *normal* assessment of the eye?

   a. The patient's eyes should not converge when you move your finger toward his/her nose.

   b. The patient's pupils should be black, equal in size, round and smooth.

   c. The pupils should be pale and cloudy in older adults.

   d. The patient's pupils should dilate when looking at a near object and constrict when looking at a distant object.

2. Which of the following assessment measures is used to assess the location, shape, size, and density of tissues?

   a. observation

   b. palpation

   c. percussion

   d. auscultation

3. When percussing the stomach, which of the following sounds would most likely be heard?

   a. tympany

   b. hyperresonance

   c. dullness

   d. flatness

4. A patient who presents with a dusky, bluish skin color is experiencing which of the following conditions?

   a. flushing

   b. jaundice

   c. cyanosis

   d. pallor

5. Which of the following is a *normal* finding when assessing internal eye structures?

   a. a uniform yellow reflex

   b. a clear, reddish optic nerve disc

   c. dark red arteries and light red veins

   d. a reddish retina

6. Which of the following are soft and low-pitched sounds, and are heard best over the base of the lungs during inspiration?

   a. bronchial sounds

   b. vesicular breath sounds

   c. bronchovesicular sounds

   d. adventitious breath sounds

7. A soft, high-pitched, flat sound that is usually percussed over muscle tissue is which of the following?

   a. flatness

   b. resonance

   c. hyperresonance

   d. dullness

8. Which of the following conditions would be a *normal* finding when palpating the skin of a patient?

   a. The skin is cool and dry.

   b. When picked up in a fold, the skin fold slowly returns to normal.

   c. The skin is taut and moist to touch.

   d. The texture of the skin varies from smooth and soft to rough and dry.

9. Which of the following eye characteristics is tested by assessing the eight cardinal fields of vision for coordination and alignment?

   a. visual acuity

   b. peripheral vision

   c. extraocular movements

   d. convergence

10. When assessing the ear canal and tympanic membrane with an otoscope, which of the following findings would be considered *normal*?

    a. The tympanic membrane should be translucent, shiny, and gray.

    b. The ear canal should be rough and pinkish in color.

    c. The tympanic membrane should be reddish in color.

    d. The ear canal should be smooth and white in color.

11. Mr. Rogers has been diagnosed as having a large tumor in his left lung. Which assessment technique would be used to determine the size of this tumor?

    a. auscultation

    b. palpation

    c. percussion

    d. inspection

12. A rubbing, grating sound that is loudest on the lower lateral anterior surface of the thorax and is auscultated during inspiration is known as which of the following?

    a. wheeze

    b. friction rub

    c. rhonchi

    d. crackles

13. To test the trochlear nerve of a patient, the nurse should do which of the following?

    a. Test pupillary reaction to light and ability to open and close eyelids.

    b. Test vision for acuity and visual fields.

    c. Test ocular movements in all directions.

    d. Test for downward and inward movement of the eye.

14. When a nurse asks a patient to raise her eyebrows, smile and show her teeth, and puff out her cheeks, he is most likely assessing which of the following nerves?

    a. facial

    b. vagus

    c. hypoglossal

    d. accessory

15. Which of the following is tested to evaluate the function of specific spinal cord segments?

    a. motor ability

    b. balance and gait

    c. reflexes

    d. sensory abilities

16. Which of the following assessment techniques would a nurse use to assess the thyroid gland?

    a. palpation

    b. inspection

    c. percussion

    d. auscultation

17. Which of the following is an accurate description of vesicular breath sounds?

    a. They are high-pitched, harsh sounds with expiration being longer than inspiration.

    b. They are noisy, strenuous respiration.

    c. They are high-pitched sounds heard on inspiration when there is a narrowing of the upper airway.

    d. They are soft, low-pitched sounds heard best over the base of the lungs during respiration. Inspiration is longer than expiration.

18. A weak, thready pulse found after the nurse palpates peripheral pulses may indicate which of the following conditions?

    a. hypertension and circulatory overload

    b. decreased cardiac output

    c. impaired circulation

    d. inflammation of a vein

COMPLETION

1. Identify the five purposes of performing a health assessment.

    a. _____

    b. _____

    c. _____

    d. _____

    e. _____

2. Briefly describe how the following instruments are used in a health assessment.

   a. Ophthalmoscope: _____

   _____

   _____

   b. Otoscope: _____

   _____

   _____

   c. Snellen chart: _____

   _____

   _____

   d. Nasal speculum: _____

   _____

   _____

   e. Vaginal speculum: _____

   _____

   _____

   f. Tuning fork: _____

   _____

   _____

   g. Percussion hammer: _____

   _____

   _____

3. List four factors that should be considered when deciding upon a position for physical assessment of a patient.

   a. _____

   b. _____

   c. _____

   d. _____

4. Describe how you would prepare a patient and the environment for a physical assessment.

   a. Patient: _____

   _____

   _____

   b. Environment: _____

   _____

   _____

5. Complete the chart at the bottom of the page depicting the four assessment techniques, giving a brief description of each and the types of assessment made with each technique.

Technique	Definition	Assessment/Observation
a. Inspection:		
b. Palpation:		
c. Percussion:		
d. Ascultation:		

6. List and describe the four characteristics of sound assessed by auscultation.

    a. _____

    b. _____

    c. _____

    d. _____

7. Briefly describe how you would assess a patient for the following conditions.

    a. Edema: _____

    _____

    _____

    b. Dehydration: _____

    _____

    _____

8. Describe the procedure for assessing the pupils of a patient for the following:

    a. Reaction to light: _____

    _____

    _____

    b. Accommodation: _____

    _____

    _____

    c. Convergence: _____

    _____

    _____

9. List the steps used to assess bone conduction according to Weber and Rinne.

    a. Weber: _____

    _____

    _____

    b. Rinne: _____

    _____

    _____

10. You are asked to perform a neurologic assessment on a patient. List the equipment you would assemble prior to performing the assessment. What position would your patient be placed in?

    _____

    _____

11. Give an example of a question you may ask to assess a patient's mental status in the following areas:

    a. Orientation: _____

    b. Immediate memory: _____

    c. Past memory: _____

    d. Abstract reasoning: _____

    e. Language: _____

12. Describe how you would assess a patient for the following reflexes.

    a. Biceps reflex: _____

    _____

    b. Brachioradialis or supinator reflex: _____

    _____

    c. Patellar or knee reflex: _____

    _____

    _____

    d. Achilles tendon reflex: _____

    _____

    _____

13. Complete the following paragraph by filling in the blanks with the correct word.

   During auscultation of the heart, the first heart sound heard is the (a) _____ of "lub-dub." This sound occurs when the (b) _____ and (c) _____ valves close and corresponds with the onset of (d) _____ contraction. This sound is called (e) _____ and is heard best in the (f) _____ area. The second heart sound, (g) _____, occurs at the end of (h) _____ and represents the closure of the (i) _____ and (j) _____ valves. It is the (k) _____ of "lub-dub." These two sounds occur within (l) _____ second(s) or less.

GUIDE TO CRITICAL THINKING AND DEVELOPING BLENDED SKILLS

1. Being prepared is a key factor when conducting a competent health assessment. The nurse must display developed cognitive, interpersonal, technical, and ethical skills. Describe what you would do to prepare the patient, the room, and the environment for an examination. How and why would you modify these preparations for the following patients:

   a. A patient who is comatose

   b. A patient who is uncooperative

   c. A patient who does not understand your language

   d. A small child

2. Make a list of all the instruments you would use to perform a health assessment. Arrange the instruments according to the order in which they will be used. Write a definition of each instrument and how it is to be used during the assessment. Rate yourself on your technical ability to use each instrument and technique. Practice using the instruments on a partner until you feel confident. Reflect on:

   a. How confident you need to be before you can assess a patient independently.

   b. When it is safe to "practice" on a patient.

CHAPTER 26

Safety

CHAPTER OVERVIEW

- Safety is the responsibility of all healthcare providers in every environment.

- Falls are the major safety problem in healthcare facilities as well as the leading cause of accidental death for older people.

- Patients at high risk of falling include older people and those who have previously fallen.

- Careless smoking and faulty electrical equipment are frequently implicated as causes in hospital fires.

- Hazards associated with the use of restraints include suffocation from improperly applied vests, impaired circulation, sensory deprivation, and emotional distress.

- Careful nursing assessment is the critical element in finding creative, resourceful alternatives to using restraints.

- The focus of emergency treatment of poisoning is to stabilize vital body functions, prevent the absorption of the poison, and encourage excretion of the toxic substance.

- Orientation to new surroundings, introduction to staff members, and explanations about equipment and procedures facilitate the patient's transfer to a new healthcare setting.

- An incident report must be filed when an accident occurs in a healthcare agency. The report should objectively document the circumstances of the accident.

■ Learning Checklist

Review the learning checklist at the end of the chapter in your textbook and be sure you can meet each objective.

■ Exercises

MATCHING

Match the type of poisonous agent in Part A with its common clinical manifestations, listed in Part B. List the type of emergency treatment you would use for each agent on the line provided.

PART A

a. salicylates (products containing aspirin, oil of wintergreen)

b. caustics (oven cleaner, drain openers, toilet bowl cleaners, rust removers, battery contents, hair perms)

c. hydrocarbons (gasoline, kerosene, furniture polish, lamp oil)

d. iron (vitamin preparations)

e. lead (paint chips, paint dust)

PART B

1. _____ Nausea, vomiting, diarrhea, abdominal pain, melena, hematemesis, lethargy, coma. _____

2. _____ Burning pain in mouth and throat, drooling, edema of lips and mouth, vomiting, hemoptysis, respiratory obstruction. _____

3. _____ Range from none (dose less than 150 mg) to nausea, hyperpnea, vomiting, confusion, fever, tinnitus, and coma. _____

4. _____ May be asymptomatic, anorexia, abdominal pain, encephalopathy. _____

5. _____ Gagging, coughing, choking, dyspnea, grunting, nausea, chills, fever, lethargy. _____

Match the safety precaution listed in Part B with the appropriate age group listed in Part A. Some answers may be used more than once.

PART A

a. fetus

b. infant

c. toddler and preschooler

d. school-age child

e. adolescent

f. adult

g. older adults

PART B

6. _____ This group needs assistance to evaluate activities that are potentially dangerous and to discuss specific interventions that provide for safety at home, in school, and in the neighborhood.

7. _____ Falls, fires, and motor vehicle accidents are significant hazards for this age group, and safety measures should be directed toward preventing these injuries.

8. _____ Education for this group must focus on safe driving skills, the dangers of drug and alcohol use, and formulation of a healthful lifestyle as a means of responding to the stress of daily living.

9. _____ A pregnant woman requires reinforcement about the risks associated with alcohol consumption, smoking, drug use, and exposure to dangers in the environment.

10. _____ This group needs reminders about the effect of stress on their lifestyle, (e.g., raising a family, promoting a career), which may lead to reliance on drugs and alcohol.

11. _____ Vigilant supervision by parents and guardians is required to anticipate hazardous elements and provide protection for this group, with precautionary devices.

12. _____ Safety care for this group entails never leaving them unattended, using crib rails, and monitoring objects that may be placed in the mouth and swallowed.

CORRECT THE FALSE STATEMENT

Circle the word true or false that follows the statement. If the word false has been circled, change the underlined word/words to make the statement true. Write your answer in the space provided.

1. Falls are the leading cause of accidental death in persons 79 years of age or older.

   True   False   _____

2. Fires are the leading cause of death in the United States for ages 1–34.

   True   False   _____

3. Children are most vulnerable to poisoning between the ages of 1 and 3.

   True   False   _____

4. In the United States, gunshot injuries and deaths among children and adolescents have decreased sharply since 1990.

   True   False   _____

5. More than one third of the falls in the elderly are associated with the need to urinate.

   True   False   _____

6. A person with a history of falling is at great risk to fall again.

   True   False   _____

7. Most exposures to toxic fumes occur in the workplace.

   True   False   _____

8. Asphyxiation may occur in any age group, but the incidence is greatest among older adults.

   True   False   _____

9. Keeping a gun in the home increases the risk of domestic homicide.

   True   False   _____

10. A rear-facing safety seat is recommended for infants who weigh less than 20 lb.

    True   False   _____

11. For the <u>school-age child</u>, the focus of parental responsibility is on child-proofing the environment.

    True   False   _____

12. Nurses consistently cite <u>the risk of injury to patient and self from irrational behavior</u> as the primary reason for applying restraints.

    True   False   _____

13. Using a restraint on an older person who tends to wander is <u>justified to ensure his/her safety</u>.

    True   False   _____

14. Nearly half of all drowning victims are <u>teenagers</u>.

    True   False   _____

15. The number of deaths from accidental poisoning has <u>decreased</u> over the years.

    True   False   _____

16. The correct dosage of ipecac for children over 1 year of age is <u>10 mL orally</u>.

    True   False   _____

MULTIPLE CHOICE

Circle the letter that corresponds to the best answer for each question.

1. Which of the following is the major safety problem in healthcare facilities?
   a. falls
   b. fires
   c. violence
   d. poisoning

2. When deciding whether or not to use restraints on a patient, the nurse should consider which of the following accurate statements?
   a. According to a recent study, unrestrained older patients were three times more likely to sustain fall-related injuries than restrained older patients.
   b. There are no physiologic hazards associated with the proper use of restraints on older patients.
   c. Litigation in cases of nonrestraint is uncommon.
   d. Generally, a physician's order is not necessary to apply restraints.

3. When filing an incident report, the nurse should be aware of which of the following accurate statements?
   a. The incident report becomes a part of the medical record.
   b. A physician must be present when completing an incident report.
   c. Laws governing the completion of an incident report are uniform throughout the country.
   d. The incident report is not a part of the medical record and should not be mentioned in the documentation.

4. Which of the following statements presents an accurate statistic that should be considered when planning safety for patients?
   a. Many men who batter their spouse also batter their children.
   b. Some people are more likely than others to have falls; e.g., it is not uncommon for some children to be involved in multiple mishaps resulting in fractured bones.
   c. The National Highway Traffic Safety Administration estimates that in 1993, 75% of adolescent motor vehicle fatalities resulted from alcohol-related accidents.
   d. Since older adults have more experience with their environment, they are less vulnerable to falls.

5. Which of the following statements concerning fires is accurate?
   a. Most people who die in house fires do not die from burns but from smoke inhalation.
   b. Most home fires are started by the use of candles.
   c. The majority of fatal home fires occur while people are awake.
   d. Fire is the major safety problem in hospitals and the leading cause of accidental death for the elderly at home.

6. Mrs. Nix is an 86-year-old woman admitted to the hospital in a confused and dehydrated state. Restraints were applied after she got out of bed and fell. She began to fight and was rapidly becoming exhausted. She had black and blue marks on her wrists from the restraints. Which of the following would be the most appropriate nursing intervention for Mrs. Nix?

   a. Sedate Mrs. Nix with sleeping pills and leave the restraints on.

   b. Take the restraints off and stay with Mrs. Nix and talk gently to her.

   c. Leave the restraints on and talk with Mrs. Nix, explaining that she must calm down.

   d. Talk with Mrs. Nix's family about taking her home because she is out of control.

7. Which of the following would be an alternative to the use of restraints for ensuring patient safety and preventing serious falls?

   a. Involve family in the care.

   b. Allow the patient to use the bathroom independently.

   c. Keep the patient sedated with tranquilizers.

   d. Maintain a high bed position so the patient will not attempt to get out unassisted.

COMPLETION

1. Identify two safety risks for each of the following age groups.

   a. Neonates and infants: _____

   _____

   _____

   b. Toddler and preschooler: _____

   _____

   _____

   c. School-age child: _____

   _____

   _____

   d. Adolescent: _____

   _____

   _____

   e. Adult: _____

   _____

   _____

   f. Older adult: _____

   _____

   _____

2. List two examples in which the following factors can affect safety.

   a. Developmental considerations: _____

   _____

   _____

   b. Lifestyle: _____

   _____

   _____

   c. Limitation in mobility: _____

   _____

   _____

   d. Limitation in sensory perception: _____

   _____

   _____

   e. Limitation in knowledge: _____

   _____

   _____

   f. Limitation in ability to communicate: _____

   _____

   _____

   g. Limitation in health status: _____

   _____

   _____

   h. Limitation in psychosocial state: _____

   _____

   _____

3. Briefly explain why the following information is necessary when assessing the patient for safety.

   a. The nursing history: _____

   _____

   _____

   b. Physical assessment: _____

   _____

   _____

   c. Accident-prone behavior: _____

   _____

   _____

   d. The environment: _____

   _____

   _____

4. Mrs. Vogel is a 72-year-old woman in a nursing home who has suffered a fall when getting out of bed to use the bathroom. List four characteristics that should be assessed to determine if this patient is at a greater risk for falls.

   a. _____

   b. _____

   c. _____

   d. _____

5. You are visiting a home-bound patient who is staying with her daughter, who also has a toddler at home. You notice that the house is not child-proofed and watch in horror as the toddler pulls a bottle of disinfectant out from under the sink while the mother is busy caring for her own mother. How would you go about preparing and presenting a plan for this mother to child-proof her home?

   _____

   _____

6. List three questions you would prepare for a patient to assess for hazards that may cause a child to asphyxiate or choke.

   a. _____

   b. _____

   c. _____

7. Write a sample nursing diagnosis for each of the following situations:

   a. A mother refuses to put her child in a car seat when traveling by automobile: _____

   _____

   _____

   b. An older patient has poor vision and cannot read the label on her medication bottle: _____

   _____

   _____

   c. A mother leaves her child unattended in the bathtub while she answers the phone: _____

   _____

   _____

   d. A patient admits she is "clumsy" and has fallen several times in the past few years: _____

   _____

   _____

   e. The windows and doors do not operate properly in the home of an older couple who cannot afford repairs: _____

   _____

   _____

8. List three opportunities a nurse can use to teach students about safety.

   a. _____

   b. _____

   c. _____

9. List five risks associated with the use of restraints.

   a. _____

   b. _____

   c. _____

   d. _____

   e. _____

10. Mrs. Bender is a patient who has been placed in restraints as a protective measure against falling after other methods had failed. She refused to listen to information about the dangers of falling and repeatedly attempted to go to the bathroom on her own. How would you document the use of restraints on this patient?

_____

_____

_____

11. List the information that should be included on an incident report, when it should be filled out, and who is responsible for recording the accident.

_____

_____

13. List DiBartolo's RESTRAINT protocol on the lines provided below.

a. R _____

b. E _____

c. S _____

d. T _____

e. R _____

f. A _____

g. I _____

h. N _____

i. T _____

GUIDE TO CRITICAL THINKING AND DEVELOPING BLENDED SKILLS

1. Visit the homes of friends or relatives who have children of different ages living with them. Ask for permission to inspect their home for safety features that are appropriate to the ages of the children. Check for poison control, fire prevention, fall protection, burns and shock protection, and so on. Share your results with the family, and explain to them what they need to do (if anything) to improve safety in their home. Reflect on the importance different families attach to safety and its implication for your nursing practice.

2. There is a tendency to take safety measures for granted. Draw on your experiences in conversations with nurses to identify safety risks for both nurses and patients in different practice settings. What can you do to minimize these risks?

CHAPTER 27

Asepsis

CHAPTER OVERVIEW

- The infection chain consists of six components and can be interrupted by measures that halt the spread of disease.

- The stage of an infection and the patient's response influence the extent and type of nursing care provided.

- Sterilization and disinfection may be accomplished by physical or chemical means, based on the nature and number of organisms, the type and intended use of equipment, and the availability and practicality of the means.

- Handwashing is the single most effective way to prevent the spread of infection and decrease the incidence of nosocomial infection.

- The most common nosocomial infections are urinary tract infections, surgical wound infections, and pneumonia.

- Medical asepsis, or clean technique, is concerned with reducing the number of pathogens.

- Surgical asepsis, or sterile technique, includes practices that keep objects and areas free of microorganisms.

- Isolation procedures develop barriers that prevent the transmission of pathogens and break the infection cycle.

- The category-specific and disease-specific isolation systems require that an infectious disease be diagnosed before initiating the appropriate infection-control techniques.

- CDC recommendations for universal precautions state that healthcare workers use gloves, gowns, masks, and protective eyewear when exposure to blood, semen, vaginal secretions, or body fluids is likely. All patients should be considered potentially infected.

- The body substance isolation system considers all body substances potentially infective and advocates consistent use of barriers whenever healthcare personnel have contact with moist body substances, mucous membranes, and nonintact skin.

- The recently revised CDC guideline recognizes the importance of all body fluid secretions and excretions in transmitting nosocomial infections and consists of Standard Precautions and Transmission-Based Precautions.

- Multidrug-resistant tuberculosis requires the use of a type N95 particulate respirator to protect the caregiver from droplet infection.

■ Learning Checklist

Review the learning checklist at the end of the chapter in your textbook and be sure you can meet each objective.

■ Exercises

MATCHING

Match the terms in Part A with their definitions listed in Part B.

PART A

a. infection

b. pathogen

c. bacteria

d. gram-positive bacteria

e. gram-negative bacteria

f. aerobic bacteria

g. anaerobic bacteria

h. host

i. fungi

j. normal flora

k. opportunists

l. virus

m. antigen

n. antibody

PART B

1. _____ Bacteria that are potentially harmful.

2. _____ Bacteria that require oxygen to live.

3. _____ A disease state that results from the presence of pathogens in or on the body.

4. _____ A disease-producing microorganism.

5. _____ Microorganisms that commonly inhabit various body sites and are part of the body's natural defense system.

6. _____ Plant-like organisms that can cause infection.

7. _____ An invading foreign protein such as bacteria, or, in some cases, the body's own proteins.

8. _____ Most significant and commonly observed infection-causing agents in healthcare institutions.

9. _____ Bacteria that have chemically more complex cell walls and can be decolorized by alcohol.

10. _____ Bacteria that can live without oxygen.

11. _____ Bacteria that have thick cell walls that resist colorization and are stained violet.

12. _____ The body responds to an antigen by producing this.

Match the diseases in Part B with their mode of transmission listed in Part A. Give an example of how the diseases are transmitted on the line provided. Answers may be used more than once.

PART A

a. direct contact

b. indirect contact

c. vehicle

d. airborne

e. vector

PART B

13. _____ AIDS _____

14. _____ Lyme disease _____

15. _____ Tuberculosis _____

16. _____ Wound infection _____

17. _____ Hepatitis _____

18. _____ Abscess _____

19. _____ Boil _____

Match the type of infection in Part A with its definition listed in Part B.

PART A

a. nosocomial

b. exogenous

c. endogenous

d. iatrogenic

PART B

20. _____ An infection that occurs as a result of treatment or diagnostic procedure.

21. _____ A hospital-acquired infection.

22. _____ An infection in which the causative organism is normally harbored within the patient.

23. _____ An infection caused by an organism acquired from other persons.

CORRECT THE FALSE STATEMENTS

Circle the word true or false that follows the statement. If the word false has been circled, change the underlined word/words to make the statement true. Place your answer in the space provided.

1. Gram-negative bacteria have chemically complex walls and can be decolorized by alcohol.

    True   False   _____

    _____

2. Surgical asepsis involves procedures and practices that reduce the number and transfer of pathogens.

    True   False   _____

    _____

3. At least <u>25%</u> of all people admitted to a hospital contract a nosocomial infection.

   True   False   _____

4. Methicillin-resistant *S. aureus* and vancomycin-resistant enterococcus are most often transmitted <u>by the hands of healthcare providers</u>.

   True   False   _____

5. <u>Wearing gloves</u> is the most effective way to help prevent the spread of organisms.

   True   False   _____

6. <u>Resident bacteria</u>, normally picked up by the hands in the usual activities of daily living, are relatively few on clean and exposed areas of the skin.

   True   False   _____

7. <u>Nonantimicrobial agents</u> are considered adequate for routine mechanical cleansing of the hands and removal of most transient microorganisms.

   True   False   _____

8. Effective handwashing requires at least a <u>10- to 15-second</u> scrub with plain soap or disinfectant and water.

   True   False   _____

9. Wearing gloves <u>eliminates</u> the need for handwashing.

   True   False   _____

10. <u>Sterilization</u> is the process by which all microorganisms, including spores, are destroyed.

    True   False   _____

11. In a home environment, contaminated items may be disinfected by placing them in boiling water for <u>10 minutes</u>.

    True   False   _____

12. When observing <u>medical asepsis</u>, areas are considered contaminated if they are touched by any object that is not also sterile.

    True   False   _____

13. Using <u>body substance isolation precautions</u> eliminates the need for category-specific or disease-specific systems except for certain airborne diseases that require special precautions.

    True   False   _____

MULTIPLE CHOICE

1. Bacteria that are spherical in shape belong to which of the following groups?
   a. bacilli
   b. cocci
   c. spirochetes
   d. vacilletes

2. Which of the following is the smallest of all microorganisms, and can be seen only through an electron microscope?
   a. cocci
   b. spirochetes
   c. fungi
   d. virus

3. When an organism is transmitted through personal contact with an inanimate object, such as contaminated blood, the route of transmission is which of the following?
   a. direct contact
   b. vectors
   c. indirect contact
   d. airborne

4. During which stage of infection is the person most infectious?
   a. incubation period
   b. prodromal stage
   c. full stage of illness
   d. convalescent period

5. Which of the following is a protective mechanism that eliminates the invading pathogen and allows for tissue repair to occur?
   a. inflammatory response
   b. immune response
   c. cellular immune response
   d. humoral immune response

6. Which of the following statements concerning nosocomial infections is accurate?
   a. At least 20% to 25% of all people admitted to a hospital contract a nosocomial infection.
   b. All nosocomial infections have an iatrogenic component.
   c. Urinary tract infections account for 75% of all nosocomial infections.
   d. Most hospital-acquired infections are caused by bacteria.

7. Which of the following statements concerning handwashing is accurate?

   a. Wearing gloves is a substitute for handwashing.

   b. According to Olsen et al. (1993), a leak in a glove occurred after 13% of exposures to patient's mucous membranes.

   c. Hands should be washed before and after gloves are applied.

   d. Gloving guarantees protection from infectious organisms.

8. Which of the following statements indicates guidelines that are followed by healthcare workers employed by a healthcare agency that observes universal precautions?

   a. Healthcare workers must use gloves, gowns, masks, and protective eyewear when exposure to blood or body fluids from infected individuals is likely.

   b. Universal precautions apply to cerebrospinal fluid, synovial fluid, pleural fluid, peritoneal fluid, pericardial fluid, and amniotic fluid.

   c. Universal precautions apply during exposure to various substances, including feces, nasal secretions, sputum, sweat, tears, urine, and vomitus.

   d. Universal precautions replace other isolation system safeguards.

9. Which of the following is a natural reservoir for tetanus?

   a. humans

   b. animals

   c. soil

   d. food

10. When handling sterile objects, the nurse should observe which of the following guidelines?

   a. Consider most solutions sterile for 24 hours after opening.

   b. Keep sterile forceps below waist level.

   c. When using a sterile drape, touch only the outer 2 inches of the drape.

   d. Once a sterile field is established, sterile supplies should not be added.

11. Mrs. Teal is to have an indwelling urinary catheter inserted. Which of the following would be the precaution taken during this procedure?

   a. surgical asepsis technique

   b. medical asepsis technique

   c. droplet precautions

   d. strict reverse isolation

12. Which of the following laboratory test results indicates the presence of an infection?

   a. a decrease in specific types of white blood cells

   b. the presence of leukocytes in the blood

   c. the presence of a pathogen in urine, blood, sputum, or other drainage cultures

   d. a white blood cell count of 8000 mm^3

COMPLETION

1. List four factors that influence an organism's potential to produce disease.

   a. _____

   b. _____

   c. _____

   d. _____

2. Give an example of a disease that is transmitted by organisms from the following reservoirs.

   a. Other humans: _____

   b. Animals: _____

   c. Soil: _____

3. List three portals of exit in the human body.

   a. _____

   b. _____

   c. _____

4. Give an example of the following means of transmission.

   a. Direct contact: _____

   b. Indirect contact: _____

   c. Vectors: _____

   d. Airborne: _____

5. Briefly describe the following body defenses against infection.

   a. Inflammatory response: _____

   _____

   _____

   b. Immune response: _____

   _____

   _____

6. List four factors that influence the susceptibility of a host.

   a. _____

   b. _____

   c. _____

   d. _____

7. Briefly describe the nurse's role in controlling or treating infection in the following stages of the nursing practice.

   a. Assessing: _____

   _____

   _____

   b. Diagnosing: _____

   _____

   _____

   c. Planning: _____

   _____

   _____

   d. Implementing: _____

   _____

   _____

   e. Evaluating: _____

   _____

   _____

8. Give two examples of how you would practice medical asepsis in the following areas.

   a. Patient's home: _____

   _____

   _____

   b. Public facilities: _____

   _____

   _____

   c. Community: _____

   _____

   _____

   d. Healthcare facility: _____

   _____

   _____

9. List three measures healthcare agencies have found to be successful in reducing the incidence of nosocomial infections.

   a. _____

   _____

   _____

   _____

   b. _____

   _____

   _____

   _____

   c. _____

   _____

   _____

   _____

10. Explain why the following factors should be considered when selecting sterilization and disinfection methods.

    a. Nature of organism present: _____

    _____

    _____

    b. Number of organisms present: _____

    _____

    _____

    c. Type of equipment: _____

    _____

    _____

d. Intended use of equipment: _____

_____

_____

e. Available means for sterilization and
disinfection: _____

_____

_____

f. Time: _____

_____

_____

11. List five guidelines for aggressive infection control
included in an advisory from the CDC to control
the spread of vancomycin-resistant enterococcus in
healthcare agencies.

a. _____

b. _____

c. _____

d. _____

e. _____

12. Describe the role of the infection control nurse in
the following situations:

a. Hospital: _____

_____

_____

b. Home care setting: _____

_____

_____

13. List the six components of an infection cycle.

a. _____

b. _____

c. _____

d. _____

e. _____

f. _____

14. Mr. Zelen is a 35-year-old fireman who sustained
third-degree burns on his upper body.

a. Write a nursing diagnosis that relates to his
increased risk for skin infection: _____

_____

_____

_____

b. Describe how the nurse can help to control or
prevent infection for this patient: _____

_____

_____

_____

15. When working in the emergency room, a patient
you are treating for lacerations tells you that he
was recently diagnosed with TB. Would you use
different precautions for this patient than another
ER patient? Why?

_____

_____

_____

GUIDE TO CRITICAL THINKING AND DEVELOPING BLENDED SKILLS

1. Try to imagine what it must feel like to be in strict
isolation. Then interview a patient whose medical
condition necessitated the use of isolation
precautions. Find out how it felt to be isolated and,
in some cases, feared by healthcare workers. See if
anything was done to help alleviate the
disorientation and meet his basic needs of love and
belonging. What did you learn to direct your future
nursing care for patients in isolation?

2. A nurse is obligated to provide nursing care to all
patients regardless of race, creed, religion, etc.
Should this code also include "regardless of the
medical condition of the patient"? Should nurses
be able to choose whether or not to take care of a
patient who has a contagious disease? Do you
believe the precautions being taken with these
patients are adequate protection for the healthcare
provider? Should there be consequences for medical
personnel who refuse to take care of these patients?
Share your responses with your classmates and see
if you agree.

CHAPTER 28

Medications

CHAPTER OVERVIEW

- Medications have several names. The nurse should be aware of a drug's generic and trade names. Drugs can be classified by body system and by the symptom they relieve (clinical indication).

- Drugs are available in many forms. Some drugs are supplied in several preparations; others are available in only one form.

- Factors that influence drug absorption include route of administration, local conditions at the site of administration, drug solubility, pH, and drug dosage.

- Variables that influence the action of medications are age, weight, sex, genetic factors, psychologic factors, illness, environment, and time of administration.

- Known adverse drug effects include iatrogenic disease, drug allergy, drug tolerance, cumulative effect, idiosyncratic reaction, and drug interactions.

- Assessment of patients receiving medications includes obtaining a comprehensive medication history.

- Components of a medication order are patient's name, date and time order is written, name of the drug, dosage, route, frequency, and signature of the prescriber. The nurse questions any unclear medication order before the order is implemented.

- Pediatric dosages are calculated by the child's weight or body surface area.

- The nurse observes the *five rights* and *three checks* in medication preparation and administration. The nurse who prepares a medication administers the medication. The medication area is locked when not in use.

- The nurse identifies the patient correctly before administering a medication and remains with the patient until the medication is taken. The nurse records the medication on the patient's record as soon as possible after administration.

- Selection of equipment for a parenteral injection is based on the route of administration, viscosity of the drug, quantity to be administered, type of medication, and patient's body size.

- After use, needles should never be recapped and are placed in a puncture-resistant container. Most needlestick injuries occur during recapping. Needleless equipment effectively prevents needlestick injuries.

- Sterile equipment is used to prepare a drug for injection.

- A vial of unmodified insulin should never be contaminated with modified insulin when preparing two insulins to be mixed in the same syringe.

- Proper site selection for an intramuscular injection should include palpation of anatomic landmarks. The Z-track method for an intramuscular injection is safer and less painful for most adults.

- Intravenous medications can be administered as a continuous infusion, as a bolus, or intermittently. A bolus dose and an intermittent infusion may be administered through the primary intravenous line or through a heparin lock. The nurse checks the placement of a heparin lock before administering any medication.

- Topical medications are applied to the skin and mucous membranes primarily for their local effects, although some systemic effects may occur.

■ Learning Checklist

Review the learning checklist at the end of the chapter in your textbook and be sure you can meet each objective.

■ Exercises

MATCHING

Match the sites for injecting intramuscular medications listed in Part A with the definition of the site listed in Part B.

PART A

a. ventrogluteal site
b. dorsogluteal site
c. vastus lateralis site
d. rectus femoris site
e. deltoid muscle site

PART B

1. _____ Posterior superior iliac spine and greater trochanter represent the anatomic landmarks.

2. _____ Located in the lateral aspect of the upper arm.

3. _____ Involves the gluteus medius and gluteus minimus muscles in the hip area.

4. _____ Bordered by the midanterior thigh on the front of the leg and the midlateral thigh on the side.

5. _____ Located on the anterior part of the thigh.

Match the types of drug preparations in Part A with their descriptions listed in Part B.

PART A

a. capsule
b. elixir
c. liniment
d. lotion
e. ointment
f. tablet
g. pill
h. powder
i. solution
j. suppository
k. suspension
l. syrup

PART B

6. _____ Small, solid dose of medication; compressed or molded; may be any size or shape, or enteric coated.

7. _____ Powder or gel form of an active drug enclosed in a gelatinous container.

8. _____ Medication mixed with alcohol, oil, or soap, which is rubbed on the skin.

9. _____ Finely divided, undissolved particles in a liquid medium; should be shaken before use.

10. _____ Medication in a clear liquid containing water, alcohol, sweeteners, and flavoring.

11. _____ An easily melted medication preparation in a firm base, such as gelatin, that is inserted into the body.

12. _____ Drug particles in a solution for topical use.

13. _____ Mixture of a powdered drug with a cohesive material; may be round or oval.

14. _____ A drug dissolved in another substance.

15. _____ Single drug or mixture of finely ground drugs.

16. _____ Medication combined with water and sugar solution.

Match the types of injections listed in Part A with their injection site listed in Part B.

PART A

a. subcutaneous injection
b. intramuscular injection
c. intradermal injection
d. intravenous injection
e. intraarterial injection
f. intracardial injection
g. intraperitoneal injection
h. intraspinal injection
i. intraosseous injection

PART B

17. _____ Corium

18. _____ Bone

19. _____ Muscle tissue

20. _____ Artery

21. _____ Heart tissue

22. _____ Vein

23. _____ Peritoneal cavity

24. _____ Subcutaneous tissue

Match the drug effect listed in Part A with its description, listed in Part B.

PART A

a. drug allergy

b. anaphylactic reaction

c. cumulative effect

d. idiosyncratic effect

e. antagonist effect

f. synergistic effect

g. drug tolerance

h. iatrogenic effect

PART B

25. _____ The combined effect of two or more drugs acting simultaneously that produces an effect less than that of each drug alone.

26. _____ Any abnormal or peculiar response to a drug that may manifest itself by overresponse, underresponse, or response different from the expected outcome.

27. _____ Occurs in a person who has been previously exposed to the drug and has developed antibodies.

28. _____ Occurs when the body becomes accustomed to a particular drug over a period of time.

29. _____ The combined effect of two drugs acting simultaneously that produces an effect greater than that of each drug alone.

30. _____ A life-threatening immediate reaction to a drug that results in respiratory distress, sudden severe bronchospasm, and cardiovascular collapse.

31. _____ Occurs when the body cannot metabolize one dose of a drug before another dose is administered.

MULTIPLE CHOICE

Circle the letter that corresponds to the best answer for each question.

1. Which of the following is the name assigned to a drug by the manufacturer that first develops it?
   a. trade name
   b. official name
   c. chemical name
   d. generic name

2. Most drugs are excreted through which of the following organs?
   a. kidneys
   b. lungs
   c. intestines
   d. skin

3. Which of the following acts designated the United States Pharmacopeia and the National Formulary as official standards of drugs and empowered the federal government to enforce these standards?
   a. Federal Food, Drug, and Cosmetic Act
   b. Food and Drug Administration
   c. Pure Food and Drug Act
   d. Comprehensive Drug Abuse Prevention and Control Act

4. Which of the following statements about patient medications is accurate?
   a. Safe practice dictates that a nurse follow written or verbal orders.
   b. In most settings, student nurses are permitted to accept verbal orders from a physician.
   c. When a patient is admitted to a hospital, all drugs that the physician may have ordered while the patient was at home are continued.
   d. Upon admittance to a hospital, all patient medications from home should be sent home with the family or placed in safe-keeping.

5. Which of the following types of medication orders would a physician prescribe for "as needed" pain medication?
   a. standing order
   b. PRN order
   c. single order
   d. stat order

6. A nurse suspects a drug she administered to her patient is in error. Who is legally responsible for the error?

   a. nurse

   b. physician

   c. hospital

   d. pharmacist

7. Which of the following measurement systems uses a grain as the basic unit of weight?

   a. metric

   b. apothecary

   c. household

   d. decimal

8. If a nurse is preparing medication for her patient and is called away to an emergency situation, which of the following should she do?

   a. Have another nurse guard the preparations.

   b. Put the meds back in the containers.

   c. Have another nurse finish preparing and administering the meds.

   d. Lock the medications in a room and finish them when she returns.

9. Before administering a drug to a patient, the nurse should identify the patient by doing which of the following?

   a. Call the patient by name.

   b. Check the patient's ID bracelet.

   c. Check the patient's record.

   d. Check the patient's name with family or significant others.

10. Which means of drug administration would be used in an emergency to achieve rapid absorption and quicker results?

    a. injection

    b. oral

    c. patch

    d. inhalation

11. Which of the following sites is recommended for both adults and children over 7 months of age as a safe site for the majority of intramuscular injections?

    a. vastus lateralis site

    b. deltoid muscle site

    c. ventrogluteal site

    d. dorsogluteal site

12. Mrs. Harris is a 78-year-old woman admitted to your unit after experiencing symptoms of stroke. When administering the medication prescribed for Mrs. Harris, the nurse should be aware that this patient has an increased possibility of drug toxicity due to which of the following age-related factors?

    a. Decreased adipose tissue and increased total body fluid in proportion to the total body mass.

    b. Increased number of protein-binding sites.

    c. Increased kidney function resulting in excessive filtration and excretion.

    d. Decline in liver function and production of enzymes needed for drug metabolism.

13. To convert 0.8 grams to milligrams, the nurse should do which of the following?

    a. Move the decimal point 2 places to the right.

    b. Move the decimal point 3 places to the right.

    c. Move the decimal point 2 places to the left.

    d. Move the decimal point 3 places to the left.

14. Mr. Downs is given a dose of gentamycin and has an immediate reaction of hypotension, bronchospasms, and rapid, thready pulse. Which of the following would be the drugs of choice for this situation?

    a. antibiotic, antihistamines, and Isuprel

    b. bronchodilators, antihistamines, and vasodilators

    c. epinephrine, antihistamines, and bronchodilators

    d. antihistamines, vasodilators, and bronchoconstrictors

15. Mrs. Banks has an order for Chloromycetin 500 mg q 6 hours. The drug comes in 250-mg capsules. Which of the following would be the correct dosage?

    a. 1 tab

    b. 2 tabs

    c. 3 tabs

    d. 4 tabs

16. George Riley is a 46-year-old man in the hospital for COPD. He has an order for penicillin to be given intramuscularly. Which of the following would be the correct angle to use for injection at the dorsogluteal site?

    a. 45-degree angle

    b. 60-degree angle

    c. 75-degree angle

    d. 90-degree angle

17. An oral medication has been ordered for Mr. Moran. He has a nasogastric tube in place. Which of the following nursing activities would increase the safety of medication administration?

    a. Check the tube placement prior to administration.

    b. Have Mr. Moran swallow the pills around the tube.

    c. Flush the tube with 30 to 40 mL saline prior to medication administration.

    d. Bring the liquids to room temperature before administration.

18. When giving an intramuscular injection using the Z-track technique, the nurse should use which of the following recommended techniques?

    a. Use a needle with a minimum length of 1 inch.

    b. Apply pressure to the injection site.

    c. Inject the medication quickly, and steadily withdraw the needle.

    d. Do not massage the site because it may cause irritation.

COMPLETION

1. List three categories for drug classification.

    a. _____

    b. _____

    c. _____

2. Explain the following processes by which drugs alter cell physiology.

    a. Drug-receptor interactions: _____

    _____

    b. Drug-enzyme interactions: _____

    _____

3. Briefly describe how the following factors influence the absorption of a drug.

    a. Route of administration: _____

    _____

    _____

    b. Drug solubility: _____

    _____

    c. pH: _____

    _____

    d. Local conditions at the site of administration:

    _____

    e. Drug dosage: _____

    _____

4. Give an example of how the following factors affect drug action.

    a. Developmental stage of patient: _____

    _____

    b. Weight: _____

    _____

    c. Sex: _____

    _____

    d. Genetic and cultural factors: _____

    _____

    e. Psychologic factors: _____

    _____

    f. Pathology: _____

    _____

    g. Environment: _____

    _____

    h. Time of administration: _____

    _____

    _____

5. List the seven parts of a medication order.

a. _____

b. _____

c. _____

d. _____

e. _____

f. _____

g. _____

6. Give three examples of situations in which you would question a medical order.

a. _____

b. _____

c. _____

7. Briefly describe the following three types of medication supply systems.

a. Stock supply system: _____

_____

_____

b. Individual supply system: _____

_____

_____

c. Unit dose system: _____

_____

_____

8. List the three checks and five rights when administering medication.

a. Three checks: _____

_____

_____

b. Five rights: _____

_____

_____

_____

9. Your patient tells you that she refuses to take the medication prescribed for her because it tastes "disgusting." List three techniques you could use to mask the taste.

a. _____

b. _____

c. _____

10. Explain how the following factors would affect the type of equipment a nurse would choose for an injection.

a. Route of administration: _____

_____

_____

b. Viscosity of the solution: _____

_____

_____

c. Quantity to be administered: _____

_____

_____

d. Body size: _____

_____

_____

e. Type of medication: _____

_____

_____

11. List four steps that should be followed when a medication error occurs.

a. _____

b. _____

c. _____

d. _____

12. Describe the use of the following types of pre-packaged medications.

a. Ampules: _____

b. Vials: _____

c. Prefilled cartridges: _____

13. A physician has ordered medications in certain amounts. You have them on hand, but in different quantities. Make the necessary conversions and state what you will give to each patient.

    a. Order: Gentamicin 60 mg. On hand: gentamicin 80 mg/2 cc.

    Give patient: _____

    b. Order: aspirin gr V. On hand: aspirin 300 mg/tab.

    Give patient: _____

    c. Order: Mestinon 30 mg. On hand: Mestinon 60 mg/tab.

    Give patient: _____

    d. Order: amitriptyline 75 mg. On hand: amitriptyline 25 mg/tab.

    Give patient: _____

    e. Order: phenylbutazone 250 mg. On hand: phenylbutazone 500 mg/tab.

    Give patient: _____

    f. Order: ProBanthine 15 mg. On hand: ProBanthine 5 mg/tab.

    Give patient: _____

    g. Order: Penicillin V 250 mg. On hand: Penicillin V 500 mg/tab.

    Give patient: _____

    h. Order: Lanoxin 0.125 mg. On hand: Lanoxin 0.250 mg/tab.

    Give patient: _____

    i. Order: metaproterenol sulfate 20 mg. On hand: metaproterenol sulfate 10 mg/tab.

    Give patient: _____

    j. Order: ACTH 40 mg. On hand: ACTH 10 mg/cc

    Give patient: _____

14. You are preparing Jim Toole for discharge. He will be taking the following medications at home. Use the chart below to identify the information you will need to teach him about these medications. Use a pharmacology text to look up Xanax, Zantac, and Cipro.

Method	Xanax	Zantac	Cipro
Dosage			
Route of administration			
Frequency/schedule			
Desired effects			
Possible adverse effects			
PS&S of toxic drug effects			
Special instructions			
Recommended course of action with problems			

15. Transcribe the following medication orders on the patient medication record and sign for the medications you would administer in a 24-hour period. Be prepared to discuss administration guidelines.

Tenormin, 50 mg, PO od

Hydrodiuril, 50 mg, PO od

NPH Insulin U-100, 45 units SQ daily in AM

Regular Insulin U-100, 10 units SQ stat

Cipro, 500 mg, PO q 12 h

Timoptic 0.25% gtt OD bid

Dalmane, 30 mg, po hs, prn

Nitro-paste 1/2 inch, q 8 h to chest wall

Tylenol with codeine #2, PO q 4 h, prn

Colace, l00 mg, PO od

Medical Administration Record

ORD DATE	PRN MEDS.		
		Date	
		Time	
		Init / Site	
		Date	
		Time	
		Init / Site	

SINGLE ORDERS—PREOPERATIVES

ORD DATE	MEDICATION—DOSAGE—ROUTE OF ADMIN	DATE/TIME	SITE/INITITALS

INJECTION SITES MUST BE CHARTED

ORD DATE	ROUTINE MEDICATIONS MEDICATION—DOSAGE—ROUTE OF ADMIN	HR	DATE/TIME							

GUIDE TO CRITICAL THINKING AND DEVELOPING BLENDED SKILLS

1. Think about your responsibilities when administering medication and then describe how you would respond in the following situations:

   a. A physician who is in a hurry prescribes a medication for your patient. After he leaves, you read the order and don't understand why your patient would need the medication prescribed. Because you are legally responsible for medications administered, what would you do?

   b. You bring a medication to a patient who tells you "That's not my pill." What would you do?

2. Medication errors are not uncommon and may be lethal. Interview several nurses about their experiences with errors and what contributes to medication errors. Think about how nurses individually and collectively can act to reduce errors. Develop a plan with your classmates to help minimize these errors.

CHAPTER 29

Perioperative Nursing

CHAPTER OVERVIEW

- Surgery is a stressful time for the patient and family, imposing physical and psychosocial alterations and adaptations.

- The time before, during, and after surgery is called the perioperative period; it is divided into preoperative, intraoperative, and postoperative phases.

- Surgical procedures are categorized by urgency, risk, and purpose.

- Anesthesia may be general or regional. General anesthesia is given to induce narcosis, loss of reflexes, and relaxation of skeletal muscles; regional anesthesia produces sensory loss but the patient remains awake.

- Patients agree to surgery by signing an informed consent form.

- Preoperative assessment identifies physical and psychosocial risk factors and strengths.

- Preoperative nursing interventions to prepare the patient for the intraoperative and postoperative phases include therapeutic communications, preoperative teaching, and physical preparation.

- Intraoperative nursing roles are either as a scrub nurse or as a circulating nurse; each has specific patient responsibilities.

- Immediate postoperative nursing care in the postanesthesia recovery area focuses on assessing and monitoring to prevent complications from anesthesia or surgery.

- Ongoing postoperative nursing care is planned to facilitate recovery from surgery and coping with alterations; both the patient and the family are part of care.

- Ambulatory surgery is provided on an outpatient basis; preoperative assessment and teaching are critical elements in safe surgery and recovery.

- A wound is a disruption in the normal integrity of the skin.

- Wound healing is influenced by a variety of factors, including state of health; nature of the wound; age; and whether healing is by primary, secondary, or tertiary intention.

- Providing wound care requires knowledge and skill in assessing for complications, in using various supplies throughout the healing process, and in teaching patients or caregivers to provide self-care at home.

- The nursing process is used throughout the perioperative period to provide knowledgeable, holistic, individualized patient care.

■ Learning Checklist

Review the learning checklist at the end of the chapter in your textbook and be sure you can meet each objective.

■ Exercises

MATCHING

Match the phase of the perioperative period listed in Part A with the appropriate action performed in that phase, listed in Part B. Answers may be used more than once.

PART A

a. preoperative phase

b. intraoperative phase

c. postoperative phase

PART B

1. _____ The nurse prepares the patient for home care.

2. _____ The physician informs the patient that surgical intervention is necessary.

3. _____ The patient is transferred to the recovery room.

4. _____ The patient is admitted to the recovery area.

5. _____ The patient begins to emerge from anesthesia.

6. _____ Screening tests are scheduled for the patient prior to surgery.

7. _____ The patient participates in a rehabilitation program after surgery.

Match the type of drug listed in Part A with its surgical risk, listed in Part B.

PART A

a. anticoagulants

b. diuretics

c. tranquilizers

d. adrenal steroids

e. antibiotics

PART B

8. _____ Abrupt withdrawal may cause cardiovascular collapse in long-term users.

9. _____ May precipitate hemorrhage.

10. _____ Those in the mycin group, when combined with certain muscle relaxants used during surgery, can cause respiratory paralysis.

11. _____ May cause electrolyte imbalance, with resulting respiratory depression from anesthesia.

Match the type of nurse listed in Part A, with the role he/she performs, listed in Part B. Answers may be used more than once.

PART A

a. scrub nurse

b. circulating nurse

c. RNFA

d. APN

e. PA

PART B

12. _____ Member of the sterile team who maintains surgical asepsis while draping and handling instruments and supplies.

13. _____ Actively assists the surgeon by providing exposure, hemostasis, and wound closure.

14. _____ Coordinates care activities, collaborates with physicians and nurses in all phases of perioperative and postanesthesia care.

15. _____ Assesses the patient on admission to the operating room and collaborates in safely positioning the patient on the operating bed.

16. _____ Integrates case management, critical paths, and research into care of the surgical patient.

17. _____ Assists with monitoring the patient during surgery, provides additional supplies, and maintains environmental safety.

MULTIPLE CHOICE

Circle the letter that corresponds to the best choice for each question.

1. Which of the following types of anesthesia is administered by injecting a local anesthetic around a nerve trunk supplying the area of surgery?

   a. nerve block

   b. subdural block

   c. surface anesthesia

   d. local infiltration with lidocaine

2. When obtaining a consent form from a patient scheduled to undergo surgery, the nurse should consider which of the following facts?

   a. A consent form is legal, even if the patient is confused or sedated.

   b. The form that is signed is not a legal document and would not hold up in court.

   c. In emergency situations, the doctor may obtain consent over the telephone.

   d. The responsibility for securing informed consent from the patient lies with the nurse.

3. A 9-month-old baby is scheduled for heart surgery. When preparing this patient for surgery, the nurse should consider which of the following surgical risks associated with infants?

   a. prolonged wound healing

   b. potential hypothermia or hyperthermia

   c. congestive heart failure

   d. gastrointestinal upset

4. Mr. Lemke is a 42-year-old man scheduled for elective hernia surgery. While taking a medical history for Mr. Lemke, you find out he is taking antibiotics for an infection. To which of the following surgical risks would Mr. Lemke be predisposed due to his use of antibiotics, if the surgery were performed?

    a. hemorrhage

    b. electrolyte imbalances

    c. cardiovascular collapse

    d. respiratory paralysis

5. When preparing a patient who has diabetes mellitus for surgery, the nurse should be aware of which of the following potential surgical risks associated with this disease?

    a. fluid and electrolyte imbalance

    b. slow wound healing

    c. respiratory depression from anesthesia

    d. altered metabolism and excretion of drugs

6. Mr. Pete is an obese 62-year-old man scheduled for heart surgery. Which of the following surgical risks related to obesity should be considered when performing an assessment for this patient?

    a. delayed wound healing and wound infection

    b. alterations in fluid and electrolyte balance

    c. respiratory distress

    d. hemorrhage

7. When teaching a postoperative patient about pain control, the nurse should consider which of the following statements?

    a. When giving pain medication prn, the patient should ask for the medication when the pain becomes severe.

    b. The nurse is responsible for ordering and administering pain medications.

    c. Medications for pain usually are given by injection for the first few days or as long as the patient is NPO.

    d. Alternate pain control methods, such as TENS and PCA, should not be used after surgery.

8. To prevent postoperative complications, which of the following measures should be taken after surgery?

    a. The patient should be instructed to avoid coughing possible to minimize damage to the incision.

    b. The patient should take shallow breaths to prevent collapse of the alveoli.

    c. The patient should be instructed to do leg exercises to increase venous return.

    d. The patient should not be turned in bed until the incision is no longer painful.

9. Which of the following is the most common postanesthesia recovery emergency?

    a. respiratory obstruction

    b. cardiac distress

    c. wound infection

    d. dehydration

10. Mr. Fischer has returned to your unit after cardiac surgery. Which of the following interventions would be appropriate to prevent cardiovascular complications for Mr. Fischer?

    a. Position Mr. Fischer in bed with pillows placed under his knees to hasten venous return.

    b. Keep Mr. Fischer from ambulating until the day after surgery.

    c. Implement leg exercises and turn in bed every two hours.

    d. Keep Mr. Fischer cool and uncovered to prevent elevated temperature.

11. Which of the following interventions should be carried out by the nurse when a postoperative patient is in shock?

    a. Remove extra covering on the patient to keep temperature down.

    b. Place the patient in a flat position with legs elevated 45 degrees.

    c. Do not administer any further medication.

    d. Place the patient in the Trendelenburg or "shock" position.

12. Which of the following is a recommended physical preparation for a patient undergoing surgery?

    a. Shave the area of the incision with a razor.

    b. Empty the patient's bowel of feces.

    c. Do not allow the patient to eat or drink anything for 8 to 12 hours before the surgery.

    d. Be sure the patient is well-nourished and hydrated.

13. Which of the following preoperative medications would be prescribed to decrease pulmonary and oral secretions and prevent laryngospasms?

    a. narcotic analgesics

    b. anticholinergics

    c. neuroleptanalgesic agents

    d. histamine-receptor antihistaminics

14. Which of the following positions would be used in minimally invasive surgery of the lower abdomen or pelvis?

    a. Trendelenburg's position

    b. Sims' position

    c. lithotomy position

    d. prone position

15. Which of the following actions would be an appropriate reaction to a patient experiencing pulmonary embolus?

    a. Try to overhydrate the patient with fluids.

    b. Instruct the patient to simulate Valsalva's maneuver.

    c. Place the patient in the semi-Fowler's position.

    d. Assist the patient to ambulate every 2 to 3 hours.

16. Your postsurgical patient is experiencing decreased lung sounds, dyspnea, cyanosis, crackles, restlessness, and apprehension. Which of the following conditions would you diagnose?

    a. atelectasis

    b. pneumonia

    c. pulmonary embolus

    d. thrombophlebitis

COMPLETION

1. Briefly describe the time period for the following stages of the perioperative period.

    a. Preoperative phase: _____

    _____

    _____

    b. Intraoperative phase: _____

    _____

    _____

    c. Postoperative phase: _____

    _____

    _____

2. Give a brief description of the following types of surgery.

    a. Based on urgency: _____

    _____

    _____

    b. Based on degree of risk: _____

    _____

    _____

    c. Based on purpose: _____

    _____

    _____

3. Describe the following three phases of anesthesia.

    a. Induction: _____

    b. Maintenance: _____

    c. Emergence: _____

4. Your patient is undergoing surgery to remove a lump from her breast. List four areas of information that should be given to the patient when securing informed consent.

    a. _____

    b. _____

    c. _____

    d. _____

5. Indicate how each of the following diseases places the patient at greater risk for postoperative complications.

    a. Cardiovascular disease: _____

    _____

    _____

    b. Pulmonary disorders: _____

    _____

    _____

    c. Kidney and liver function disorders: _____

    _____

    _____

    d. Metabolic disorders: _____

    _____

    _____

6. Explain how you would help your patient overcome the following fears experienced in the preoperative phase.

    a. Fear of the unknown: _____

    _____

    _____

    b. Fear of pain and death: _____

    _____

    _____

    c. Fear of changes in body image and self-concept:

    _____

    _____

7. Describe the nurse's role in providing screening tests for the preoperative patient: _____

    _____

    _____

8. Describe how you would prepare a preoperative patient for the following conditions.

    a. Surgical events and sensations: _____

    _____

    _____

    b. Pain management: _____

    _____

    _____

9. Describe how you would prepare a patient on the day of surgery in the following areas.

    a. Hygiene and skin preparation: _____

    _____

    _____

    b. Elimination: _____

    _____

    _____

    c. Nutrition and fluids: _____

    _____

    _____

    d. Rest and sleep: _____

    _____

    _____

10. Give three examples of expected outcomes for a patient during the intraoperative phase.

    a. _____

    b. _____

    c. _____

11. List the five phases that signify the return of CNS function.

    a. _____

    b. _____

    c. _____

    d. _____

    e. _____

12. Prepare a teaching plan for a postoperative patient who is moving into a home-healthcare setting. Include the family in your planning: _____

    _____

    _____

    _____

13. Give an example of how the following factors may present a greater surgical risk for some clients.

    a. Developmental considerations: _____

    b. Medical history: _____

    c. Medications: _____

    d. Previous surgery: _____

    e. Perceptions and knowledge of surgery: _____

    f. Lifestyle: _____

    g. Nutrition: _____

    h. Use of alcohol, illicit drugs, nicotine: _____

    i. Activities of daily living: _____

    j. Occupation: _____

    k. Coping patterns: _____

    l. Support systems: _____

    m. Sociocultural needs: _____

14. Explain what a nurse in the PACU would assess when checking a patient in the postoperative phase using the following guidelines.

    a. Vital signs: _____

    b. Color and temperature of skin: _____

    c. Level of consciousness: _____

    d. Intravenous fluids: _____

    e. Surgical site: _____

    f. Other tubes: _____

    g. Comfort level: _____

    h. Position and safety: _____

    i. Comfort: _____

15. Give an example of two nursing interventions you would institute for a postoperative patient to help alleviate the following problems that interfere with comfort.

    a. Nausea and vomiting: _____

    _____

    _____

    b. Thirst: _____

    _____

    _____

c. Hiccups: _____

_____

_____

d. Surgical pain: _____

_____

_____

GUIDE TO CRITICAL THINKING AND DEVELOPING BLENDED SKILLS

1. Prepare a preoperative assessment for the patients described below. Develop a nursing care plan for each patient based on the data collected. Be sure to include preoperative care, intraoperative care, and postoperative care in your planning.

   a. A 52-year-old male patient who smokes a pack of cigarettes a day is scheduled to undergo heart bypass surgery. The patient is overweight and admits that he rarely finds time to exercise.

   b. A 35-year-old female patient is scheduled to undergo surgery for the removal of a tumor in her colon. She underwent radiation therapy 6 weeks before the surgery date. The patient has a family history of colon cancer.

   Reflect on how individual differences in patients influence their need for nursing and nursing's perioperative priorities.

2. Make a list of common postoperative complications. Describe how you would monitor the patient for these complications and what nursing measures you would take to prevent them. Be sure to include cardiovascular complications, shock, hemorrhage, thrombophlebitis, respiratory complications, pneumonia, atelectasis, and wound complications. Think of personal and system variables that might influence your effectiveness.

UNIT VII

Promoting Healthy Psychosocial Reponses

CHAPTER 30

Self-Concept

CHAPTER OVERVIEW

- Self-concept is the mental image or picture of self. It has the power to encourage or thwart personal growth and development.

- Included in the notion of self-concept are body image ("how I experience my body"); subjective self ("how I see myself"); ideal self ("the self I want to be"); and social self ("the way I feel others see me").

- It is helpful to explore the self-concept by assessing self-knowledge, self-expectations, and self-evaluation or self-esteem. Self-esteem is a measure of a person's satisfaction with his or her significance, competence, virtue, and power.

- Self-concept is a social creation. An infant, born without a self-concept, develops positive feelings about self if basic needs are met and warmth and affection are experienced.

- A positive self-concept is characterized by stable and diversified self-knowledge, realistic self-expectations, and positive self-evaluation and acceptance of self.

- High self-esteem is characterized by positive expectations of the future, ability to approach others freely because of a history of being well received and successful, and ability to approach new tasks and situations freely, confident of own ability to get along.

- Life experiences both affect and are affected by a person's self-concept. Key factors influencing self-concept are developmental state, culture, internal and external resources, history of success and failure, stressors, and illness or trauma.

- Nurses who wish to meet the self-concept needs of patients effectively need to be comfortable with themselves and their own abilities and needs before they can interact therapeutically with patients. It is important for nurses to role-model positive self-concept behaviors.

- Because a patient may offer the responses the interviewer wants rather than what is really felt,

patient responses should be evaluated in relation to observations the nurse makes of the patient's behaviors.

- Nursing diagnoses may be written specifically addressing disturbances in self-concept (disturbances in self-concept, body image, self-esteem, role competence, and personal identity), or identifying the effect these disturbances have on other areas of human functioning (e.g., coping, health maintenance, powerlessness).

■ Learning Checklist

Review the learning checklist at the end of the chapter in your textbook and be sure you can meet each objective.

■ Exercises

MATCHING

Match the definition in Part B with the term listed in Part A.

PART A

a. self-esteem

b. self-actualization

c. self-concept

d. body image

e. self-knowledge

f. self-expectations

g. self-evaluation

h. personal identity

PART B

1. _____ The need to feel good about oneself and believe others also hold one in high regard.

2. _____ How I experience my body.

3. _____ Describes an individual's conscious sense of who he or she is.

4. _____ Includes basic facts, which place that person in social groups, and a listing of qualities or traits, which describe typical behaviors, feelings, moods, and other characteristics.

5. _____ These flow from the ideal self, the self one wants to be or thinks one should be.

6. _____ The mental image or picture of self.

7. _____ The assessment of how well I like myself.

Match the examples of high-risk factors for self-concept disturbances in Part B with the factors listed in Part A. Some answers may be used more than once.

PART A

a. personal identity disturbances

b. body image disturbances

c. self-esteem disturbances

d. altered role performance

PART B

8. _____ A 55-year-old executive is laid off from his job due to cutbacks.

9. _____ A 45-year-old woman undergoes a radical mastectomy.

10. _____ A 30-year-old woman finds herself in a relationship with an abusive husband.

11. _____ An exchange student from France attends high school in America to learn a new language and customs.

12. _____ A new mother discovers she is terrified of taking care of her newborn son on her own.

13. _____ An 11-year-old girl starts menstruating and developing earlier than her peers.

14. _____ A 65-year-old retired lawyer regrets that he was unable to become a judge as he had always dreamed of doing.

15. _____ An athlete loses his pitching arm to cancer.

16. _____ A 38-year-old woman who is recently divorced is lost without her husband.

MULTIPLE CHOICE

Circle the letter that corresponds to the best choice for each question.

1. When children identify sports figures as their heroes, they are experiencing which of the following aspects of self-concept?
   a. self-knowledge
   b. self-expectations
   c. self-evaluation
   d. self-actualization

2. The need to reach one's potential through full development of one's unique capability is known as which of the following?
   a. self-actualization
   b. self-concept
   c. self-esteem
   d. ideal self

3. A child is able to learn self-recognition in which of the following stages of childhood?
   a. infancy
   b. 18 months
   c. 3 years
   d. 6 to 7 years

4. A student nurse who has not maintained healthy relationships with her peers would be at risk for which of the following self-concept disturbances?
   a. personal identity disturbance
   b. body image disturbance
   c. self-esteem disturbance
   d. altered role performance

5. When a nurse asks a patient to describe her personal characteristics and traits, she is most likely assessing the patient for which of the following self-concept factors?
   a. body image
   b. role performance
   c. self-esteem
   d. personal identity

6. Which of the following questions would you expect
to find on a self-concept assessment related to body
image?

   a. Do you like who you are?

   b. Who has influenced you the most growing up?

   c. How do you feel about any physical changes you
   noticed recently?

   d. Who would you most like to be?

7. Which of the following questions would best relate
to self-identity on a focused self-concept
assessment?

   a. Who would you like to be?

   b. What do you like most about your body?

   c. What are your personal strengths?

   d. Do you like being a teacher?

8. Which of the following nursing diagnoses lacks a
self-concept disturbance etiology?

   a. Self-care deficit related to dysfunctional grieving.

   b. Noncompliance related to low self-esteem.

   c. Posttrauma response related to disturbance in
   personal identity.

   d. Altered health maintenance related to altered
   role performance.

9. Which of the following questions would provide
the healthcare worker with the information needed
first when assessing self-concept?

   a. How would you describe yourself to others?

   b. Do you like yourself?

   c. What do you see yourself doing five years from
   now?

   d. What are some of your personal strengths?

COMPLETION

1. What measure could you as a nurse employ to
promote self-esteem in older adults?

   _____

   _____

2. Reflect on your own personal self-concept and
how it affects the way you live your life. Keeping
this in mind, explain how you would answer the
following questions.

   a. Who am I? _____

   _____

   _____

   b. Who or what do I want to be?

   _____

   _____

   c. How well do I like me? _____

   _____

   _____

3. Give an example of a question you might use to
assess a patient for the following concepts.

   a. Significance: _____

   b. Competence: _____

   c. Virtue: _____

   d. Power: _____

4. Give a personal example of how each of the
following factors may have influenced your self-
concept.

   a. Developmental considerations: _____

   _____

   _____

   b. Culture: _____

   _____

   _____

   c. Internal or external resources: _____

   _____

   _____

   d. History of success or failure: _____

   _____

   _____

   e. Stressors: _____

   _____

   _____

   f. Aging, illness, or trauma: _____

   _____

   _____

5. List one example from your experience as a nurse that exemplifies the use of the following strategies for developing self esteem into your practice.

   a. Dispel the myth that it is necessary to know all there is to know about nursing to be a good nurse: _____

   _____

   _____

   b. Realistically evaluate strengths and weaknesses:

   _____

   _____

   c. Accentuate the positive: _____

   _____

   _____

   d. Develop a conscious plan for changing weaknesses into strengths: _____

   _____

   _____

   e. Work to develop team self-esteem: _____

   _____

   _____

   f. Actively demonstrate your commitment to nursing and concern about nursing's public image: _____

   _____

   _____

6. Describe how you would record a self-concept assessment, using your own personal strengths as an example: _____

   _____

   _____

7. Give an example of an interview question you could use to assess self-concept in the following areas.

   a. Personal identity: _____

   b. Patient strengths: _____

   c. Body image: _____

   d. Self-esteem: _____

   e. Role performance: _____

8. Write a sample nursing diagnosis and goal for the following disturbances in self-concept.

   a. A 42-year-old woman is anxious about disfigurement from her mastectomy.

   Diagnosis: _____

   Patient goal: _____

   _____

   _____

   b. A teen is anxious about being able to cope with pregnancy.

   Diagnosis: _____

   Patient goal: _____

   _____

   _____

   c. A 76-year-old man stops taking care of his physical needs because he doesn't care to go on with life without his recently deceased spouse.

   Diagnosis: _____

   Patient goal: _____

   _____

   _____

   d. A parent doesn't know how to teach a child who is being ridiculed by his peers in school how to establish self-esteem.

   Diagnosis: _____

   Patient goal: _____

   _____

   _____

   e. A battered woman feels her situation is hopeless, and that she deserves to be abused because she is so weak.

   Diagnosis: _____

   Patient goal: _____

   _____

   _____

f. A woman, post hysterectomy, feels she can no longer have a sexual relationship with her husband.

Diagnosis: _____

Patient goal: _____

_____

_____

9. Describe three strategies nurses can use to help patients identify and use personal strengths.

a. _____

b. _____

c. _____

10. Give three examples of how nurses can help patients maintain a sense of self and worth.

a. _____

b. _____

c. _____

11. Describe nursing strategies to develop self-esteem that you might use to meet the needs of the following elderly patients with disturbances in self-concept.

a. An 88-year-old woman, newly admitted to a nursing home, who states she has lost all sense of self. Self-identity disturbance:

_____

_____

b. A 75-year-old man with crippling arthritis who tells you that he no longer recognizes himself when he looks in the mirror. Body image disturbance:

_____

_____

c. A 62-year-old man who is recovering from a stroke that has paralyzed his right side states: "I don't know if I can live like this." Self-esteem disturbance:

_____

_____

d. A 67-year-old woman who complains that she no longer has the patience to babysit for her grandchildren whom she loves. Role performance disturbance:

_____

_____

GUIDE TO CRITICAL THINKING AND DEVELOPING BLENDED SKILLS

1. There are many factors that influence the self-concept of patients, including developmental considerations, culture, internal or external sources, history of success or failure, stressors, and aging, illness, or trauma. Interview several patients to find out how these factors have influenced their self-concept. Once you've identified these factors, write a nursing diagnosis for each patient and develop patient health goals where appropriate.

2. Would you describe yourself as having high or low self-concept? Ask your friends if they agree with your assessment. How might your self-concept influence the relationship you establish with patients and colleagues?

PATIENT CARE STUDY

Read the following patient care study and use your nursing process skills to answer the questions below.

An English teacher asks you, the school nurse, to see one of her students whose grades have recently dropped and who no longer seems to be interested in school or anything else. "She was one of my best students, and I can't figure out what's going on. She seems reluctant to talk about this change." When Julie, a 16-year-old junior, walks into your office, you are immediately struck by her stooped posture, unstyled hair, and sloppy appearance. Julie is attractive, but at 5 feet, 3 inches and 150 pounds, she is overweight. Although Julie is initially reluctant to talk, she breaks down at one point and confides that for the first time in her life she feels "absolutely awful" about herself. "I've always concentrated on getting good grades and achieved this easily. But right now, this doesn't seem so important. I don't have any friends. All I hear the girls talking about is boys, and I was never even asked out by a boy, which I guess isn't surprising. Look at me...." After a few questions, it becomes clear that Julie has new expectations for herself based on what she observes in her peers, and she finds herself falling far short of her new, ideal self. Julie admits that in the past, once she set a goal for herself, she was always able to achieve it because she is strongly self-motivated. Although she has withdrawn from her parents and teachers, she admits that she does know adults she can trust who have been a big support to her in the past. "If only I could become the kind of teenager other kids like and have lots of friends!"

1. Identify pertinent patient data by placing a single underline beneath the objective data in the case study and a double underline beneath the subjective data.

2. Complete the Nursing Process Worksheet on the next page to develop a three-part diagnostic statement and related plan of care for this patient.

3. Write down the patient and personal nursing strengths you hope to draw upon as you assist this patient to better health.

   Patient strengths: _____

   Personal strengths: _____

4. Pretend that you are performing a nursing assessment of this patient after the plan of care has been implemented. Document your findings below.

NURSING PROCESS WORKSHEET

Health Problem (Title)	Expected Outcome

Related to

↓

Etiology (Related Factors)	Nursing Interventions**

As Manifested by

↓

Signs and Symptoms (Defining Characteristics)	Evaluative Statement

*More than one patient goal may be appropriate. For the purposes of this exercise, develop the one patient goal that demonstrates a direct resolution of the patient problem identified in the nursing diagnosis.
**Be sure you are able to list the scientific rationale for each nursing intervention you ordered.

CHAPTER 31

Stress and Adaptation

CHAPTER OVERVIEW

- Homeostasis, or a healthy, balanced state, is maintained by various physiologic and psychologic mechanisms. Physiologic mechanisms are largely involuntary responses of the autonomic and endocrine systems, necessary to health maintenance. Psychologic balance is maintained through the use of coping or defense mechanisms.

- Stress, stressors, and adaptation are all interrelated parts of a process. *Stressors* (a challenge, a danger, or a threat) cause *stress* (a change in the balanced state). A person *adapts* through a series of responses. Each component is highly individualized and holistic in effect.

- Stress may be developmental or situational; stressors may be physiologic or psychosocial. Physiologic stressors have both a general and a specific effect. Psychosocial stressors affect us constantly in day-to-day living.

- The relation between physical and emotional stress is illustrated by the mind–body interaction, in which the perception of a threat on an emotional level results in the fight-or-flight response by the body. Resulting illnesses are called psychosomatic disorders.

- The LAS is a localized body response to traumatic or pathologic stress that helps to maintain homeostasis and adaptation. Two examples of the LAS are the reflex pain response and the inflammatory response.

- The inflammatory response occurs in response to injury or infection, serving to prevent the spread of infection and promote wound healing through regeneration of tissue or formation of scar.

- The GAS is a biochemical model that describes the body's general response to stress. There are three stages to the GAS: alarm reaction, stage of resistance, and stage of exhaustion. The stages occur in response to both physical and emotional stress.

- The most common psychologic response to stress is anxiety. Anxiety, precipitated by new experiences and the unknown, is a threat to self-esteem and identity. Anxiety has four levels: mild, moderate, severe, and panic.

- Coping mechanisms are largely unconscious methods of attempting to adapt to stress.

- Higher levels of stress may require psychologic adaptation by coping with task-oriented reactions (attack, withdrawal, or compromise behavior) or defense mechanisms. Many of these behaviors are learned, based on past experiences and sociocultural environment.

- Stress can interfere with basic need attainment, disrupting homeostasis and causing illness.

- Stress can promote health and learning, but the stress of illness imposes additional burdens on a person who is out of balance. Adaptation to illness involves general tasks and illness-related tasks. Nursing interventions to reduce the stress of illness must be individualized and holistic.

- Stress affects the family as well as the individual. Families use varied coping methods and provide an important support system for the ill person.

- Prolonged stress affects both physical and mental health.

- Crisis results from ineffective coping, leading to severe anxiety, disorganized behavior, and malfunction.

- Nurses can promote health by teaching stress reduction teaching methods, including healthy lifestyle, support groups, stress management techniques, and crisis intervention.

- Nursing is a stressful occupation. Nurses may become overwhelmed by the demands made on them and may develop symptoms of burnout. They can practice stress management techniques both on and off the job to help prevent stress and to improve career satisfaction.

■ Learning Checklist

Review the learning checklist at the end of the chapter in your textbook and be sure you can meet each objective.

■ Exercises

MATCHING

Match the type of defense mechanism listed in Part A with its example listed in Part B.

PART A

a. compensation
b. denial
c. displacement
d. introjection
e. projection
f. rationalization
g. reaction formation
h. regression
i. repression
j. sublimation
k. suppression
l. undoing

PART B

1. _____ A patient bangs his hand on the bed tray over frustration with his rehabilitation progress.

2. _____ A patient doesn't remember striking a nurse during a painful procedure.

3. __a__ A patient who screamed at a nurse in anger over a lack of privacy, gives the nurse a box of candy.

4. __e__ A patient who continually forgets to take his medications complains that "there are too many pills to take."

5. __b__ A patient refuses to accept her diagnosis of cancer.

6. _____ A patient who has sexual feelings for a nurse accuses her of sexual harassment.

7. _____ A patient who is unable to stop smoking becomes a fitness fanatic.

8. _____ A patient adopts his spiritual director's philosophy of life.

9. _____ A patient who secretly admires her doctor's medical ability questions his competency.

10. _____ A nursing home patient who is depressed becomes incontinent.

11. _____ A wheelchair-bound patient becomes involved in wheelchair races.

Match the homeostatic regulators of the body listed in Part A with their action listed in Part B.

PART A

a. parasympathetic
b. sympathetic
c. pituitary
d. adrenals
e. thyroid
f. cardiovascular
g. renal
h. respiratory
i. gastrointestinal

PART B

12. _____ Secretes adrenocorticotropic hormone and thyroid-stimulating hormone.

13. _____ Takes in food and fluids and eliminates waste products.

14. _____ Functions under stress conditions to bring about the fight-or-flight response.

15. _____ Regulates intake and output of oxygen and carbon dioxide.

16. _____ Functions under normal conditions and at rest.

17. _____ Secretes thyroid hormone and calcitonin.

18. _____ Serves as a transport system and pump.

19. _____ Filters, excretes, and reabsorbs metabolic products and water.

MULTIPLE CHOICE

Circle the letter that corresponds to the best choice for each question.

1. Which of the following describes the change that takes place as a result of a response to a stressor?
   a. adaptation
   b. stress
   c. defense mechanism
   d. anxiety

2. The primary controller of homeostatic mechanisms is which of the following systems?

    a. respiratory

    b. cardiovascular

    c. autonomic

    d. gastrointestinal

3. In which of the stages of the GAS does the body attempt to adapt to the stressor?

    a. alarm reaction

    b. resistance

    c. exhaustion

4. A patient who responds to bad news concerning his lab reports by crying uncontrollably is handling stress by using which of the following?

    a. adaptation technique

    b. coping mechanism

    c. withdrawal behavior

    d. defense mechanism

5. Which of the following statements concerning interactions with basic human needs is accurate?

    a. As a person strives to meet basic human needs at each level, stress can serve as either a stimulus or barrier.

    b. Basic human needs and responses to stress are generalized.

    c. Basic human needs and responses to stress are unaffected by sociocultural backgrounds, priorities and past experiences.

    d. Stress affects all people in their attainment of basic human needs in the same manner.

6. When a patient is withdrawn and isolated, he is most likely suffering from which of the following stressors on basic human needs?

    a. physiologic needs

    b. safety and security needs

    c. self-esteem needs

    d. love and belonging needs

7. Which of the following reactions would be considered anxiety due to a psychologic response?

    a. tremors

    b. sleep disturbances

    c. expressions of anger

    d. withdrawal from interactions with others

8. When physiologic mechanisms within the body respond to internal changes to maintain an essential balance, which of the following processes has occurred?

    a. stress

    b. self-regulation

    c. homeostasis

    d. fight-or-flight response

9. You respond to an approaching examination with a rapidly beating heart and shaking hands. This is the result of what type of response?

    a. coping mechanism

    b. stress adaptation

    c. defense mechanism

    d. mind–body interaction

10. Which of the following phrases best illustrates the panic level of anxiety?

    a. loss of control and rational thought

    b. increased alertness and motivated learning

    c. narrow focus on specific detail

    d. narrow perception field

11. When nurses become overwhelmed in their jobs and develop symptoms of anxiety and stress, they are experiencing which of the following conditions?

    a. culture shock

    b. adaptation syndrome

    c. ineffective coping

    d. burnout

12. Which of the following best illustrates a general task for a patient adapting to acute and chronic illness?

    a. maintain self-esteem

    b. handle pain

    c. carry out medical treatment

    d. confront family problems

13. Which of the following is the most common response to stress?

    a. anger

    b. anxiety

    c. despair

    d. depression

COMPLETION

1. Briefly describe the following adaptive responses to stress, and give an example of each response.

   a. Mind–body interaction: _____

   _____

   _____

   b. Local adaptation syndrome: _____

   _____

   _____

   c. General adaptation syndrome: _____

   _____

   _____

2. Describe the three stages of the inflammatory response.

   a. _____

   b. _____

   c. _____

3. List three variables on which the length of the alarm stage depends.

   a. _____

   b. _____

   c. _____

4. Describe the following types of anxiety. Can you think of any examples in your practice in which you experienced any of these levels of anxiety?

   a. Mild anxiety: _____

   _____

   _____

   b. Moderate anxiety: _____

   _____

   _____

   c. Severe anxiety: _____

   _____

   _____

   d. Panic: _____

   _____

   _____

5. Give an example of a situation in which you experienced the following coping mechanisms personally or witnessed them in a friend, relative, or patient.

   a. Attack behavior: _____

   b. Withdrawal behavior: _____

   c. Compromise behavior: _____

6. List three examples of situations in which stress may have a positive impact on an individual.

   a. _____

   b. _____

   c. _____

7. Give three examples of the following sources of stress.

   a. Developmental stress: _____

   _____

   _____

   b. Situational stress: _____

   _____

   _____

8. An 18-year-old male is admitted to your unit with a broken leg and facial lacerations following an automobile accident. Give an example of two questions a nurse may ask during the nursing history to assess this patient for anxiety.

   a. _____

   b. _____

9. You are a visiting nurse for a patient recovering from a stroke who is being taken care of by her daughter-in-law, who is also the mother of 2-year-old twins. During your visit, you notice that your patient's daughter is restless and unfocused. She admits having resumed her smoking habit. You suspect she is suffering from caregiver burden. How would you plan and implement care to help relieve her stress? _____

   _____

   _____

10. Briefly describe how the following components can help reduce stress.

    a. Exercise: _____

    b. Rest and sleep: _____

    c. Nutrition: _____

11. List the five steps of the problem-solving technique used in crisis intervention.

    a. _____

    b. _____

    c. _____

    d. _____

    e. _____

12. List four personal factors that affect stress.

    a. _____

    b. _____

    c. _____

    d. _____

13. Give three examples of how a family can help a patient manage stress.

    a. _____

    b. _____

    c. _____

GUIDE TO CRITICAL THINKING AND DEVELOPING BLENDED SKILLS

1. Describe the nursing interventions you would use to relieve the stress of the following patients:

    a. A 42-year-old man with a wife and three children is being treated for an ulcer. He recently lost his job and is having a hard time finding a new one. He doesn't know if he can make his mortgage and school payments.

    b. A 16-year-old male patient is admitted to a unit for drug rehabilitation. He put pressure on himself to be the best in sports and school work and stated he couldn't handle the stress without getting high.

    How would you use your knowledge of the patients to individualize the plan of care?

2. Think of a period in your life when you were under a considerable amount of stress, such as during exams, following a death, or during an illness. How did the stress affect you physically? Did it alter your health state? What did you do to compensate for the effects of stress on your body? How can you use this information in care of patients?

PATIENT CARE STUDY

1. Read the following patient care study and use your nursing process skills to answer the questions below.

Tisha Brent, age 52, comes to the local clinic for feelings of nervousness and an inability to sleep. During the health history, she states that "this past year has been almost more than I could stand," adding that in one year her grandmother and father died, her husband was diagnosed with cancer, her daughter got a divorce, and her son became depressed and unable to work. She believes herself to be "the strong person in the family; the one who always takes care of everyone else."

Mrs. Brent works full time as a social worker, but is finding it more and more difficult to help others because of her own worries. She tells you that she rarely sees her friends anymore because she must care for her husband. She also says that she has no appetite, cries often, and sometimes has trouble catching her breath. Findings from the physical assessment included a weight loss of 10 pounds in the past 3 months (with weight 5% below normal for height), tachycardia, slightly elevated blood pressure, and hand tremors.

    a. What additional questions might you ask to complete the health history?

    b. What physical manifestations of stress might be elicited during the health history and physical assessment?

    c. List nursing diagnoses obtained from your data.

    d. List expected outcomes for Mrs. Brent.

    e. Mrs. Brent is diagnosed as being in crisis. What does this mean?

f. What are the steps of crisis intervention that may be used with Mrs. Brent?

g. What would you teach Mrs. Brent about reducing stress through healthy activities of daily living?

Exercise: _____

Rest and sleep: _____

Nutrition: _____

h. How would you know if Mrs. Brent had decreased her level of stress and increased her ability to cope with stressors?

CHAPTER 32

Loss, Grief, and Dying

CHAPTER OVERVIEW

- Everyone experiences losses at various points in the life continuum. Such losses can be actual, perceived, physical, psychologic, or anticipatory. Loss can have an effect on the developmental stages of the human life span, especially in children.

- Grief is the emotional response to loss, and grief reactions can be divided into identifiable stages. Grief can be manifested both emotionally and physically, and grief reactions are influenced by development, family and socioeconomic factors, and religious and cultural influences.

- Like grief, dying can be broken down into identifiable and overlapping stages.

- Nurses should be familiar with the clinical signs of approaching or impending death and three definitions of death.

- Patients and families increasingly look to nurses for information, advice, and support when making end-of-life treatment decisions. Nurses need to recognize the ethical, spiritual, and legal ramifications of these decisions.

- Stage of development, family, socioeconomic factors, culture, religion, and the cause of death can all influence an individual's experience of loss, grief, and dying.

- Dying patients have various needs, ranging from the need for open communication to physiologic, psychologic, and spiritual needs. They should maintain self-care as long as possible.

- Families of dying patients also need open communication, and may want to assist the nurse in providing care. This is considered a healthy experience for both the patient and family members.

- The nurse should provide emotional support for the grieving family by being an attentive, nonjudgmental listener and a good communicator.

- The nurse has specific responsibilities at the time of a patient's death, including ensuring that a death certificate is issued, caring for the body, placing identification tags on the shroud and body, ensuring that the body is discharged to the proper party, and caring for the family.

- The nurse should provide care to other patients who are affected by the loss.

■ Learning Checklist

Review the learning checklist at the end of the chapter in your textbook and be sure you can meet each objective.

■ Exercises

MATCHING

Match the term in Part A with the appropriate definition listed in Part B.

PART A

a. actual loss

b. perceived loss

c. physical loss

d. psychologic loss

e. anticipatory loss

f. grief

g. bereavement

h. mourning

PART B

1. _____ The period of acceptance of loss during which the person learns to deal with the loss.

2. _____ A type of loss in which a person displays loss and grief behaviors for a loss that has yet to take place.

3. _____ A type of loss that can be recognized by others as well as by the person sustaining the loss.

4. _____ The state of grieving during which a person goes through grief reaction.

5. _____ A type of loss that is felt by the individual but is intangible to others, such as loss of youth or financial independence.

6. _____ A type of loss that may be caused by an altered self-image and inability to return to work.

7. _____ A type of loss that is tangible, such as the loss of a limb or organ.

Match Engel's six stages of grief listed in Part A with the appropriate conversation that may occur during each stage listed in Part B.

PART A

a. shock and disbelief

b. developing awareness

c. restitution

d. resolving the loss

e. idealization

f. outcome

PART B

8. _____ "I know I won't be having Sunday dinner with my mother anymore. Maybe my husband and I can eat out this Sunday."

9. _____ "I can't believe my mother died of breast cancer; she was never seriously ill in her life."

10. _____ "My mother was the perfect parent. I wish I could be more like her with my kids."

11. _____ "Every time I think of my mother, I can't help but cry."

12. _____ "I've been attending Mass every morning to pray for my mother's soul and to help me get over her death."

13. _____ "I miss my mother, but at least now I can accept her death and try to get on with my life."

CORRECT THE FALSE STATEMENTS

Circle the word true or false that follows the statement. If the word false has been circled, change the underlined word/words to make the statement true. Place your answer in the space provided.

1. A person experiencing <u>abbreviated grief</u> may have trouble expressing feelings of loss or may deny them.

   True   False   _____

2. In the <u>denial and isolation</u> stage of dying, the patient expresses rage and hostility, and adopts a "why me?" attitude.

   True   False   _____

3. In the case of a terminal illness, the <u>physician</u> is usually responsible for deciding what and how much the patient should be told.

   True   False   _____

4. A <u>living will</u> appoints an agent the person trusts to make decisions in the event of the appointing person's subsequent incapacity.

   True   False   _____

5. The <u>Patient Self-Determination Act of 1990</u> requires all hospitals to inform their patients of advance directives.

   True   False   _____

6. A <u>slow-code</u> may be written on the chart of a terminally ill patient if the patient or family has expressed a wish that there be no attempts to resuscitate the patient in the event of cardiopulmonary failure.

   True   False   _____

7. <u>Terminal weaning</u> is the gradual withdrawal of mechanical ventilation from a patient with a terminal illness or an irreversible condition with poor prognosis.

   True   False   _____

8. The <u>nurse</u> assumes responsibility for handling and filing the death certificate with proper authorities.

   True   False   _____

9. After the patient has been pronounced dead, the <u>physician</u> is responsible for preparing the body for discharge.

   True   False   _____

10. After the death of a patient, <u>the nurse is always responsible</u> for washing the body.

   True   False   _____

11. After the death of a patient, the nurse should place an identification tag on the <u>shroud or garment the body is clothed in and the ankle.</u>

   True   False   _____

MULTIPLE CHOICE

Circle the letter that corresponds to the best answer for each question.

1. Which of the following stages of grief, according to Engel, involve the rituals surrounding loss, including funeral services?

   a. shock and disbelief

   b. developing awareness

   c. restitution

   d. resolving the loss

2. The husband of a patient who has died is unable to express his feelings of loss and at times denies them. His bereavement has extended over a lengthy period. Which of the following types of grief would the husband be experiencing?

   a. anticipatory grief

   b. inhibited grief

   c. normal grief

   d. unresolved grief

3. A patient who has been treated in the emergency room for gunshot wounds dies in intensive care 15 hours later. Which of the following statements concerning the need for an autopsy would apply to this patient?

   a. The closest surviving family member should be consulted to determine whether or not an autopsy should be performed.

   b. The coroner must be notified to determine the need for an autopsy.

   c. The physician should be present to prepare the patient for an autopsy.

   d. An autopsy should not be performed since the nature of death has been established.

4. Mr. Cooney is an 85-year-old male patient in advanced stages of pneumonia with a no-code order in his chart. Which of the following nursing care actions will help establish a trusting nurse–patient relationship?

   a. The nurse should not express his own fears about death in order to better concentrate on the patient's needs.

   b. The nurse should reduce verbal and nonverbal contact with the patient to avoid confusing him.

   c. The nurse should encourage family members to assist in his nursing care.

   d. The nurse should arrange a visit from a spiritual advisor against the patient's wishes to provide hope in the face of death.

5. A nurse informs a new mother that there is nothing more that can be done medically for her premature infant, who is expected to die. Which of the following types of grief might the mother be experiencing?

   a. anticipatory grief

   b. inhibited grief

   c. unresolved grief

   d. dysfunctional grief

6. According to Engel (1964), the exaggeration of the good qualities of the person or object lost followed by acceptance of the loss is which of the following?

   a. restitution

   b. awareness

   c. outcome

   d. idealization

7. Prior to the death of her husband, Mrs. Sardi complained of frequent headaches and loss of appetite. No medical cause was found. Mrs. Sardi probably was experiencing which type of grief?

   a. abbreviated grief

   b. anticipatory grief

   c. unresolved grief

   d. inhibited grief

8. Which of the following diagnoses specifically addresses human response to loss and impending death in the problem statement?

   a. Dysfunctional grieving related to loss of partner.

   b. Anxiety related to unknown reaction to stages of death.

   c. Self-care deficit related to weakness.

   d. Altered comfort related to complications of chemotherapy for end-stage liver cancer.

COMPLETION

1. List two nursing responsibilities that should be carried out after the death of a patient in each of the following areas.

   a. Care of the body: _____

   _____

   b. Care of the family: _____

   _____

   c. Discharging legal responsibilities: _____

   _____

2. Describe the following three definitions of death:

   a. Heart-lung death: _____

   _____

   b. Whole brain death: _____

   _____

   c. Higher brain death: _____

   _____

   _____

3. Briefly describe the following stages of dying, according to Kubler-Ross.

   a. Denial and isolation: _____

   _____

   b. Anger: _____

   _____

   c. Bargaining: _____

   _____

   d. Depression: _____

   _____

   e. Acceptance: _____

   _____

4. Your patient is a 50-year-old woman newly diagnosed with terminal uterine cancer. What information should be provided to her regarding her condition? _____

   _____

   _____

5. List the clinical signs of impending death: _____

   _____

   _____

6. How would you respond to a patient dying of AIDS, who says to you "Nurse, please help me die"? _____

   _____

   _____

7. Describe the role of the nurse in terminal weaning.

   _____

   _____

8. List three goals for nurses who wish to become effective in caring for patients experiencing loss, grief, or dying and death.

   a. _____

   b. _____

   c. _____

9. Your patient is a 62-year-old man dying of liver cancer at home with his family. List three patient goals or outcomes for this patient and his family.

   a. _____

   b. _____

   c. _____

10. List three arguments in favor of and against assisted suicide and direct voluntary euthanasia.

   a. In favor of: _____

   _____

   _____

   b. Against: _____

   _____

   _____

11. What is the role of the nurse during the following code situations:

   a. No-code: _____

   _____

   _____

   b. Comfort measures only: _____

   _____

   c. Do not hospitalize order: _____

   _____

   d. Terminal weaning: _____

   _____

   _____

12. Explain the role of the nurse in obtaining the following advance directives for a patient:

    a. Durable power of attorney: _____

    _____

    _____

    b. Living will: _____

    _____

    _____

GUIDE TO CRITICAL THINKING AND DEVELOPING BLENDED SKILLS

1. Develop nursing plans to help the following clients deal with their grief:

    a. A 22-year-old male athlete has his left leg amputated after it was crushed in a car accident.

    b. You find a 30-year-old woman crying softly in her bed after undergoing a hysterectomy.

    c. A 50-year-old woman has just been told she has a brain tumor that is inoperable.

    What knowledge and skills would you need to meet their needs effectively?

2. Think of a time when you lost someone dear to you. How did you cope with your loss? Were you aware of going through Engel's six stages of grief? How long did it take you to resolve the loss and get back to normal life activities? Interview some friends about coping with losing a loved one and compare their experiences to yours. How can you use this knowledge in your care of patients?

PATIENT CARE STUDY

Read the following patient care study and use your nursing process skills to answer the questions below.

LeRoy is a 40-year-old architect whose life partner, Michael, is dying of AIDS. Although both LeRoy and Michael did the bathhouse scene in the early 1980s and had multiple unprotected sexual encounters, they have been in a monogamous relationship for the last 14 years. Michael has been in and out of the hospital during the last 3 years and is now dying of end-stage AIDS at home. He is enrolled in a hospice program. LeRoy has been very supportive of Michael throughout the different phases of his illllness, but at present seems to be "losing it." Michael noticed that LeRoy is sleeping at odd times and seems to be losing weight. He suspects that LeRoy may be drinking more than usual and using recreational drugs. He also says that he is "acting strangely"; he seems emotionally withdrawn and unusually uncommunicative. "I don't think he's able to deal with the fact that I am dying. He won't let me talk about it at all." The hospice nurse noted that LeRoy is now rarely home when he comes to visit. When the hospice nurse called to arrange a meeting with LeRoy, LeRoy informed him that he was "managing quite well, thank you" and that he had no concerns or problems to discuss.

1. Identify pertinent patient data by placing a single underline beneath the objective data in the patient care study and a double underline beneath the subjective data.

2. Complete the Nursing Process Worksheet on the next page to develop a three-part diagnostic statement and related plan of care for this patient.

3. Write down the patient and personal nursing strengths you hope to draw on as you assist this patient to better health.

    Patient strengths: _____

    _____

    _____

    Personal strengths: _____

    _____

    _____

4. Pretend that you are performing a nursing assessment of this patient after the plan of care is implemented. Document your findings below.

NURSING PROCESS WORKSHEET

Health Problem (Title)	Expected Outcome
Related to ↓	
Etiology (Related Factors)	Nursing Interventions**
As Manifested by ↓	
Signs and Symptoms (Defining Characteristics)	Evaluative Statement

*More than one patient goal may be appropriate. For the purposes of this exercise, develop the one patient goal that demonstrates a direct resolution of the patient problem identified in the nursing diagnosis.

**Be sure you are able to list the scientific rationale for each nursing intervention you ordered.

CHAPTER 33

Sensory Stimulation

CHAPTER OVERVIEW

- Sensory alterations occur when a person experiences decreased sensory input or input that is monotonous, unpatterned, or meaningless (sensory deprivation), or excessive sensory input such that the brain is unable to respond meaningfully (sensory overload).

- Responses to both sensory deprivation and overload include perceptual changes (mild to gross distortions or hallucinations); cognitive changes (decreased attention and concentration, decreased problem-solving ability); and affective changes (apathy, anxiety, fear, panic, anger, depression, and rapid mood swings).

- Patients at high risk for sensory deprivation include those experiencing decreased environmental stimuli (homebound or institutionalized patients, patients on bed rest or in isolation) and those with impaired ability to receive or process environmental stimuli (patients with sensory deficits, patients from a different culture, patients with certain affective disorders and disturbances of the nervous system, patients with bandages or casts that interfere with sense reception, patients taking medications that affect the central nervous system).

- Patients at high risk for sensory overload include acutely ill patients, patients in critical care settings, patients in pain, patients with intrusive and discomforting monitoring or treatment equipment, and patients with disturbances of the nervous system.

- Factors affecting sensory stimulation include age, culture, personality and lifestyle, stress, illness, and medication.

- A comprehensive nursing assessment of sensory functioning includes an examination of the patient for sensory deficits and manifestations of sensory deprivation or overload and an examination of the patient's environment to see if it is providing adequate sensory stimulation for healthy development.

- Nursing diagnoses may be written specifically addressing sensory/perceptual alterations (visual, auditory, olfactory, gustatory, tactile, sensory deprivation, sensory overload) or identifying the effect sensory/perceptual alterations have in other areas of human functioning (e.g., verbal communication, self-care, social interaction, thought processes).

- Small modifications in a patient's environment and in the nurse's pattern of interacting may be all that is needed to prevent sensory alterations.

- Sensory deprivation during a child's formative years may yield permanent results because sensory organs and nerve fibers need early sensory stimulation to develop normally both structurally and functionally. Parents may fail to provide a developmentally stimulating environment for their child because of lack of knowledge, decreased motivation, or inadequate resources.

- The elderly person who has multiple sensory deficits or who lives in a nonstimulating environment is at high risk for chronic sensory deprivation. Symptoms of this disorder are often mistaken for senility.

■ Learning Checklist

Review the learning checklist at the end of the chapter in your textbook and be sure you can meet each objective.

■ Exercises

MATCHING

Match the senses in Part A with their definition in Part B.

PART A

a. visual

b. auditory

c. olfactory

d. gustatory

e. tactile

f. kinesthesia

g. visceral

h. stereognosis

PART B

1. _____ The sense that perceives the solidity of objects and their size, shape, and texture.

2. _____ The sense of taste

3. _____ The sense of sight

4. _____ The sense of smell

5. _____ The sense of hearing

6. _____ The awareness of positioning of body parts and body movement

7. _____ The sense of touch

Match the examples in Part B with the appropriate stimulation listed in Part A. Some answers may be used more than once.

PART A

a. visual stimulation

b. auditory stimulation

c. gustatory/olfactory stimulation

d. tactile stimulation

PART B

8. _____ A nurse wears a brightly colored top when caring for patients confined to bed.

9. _____ A nurse collaborates with the hospital nutritionist to prepare meals with varied seasonings and textures.

10. _____ A patient confined to bed is given daily massages.

11. _____ Soft music is played in the room of a patient who has eye patches following his surgery.

12. _____ A nurse checks patient for properly fitting dentures in a long-term facility.

13. _____ A nurse hugs a depressed patient who makes the effort to bathe and dress herself.

14. _____ A nurse explains a procedure to a comatose patient.

15. _____ A nurse arranges a patient's cards in a heart shape on her walls.

MULTIPLE CHOICE

1. A patient living in a nursing home for the past 5 years no longer responds to the everyday noises outside his room. This ability to ignore continuing noise is known as which of the following?

   a. sensoristasis

   b. sensory overload

   c. adaptation

   d. stereognosis

2. Which of the following statements concerning sensory stimulation is accurate?

   a. Different personality types demand the same level of stimulation.

   b. Decreased sensory stimulation may be sought during periods of low stress.

   c. Illness does not affect the reception of sensory stimuli.

   d. An individual's culture may dictate the amount of sensory stimulation considered normal.

3. An unconscious patient is assigned to your unit. When caring for this patient, you should follow which of the following guidelines for communication?

   a. Hearing is the first sense lost in an unconscious patient; therefore, verbal communication is unnecessary.

   b. You should assume the patient can hear you, and talk with the person in a normal tone of voice.

   c. You should not touch the unconscious patient unnecessarily, because it may confuse him/her.

   d. You should keep the environmental noise level high to help stimulate the patient.

4. Which of the following is the optimal arousal state of the RAS?

   a. sensoristasis

   b. presbycusis

   c. kinesthesia

   d. stereognosis

5. Which of the following conditions occurs when the RAS is no longer able to activate the brain at a normal level and the individual hallucinates simply to maintain an optimal level of arousal?

   a. sensory overload

   b. sensory deprivation

   c. cultural care deprivation

   d. sleep deprivation

6. Your patient in a nursing home is unable to control the direction of thought content, has a decreased attention span, and is unable to concentrate. Which of the following effects of sensory deprivation might he be experiencing?

   a. perceptual response

   b. emotional response

   c. physical response

   d. cognitive response

7. Which of the following refers to impaired or absent functioning in one or more senses?

   a. sensory overload

   b. sensory deficit

   c. sensory deprivation

   d. sensory overstimulation

COMPLETION

1. List four conditions that must be present for a person to receive data necessary to experience the world.

   a. _____

   b. _____

   c. _____

   d. _____

2. Give an example of how the following factors may place a patient at high risk for sensory deprivation.

   a. Environment: _____

   _____

   _____

   b. Impaired ability to receive environmental stimuli: _____

   _____

   _____

   c. Inability to process environmental stimuli:

   _____

   _____

3. Briefly describe the following effects of sensory deprivation:

   a. Perceptual responses: _____

   _____

   _____

   b. Cognitive responses: _____

   _____

   _____

   c. Emotional responses: _____

   _____

   _____

4. List three examples of sensory overload you have observed when caring for patients on your nursing unit.

   a. _____

   b. _____

   c. _____

5. Describe the concept of cultural care deprivation, and list an example from your own experience of a patient who has experienced this alteration.

   _____

   _____

6. Give an example of sensory stimulation that could be provided for each of the following age groups:

   a. Infant: _____

   b. Adult: _____

   c. Elderly: _____

7. Give an example of two goals for patients with impaired sensory functioning.

   a. _____

   b. _____

8. You have been assigned to visit a home healthcare patient, a 75-year-old woman with diabetes living at home with her husband. When you arrive at their home, you notice the drapes are shut, the room is dark and bleak, and there are no pictures, flowers, or the like to visually stimulate the patient. The patient appears in good physical health, but slightly disoriented and confused about the date and time of day. Develop a nursing care plan for this patient with emphasis on the necessity for sensory stimulation:

_____

_____

_____

9. List four precautions you could teach a patient to avoid eye injury in the home.

a. _____

b. _____

c. _____

d. _____

10. Give two examples of suggestions for increasing environmental stimulation and role-model appropriate interactional behaviors for children in the following areas:

a. Visual: _____

_____

b. Auditory: _____

_____

c. Olfactory: _____

_____

d. Gustatory: _____

_____

e. Tactile: _____

_____

11. Give an example of how each of the following factors may influence the amount and quality of stimuli need to maintain cortical arousal.

a. Developmental considerations: _____

_____

b. Culture and lifestyle: _____

_____

c. Personality: _____

_____

d. Stress: _____

_____

e. Illness and medication: _____

_____

12. Explain how you, as a nurse, might assess a patient for the following sensory experiences:

a. Stimulation: _____

_____

b. Reception: _____

_____

c. Transmission-reception-reaction: _____

_____

13. Give three examples of how a nurse might communicate with the following patients:

a. Visually impaired patients: _____

_____

b. Hearing-impaired patients: _____

_____

c. Unconscious patients: _____

_____

GUIDE TO CRITICAL THINKING AND DEVELOPING BLENDED SKILLS

1. Test your friends' senses by trying out these tactile, gustatory and olfactory exercises:

a. Gather several items from your home/work area and place them in a paper bag. These items could include things such as a key, a cotton ball, a toothpick, a tongue depressor, and so on. Have your friends take turns feeling the objects in the bag and guessing what they are without looking at them. As an item is identified, remove it from the bag. Discuss the importance of tactile experiences to the vision-impaired client.

b. Gather several foods for your friends to taste and identify. You could use pudding, Jello, mints, chocolate, and so on. Blindfold your friends and give them a taste of each food. See how many they can identify correctly.

c. Gather items with a pungent odor for your friends to smell and identify. You could use alcohol, lemon juice, pickle juice, cinnamon, mint, and so on. See how many odors they can identify correctly.

Reflect on the role different senses play. Do you believe using only one sense at a time heightens the awareness of that sense? Relate the exercises above to the special needs of the hearing impaired, vision impaired, and the deaf.

2. Walk down a busy street in a city and try to pick out individual noises. How many noises were you able to identify? How many noises became indistinct due to sensory overload? Relate this experience to a patient in a critical care unit.

PATIENT CARE STUDY

Read the following patient care study and use your nursing process skills to answer the questions below.

Mr. Gibson, an 81-year-old married African American, with much prodding from his wife, reluctantly reports that he seems not to be hearing as well as he used to be. "I don't know what the trouble is. I'm in perfect health; always have been. More and more people just seem to be mumbling instead of talking." You notice that he is seated on the edge of his chair and bends toward you when you speak to him. His wife reports that he has stopped going out and pretty much stays in his room whenever people come to the house to visit because he is embarrassed by his inability to hear. "This is really a shame because George was always the life of the party." You ask Mr. Gibson if he has ever had his hearing evaluated and he tells you, "no," that until now he's been trying to convince himself that nothing's wrong with his hearing.

1. Identify pertinent patient data by placing a single underline beneath the objective data in the patient care study and a double underline beneath the subjective data.

2. Complete the Nursing Process Worksheet on the next page to develop a three-part diagnostic statement and related plan of care for this patient.

3. Write down the patient and personal nursing strengths you hope to draw upon as you assist this patient to better health.

Patient strengths: _____

_____

_____

Personal strengths: _____

_____

_____

4. Pretend that you are performing a nursing assessment of this patient after the plan of care is implemented. Document your findings below.

_____

_____

_____

_____

NURSING PROCESS WORKSHEET

Health Problem (Title)	Expected Outcome
Related to ↓	
Etiology (Related Factors)	**Nursing Interventions****
As Manifested by ↓	
Signs and Symptoms (Defining Characteristics)	**Evaluative Statement**

*More than one patient goal may be appropriate. For the purposes of this exercise, develop the one patient goal that demonstrates a direct resolution of the patient problem identified in the nursing diagnosis.

**Be sure you are able to list the scientific rationale for each nursing intervention you ordered.

CHAPTER 34

Sexuality

CHAPTER OVERVIEW

- Sexuality is a human component that is inadequately understood.

- Sexuality defines maleness and femaleness and is evident in behavior, physical appearance, and relationships with others.

- Nurses are concerned with patients' sexuality because individuals bring with them to a healthcare setting all aspects of what makes them human.

- A sound knowledge base of female and male reproductive anatomy and physiology, the sexual response cycle, and factors that affect sexuality is important for the nurse to be an effective teacher, counselor, and advocate in dealing with patients with sexual concerns.

- Factors that affect sexuality include developmental stage, culture, religion, ethics, lifestyle, sexual orientation, health state, and use of medications.

- Obtaining a comprehensive history and performing a physical assessment are paramount before nursing care can be planned for a patient with a sexual concern. However, the collection of a sexual history is not appropriate in all healthcare situations. Patients who should have at least a brief sexual history recorded are those with concerns of a reproductive nature, those experiencing a sexual dysfunction, and those whose illness or treatment will affect their sexual functioning.

- The physical assessment of reproductive anatomy can be stressful and uncomfortable for both male and female patients. Because the major portion of female genitalia is internal, the examination is invasive and may be frightening. The nurse should provide support and information before and during a pelvic examination to create a positive experience for the woman.

- Problems associated with sexuality are rarely simple and clear cut owing to the integral nature of sexuality. Patients may need assistance to talk through their concerns before definitive nursing diagnoses can be formulated.

- Nursing diagnoses can be written specifically to address Altered Sexuality Patterns and Sexual Dysfunction. The effect of sexual concerns on other areas of human functioning can also be identified (e.g., Body Image Disturbance, Anxiety, Impaired Adjustment).

- Nurses who are good role models in promoting healthy sexuality have developed a definition of their own sexuality, have developed a self-awareness of their beliefs, and possess a knowledge base of sexual topics and issues.

- Nursing interventions that promote healthy sexuality include establishing a trusting nurse–patient relationship, advocating for hospitalized patients' sexual needs, counseling patients regarding sexual concerns, and teaching patients about sexuality-related subjects.

- Patient education, which includes topics of self-examination, contraceptive methods, and responsible sexual expression, can be implemented in many healthcare situations.

■ Learning Checklist

Review the learning checklist at the end of the chapter in your textbook and be sure you can meet each objective.

■ Exercises

MATCHING

*Match the female reproductive organs listed in Part A
with their appropriate location depicted in Part B.*

PART A

a. bladder

b. labia minora

c. urethra

d. uterine tube

e. posterior fornix

f. body of uterus

g. vagina

h. clitoris

i. labia majora

j. symphysis pubis

k. uterine cavity (cavitas uteri)

l. ovary

m. cul-de-sac of Douglas

n. external os

o. anus

PART B

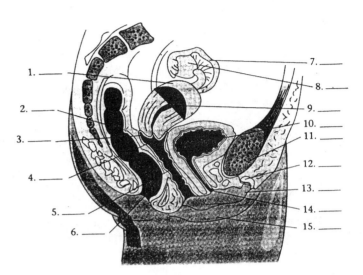

*Match the terms listed in Part A with their definition
listed in Part B.*

PART A

a. biologic sex

b. gender role

c. gender identity

d. sexual orientation

e. heterosexual

f. homosexual

g. bisexual

h. transsexual

i. transvestite

PART B

16. _____ Refers to the preferred gender of partner
of an individual.

17. _____ Term used to denote chromosomal sexual
development.

18. _____ Person of a certain biologic gender with
the feelings of the opposite sex.

19. _____ The behavior a person displays about
being male or female.

20. _____ A person who finds pleasure with both
same or opposite sex partners.

21. _____ One who experiences sexual fulfillment
with a person of the opposite gender.

22. _____ The inner sense a person has of being
male or female.

23. _____ One who experiences sexual fulfillment
with a person of the same gender.

MULTIPLE CHOICE

Circle the letter that corresponds to the best answer for each question.

1. The function of which of the following female organs is to transport a mature ovum from an ovary to the uterus?
   a. fallopian tubes
   b. ovaries
   c. uterus
   d. vagina

2. Which of the following layers of the uterus consists of tissue that thickens and sloughs off during menses?
   a. perimetrium
   b. myometrium
   c. endometrium
   d. cervix

3. During which stage of the menstrual cycle are hormones produced that encourage a fertilized egg to grow?
   a. follicular phase
   b. proliferation phase
   c. luteal phase
   d. secretory phase

4. Which of the following male organs produces the sperm?
   a. scrotum
   b. testes
   c. vas deferens
   d. penis

5. Which of the following organs is believed to act as a reservoir for sperm between ejaculations?
   a. scrotum
   b. testes
   c. epididymis
   d. vas deferens

6. What amount of sperm is dispelled by a fertile man during ejaculation?
   a. 60–100 million/mL
   b. 100–120 million/mL
   c. 120–160 million/mL
   d. 160–180 million/mL

7. The condom, cervical cap, and vaginal sponge are examples of which of the following types of contraceptives?
   a. hormonal methods
   b. barrier methods
   c. natural family planning
   d. sterilization

8. Which of the following statements about orgasm is accurate?
   a. Women who have multiple orgasms are promiscuous.
   b. A mature sexual relationship is not dependent upon a man and woman achieving simultaneous orgasm.
   c. The larger the penis, the greater the potential for achieving orgasm.
   d. The ability to achieve orgasm is the only indicator of a person's sexual responsiveness.

9. Which of the following examples best supports the diagnosis, "sexual dysfunction: dyspareunia"?
   a. Patient with a colostomy feels she is unable to have a sexual relationship with her husband because he will be repulsed by her stoma.
   b. A 50-year-old woman with a history of stroke is afraid to have sex with her partner and elevate her blood pressure.
   c. A 50-year-old woman in the process of menopause has pain and burning during intercourse.
   d. A 39-year-old alcoholic woman is no longer interested in sex with her partner.

COMPLETION

1. Give an example of an intervention for patients with the following health problems to help facilitate sexual contact with their partners.
   a. Chronic pain: _____
   b. Diabetes: _____
   c. Cardiovascular disease: _____
   d. Loss of body part: _____
   e. Spinal cord injury: _____
   f. Mental illness: _____
   g. STDs: _____

2. Briefly describe the four phases of the menstrual cycle.

   a. Follicular phase: _____

   _____

   _____

   b. Proliferation phase: _____

   _____

   _____

   c. Luteal phase: _____

   _____

   _____

   d. Secretory phase: _____

   _____

   _____

3. Briefly describe the male and female responses in the following phases of the sexual response cycle.

   a. Excitement phase: female: _____

   _____

   _____

   male: _____

   _____

   _____

   b. Plateau: female: _____

   _____

   _____

   male: _____

   _____

   _____

   c. Orgasm: female: _____

   _____

   _____

   male: _____

   _____

   _____

   d. Resolution: female: _____

   _____

   _____

male: _____

_____

_____

4. Describe Horsley's specific measures to stop harassment.

   a. Confrontation: _____

   b. Documentation: _____

   c. Written complaint: _____

   d. Government complaint: _____

5. List three general categories of patients who should have a sexual history recorded by the nurse.

   a. _____

   b. _____

   c. _____

6. List three interview questions a nurse may use during a sexual history when assessing a male for impotency.

   a. _____

   b. _____

   c. _____

7. List three major goals of patient teaching about sexuality and wellness.

   a. _____

   b. _____

   c. _____

8. Complete the following chart listing the advantages and disadvantages associated with the following contraceptive methods.

Method	Advantages	Disadvantages
a. Natural family planning		
b. Barrier Methods		
c. Intrauterine Devices		
d. Hormonal Methods		
e. Sterilization		

GUIDE TO CRITICAL THINKING AND DEVELOPING BLENDED SKILLS

1. Write down the interview questions you would use to obtain a sexual history from the following patients:

   a. An 18-year-old female victim of date rape who is brought to the ER for testing and treatment.

   b. A 48-year-old man diagnosed with prostate cancer who is seeking a prescription for Viagra.

   c. An HIV-positive female patient who has had multiple partners and who admits she probably infected other people through unsafe practices.

   d. A 5-year-old female patient who presents with soreness and redness in the genital area.

   How comfortable would you be asking these patients the necessary questions and how might you develop the skills necessary to influence the interview?

2. What knowledge and skills would you need to care for patients experiencing the following sexual dysfunctions:

   a. A man undergoing radiation treatment for colon cancer complains of impotence.

   b. A menopausal woman complains of vaginal dryness and pain during intercourse.

   c. A sexually active teenager complains of a burning sensation during urination.

PATIENT CARE STUDY

Read the following patient care study and use your nursing process skills to answer the questions below.

Anthony Piscatelli, a 6-foot-tall, muscular, healthy 19-year-old college freshman in the School of Nursing confides to his nursing advisor that "everything is great" about college life, with one exception. "All of a sudden I find myself questioning the values I learned at home about sex and marriage. My mom was really insistent that each of her sons should respect women and that intercourse was something you saved until you were ready to get married. If she told us once she told us a hundred times that we'd save ourselves, the girls in our lives, and her and dad a lot of heartache if we could just learn to control ourselves sexually. Problem is that no one here seems to subscribe to this philosophy. I feel like I'm abnormal in some way to even think like this. There's a lot of sexual activity in the dorms, and no one even thinks you're serious if you talk about virginity positively. What do you think? Did my mom sell me a bill of goods? Is it true that if you take the proper precautions, no one gets hurt and everyone has a good time?" Tony reports that he is a virgin and that he really misses his close family back home. "I do get lonely at times, and would love to just cuddle with someone or even give and get a big hug, but no one seems to understand this."

1. Identify pertinent patient data by placing a single underline beneath the objective data in the patient care study and a double underline beneath the subjective data.

2. Complete the Nursing Process Worksheet on the opposite page to develop a three-part diagnostic statement and related plan of care for this patient.

3. Write down the patient and personal nursing strengths you hope to draw upon as you assist this patient to better health.

   Patient strengths: _____

   _____

   _____

   Personal strengths: _____

   _____

   _____

4. Pretend that you are performing a nursing assessment of this patient after the plan of care is implemented. Document your findings below.

   _____

   _____

   _____

   _____

NURSING PROCESS WORKSHEET

Health Problem (Title)

Expected Outcome

Related to
↓

Etiology (Related Factors)

Nursing Interventions**

As Manifested by
↓

**Signs and Symptoms
(Defining Characteristics)**

Evaluative Statement

*More than one patient goal may be appropriate. For the purposes of this exercise, develop the one patient
goal that demonstrates a direct resolution of the patient problem identified in the nursing diagnosis.
**Be sure you are able to list the scientific rationale for each nursing intervention you ordered.

CHAPTER 35

Spirituality

CHAPTER OVERVIEW

- The tradition of nursing has always been strongly holistic and nurses have practiced nursing sensitive to the physical, psychosocial, and spiritual needs of patients.

- Spiritual needs underlying all religious traditions and common to all people include need for meaning and purpose, need for love and relatedness, and need for forgiveness.

- Spiritual beliefs and practices are associated with all aspects of a person's life: health and illness, relationships with others, daily living habits, required and prohibited behaviors, the general frame of reference for thinking about oneself and the world.

- Spiritual beliefs during illness may be an important source of support, strength, and healing but may also be a source of anxiety when they conflict with proposed medical therapy.

- It is important for the nurse to be knowledgeable about and respect the spiritual beliefs of patients.

- The nurse who demonstrates peace, inner strength, warmth, joy, caring, and creativity in interactions with others will be most effective when assisting patients to meet spiritual needs.

- A comprehensive nursing assessment of spirituality addresses spiritual beliefs and practices, the relationship between spiritual beliefs and everyday living, indicators of spiritual distress, and unmet spiritual needs.

- Nursing diagnoses may be written that specifically address spiritual distress (spiritual pain, alienation, anxiety, guilt, anger, loss, or despair) or that identify the effect of spiritual distress on other areas of human functioning (Ineffective Individual Coping, Dysfunctional Grieving, Hopelessness, Powerlessness, Self-Esteem Disturbance).

- Nursing interventions that promote spiritual health include offering a supportive presence, facilitating the patient's practice of religion, nurturing spirituality, praying with a patient, spiritual counseling, referring a patient to a religious counselor, and assisting patients to resolve conflicts between spiritual beliefs and treatment.

■ Learning Checklist

Review the learning checklist at the end of the chapter in your textbook and be sure you can meet each objective.

■ Exercises

MATCHING

Match the religions in Part A with their basic tenets listed in Part B.

PART A

a. Baha'i International Community

b. Islam

c. Protestantism

d. Roman Catholicism

e. American Muslim Mission

f. Native American Religions

g. Judaism

PART B

1. _____ Belief in Allah, one God, who is only one, all seeing, all hearing, all speaking, all knowing, all willing, all powerful.

2. _____ Worship of the one God revealed to the world through Jesus Christ. Love of neighbor is a central tenet. Other beliefs include sin, redemption, salvation, and a final accounting with God.

3. _____ Belief in a basic harmony between religion and science.

4. _____ Notion of cosmic harmony, emphasis on directly experiencing powers and visions, and a common view of the cycle of life and death. Death is not the end but a beginning of new life.

5. _____ Formation is closely bound with a divine revelation and with commitment to obedience to God's will. The Hebrew Bible is the authority,

guide, and inspiration of the many forms of this religion.

6. _____ Accept the Koran as their sacred scripture, most stress the importance of cooperation among blacks in business and education to build self-esteem.

Match the spiritual distress listed in Part A with the appropriate example listed in Part B.

PART A

a. spiritual pain

b. spiritual alienation

c. spiritual anxiety

d. spiritual guilt

e. spiritual anger

f. spiritual loss

g. spiritual despair

PART B

7. _____ A Roman Catholic college student stops going to Mass on Sundays and moves in with her boyfriend; "I really want to do this, but it still feels wrong."

8. _____ A woman cannot accept the death of her newborn infant; "How long will it hurt this bad?"

9. _____ A man with a terminal illness cannot accept his eventual death; "What kind of God are you?"

10. _____ An elderly woman with a hip replacement is confined to her home and unable to get out to her usual daily services.

11. _____ A man dying of AIDS has no friends or support system, and believes that God and humanity have abandoned him.

12. _____ A young man challenges his faith and his own belief in God.

Match the examples of a nurse's supportive presence listed in Part B with the appropriate measure listed in Part A. Answers may be used more than once.

PART A

a. facilitating the practice of religion

b. promoting meaning and purpose

c. promoting love and relatedness

d. promoting forgiveness

PART B

13. _____ A nurse attempts to meet a patient's religious dietary restrictions.

14. _____ A nurse explores with a patient the importance of learning to accept himself even with faults.

15. _____ A nurse treats her patient with respect, empathy, and genuine caring.

16. _____ A nurse explores with a patient spiritual practices from which strength and hope might be derived.

17. _____ A nurse respects a patient's need for privacy during religious prayer.

18. _____ A nurse helps a patient explore his self-expectations and determine how realistic they are.

19. _____ A nurse encourages a patient to explore her relationship with her family and identify the origin of negative beliefs about people.

MULTIPLE CHOICE

Circle the letter that corresponds to the best answer for each question.

1. Which of the following terms describes anything that pertains to a person's relationship with a nonmaterial life force or higher power?

   a. religion

   b. spirituality

   c. faith

   d. belief

2. A terminally ill patient tells you that he does not belong to an organized religion. It is safe to assume which of the following?

   a. The patient is an atheist.

   b. The patient has no belief system.

   c. The patient is an agnostic.

   d. The patient may still be deeply spiritual.

3. Which of the following statements concerning atheists and agnostics is accurate?

   a. Both deny the existence of God.

   b. Nurses should attempt to change their views and offer religious counseling.

   c. Both are guided by a philosophy of living that does not include a religious faith.

   d. Both have religious influences that are life denying.

4. In which of the following religions are women not allowed to make independent decisions and husbands must be present when consent is sought?

    a. Islam

    b. Judaism

    c. Roman Catholicism

    d. Protestantism

5. In which religion are members encouraged to obtain healthcare provided by members of the black community?

    a. Baha'i International Community

    b. American Muslim Mission

    c. Native American Religion

    d. Islam

6. According to Fish and Shelly (1978), which of the following is a spiritual need underlying all religious traditions?

    a. need for formal ceremony

    b. need for power in relationship with God

    c. need for justice

    d. need for meaning and purpose

7. When assessing a child's spiritual dimension, a nurse should be aware of which of the following basic tenets?

    a. Children do not have a definite perception of God.

    b. Children attribute to God tremendous and expansive power.

    c. Children do not experience spiritual distress.

    d. Children view God as a person with divine powers.

8. In which religion do common therapeutic measures include sucking, blowing, and drawing out with a feather fan?

    a. Native American Religion

    b. Islam

    c. Baha'i International Community

    d. Roman Catholicism

COMPLETION

1. List three spiritual needs underlying all religious traditions that are common to all people (Fish and Shelly, 1978).

    a. _____

    b. _____

    c. _____

2. List four methods that nurses can use to assist patients in meeting spiritual needs.

    a. _____

    b. _____

    c. _____

    d. _____

3. Explain how the following religious influences may affect an individual.

    a. Life-affirming influences: _____

    _____

    _____

    b. Life-denying influences: _____

    _____

    _____

4. Give two examples of practices associated with healthcare that may have religious significance to a patient.

    a. _____

    b. _____

5. Briefly describe how religious faith may affect a patient in the following areas.

    a. As a guide to daily living: _____

    _____

    _____

    b. As a source of support: _____

    _____

    _____

    c. As a source of strength and healing: _____

    _____

    d. As a source of conflict: _____

    _____

6. Give an example of how the following factors may influence a person's spirituality:

   a. Developmental considerations: _____

   _____

   _____

   b. Family: _____

   _____

   _____

   c. Ethnic background: _____

   _____

   _____

   d. Formal religion: _____

   _____

   _____

   e. Life events: _____

   _____

   _____

7. Describe how you would handle the following cases:

   a. A family who insists on care deemed medically futile for a terminally ill patient because they believe that God is going to work a miracle:

   _____

   _____

   b. Christian Scientist parents of a child needing an appendectomy who refuse to sign a consent form for surgery: _____

   _____

   _____

8. List six characteristics the religions discussed in this chapter have in common.

   a. _____

   b. _____

   c. _____

   d. _____

   e. _____

   f. _____

9. Give an example of an interview question you might use to asses a patient for the following types of spiritual distress.

   a. Spiritual pain: _____

   b. Spiritual alienation: _____

   c. Spiritual anxiety: _____

   d. Spiritual anger: _____

   e. Spiritual loss: _____

   f. Spiritual despair: _____

10. You are visiting a patient at home who is paralyzed following a car accident. She confesses to you that she feels God has abandoned her and her family, which includes two small children. Suggest a nursing diagnosis for this patient and develop a nursing care plan that includes at least two interventions to help her with her spiritual needs.

   Diagnosis: _____

   Nursing care plan: _____

   _____

   _____

   _____

11. Develop a prayer expressing a patient's needs that could be used for a patient facing surgery.

   _____

   _____

   _____

12. List four guidelines for preparing a patient's room to receive a spiritual counselor.

   a. _____

   b. _____

   c. _____

   d. _____

13. List three interventions to assist a patient with the following deficits.

   a. Deficit: Meaning and Purpose: _____

   _____

   _____

b. Deficit: Love and Relatedness: _____

_____

_____

c. Deficit: Forgiveness: _____

_____

_____

GUIDE TO CRITICAL THINKING AND DEVELOPING BLENDED SKILLS

1. How would you respond to parents who ask you to pray with them for their child's recovery from surgery? Would you feel comfortable praying with them? Do you believe nurses should pray aloud with patients and families? Write down a prayer for the sick that you can use in these situations.

2. Identify your own spiritual beliefs. How do these beliefs influence the way you carry on your daily routine in life? Do these beliefs affect the way you relate to others? In what ways might they affect the way you react to patients of different faiths?

PATIENT CARE STUDY

Read the following patient care study and use your nursing process skills to answer the questions below.

Jeffrey Stein is a 31-year-old attorney who is presently in a step-down unit following his transfer from the cardiac care unit, where he was treated for a massive heart attack. "Bad hearts run in my family, but I never thought it would happen to me. I jog several times a week and work out at the gym, eat a low fat diet, and I don't smoke." Jeffrey is 5 feet, 7 inches tall, weighs about 150 pounds, and is well-built. During his second night in the step-down unit, he is unable to sleep and tells the nurse, "I've really got a lot on my mind tonight. I can't stop thinking about how close I was to death. If I wasn't with someone who knew how to do CPR when I keeled over, I probably wouldn't be here today." Gentle questioning reveals that Mr. Stein is worried about what would have happened had he

died. "I don't think I've ever thought seriously about my mortality, and I sure don't think much about God. My parents were semi-observant Jews, but I don't go to synagogue myself. I celebrate the holidays, but that's about all. If there is a God, I wonder what he thinks about me." He asks if there is a rabbi or anyone he can talk with in the morning who could answer some questions for him and perhaps help him get himself back on track. "For the last couple of years, all I've been concerned about is paying off my school debts and making money. I guess there's a whole lot more to life, and maybe this was my invitation to sort out my priorities."

1. Identify pertinent patient data by placing a single underline beneath the objective data in the patient care study and a double underline beneath the subjective data.

2. Complete the Nursing Process Worksheet on the next page to develop a three-part diagnostic statement and related plan of care for this patient.

3. Write down the patient and personal nursing strengths you hope to draw upon as you assist this patient to better health.

   Patient strengths: _____

   _____

   _____

   Personal strengths:_____

   _____

   _____

4. Pretend that you are performing a nursing assessment of this patient after the plan of care is implemented. Document your findings below.

   _____

   _____

   _____

   _____

NURSING PROCESS WORKSHEET

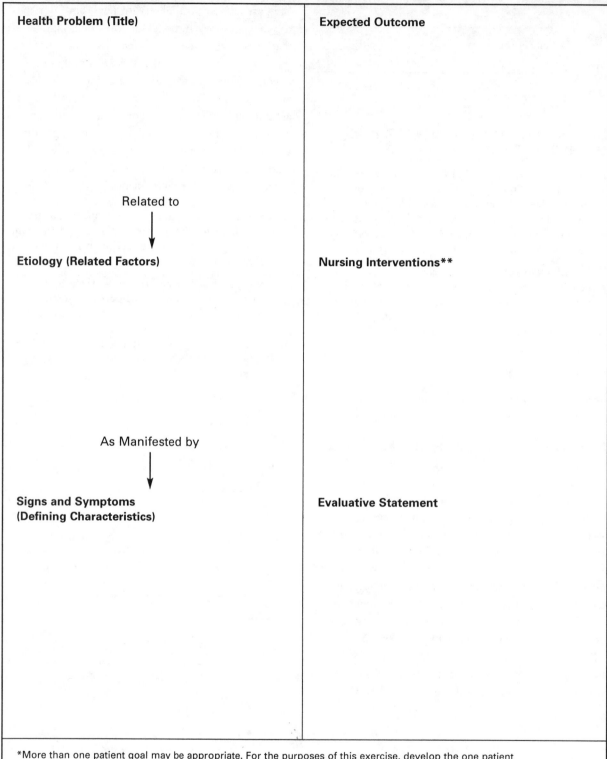

Health Problem (Title)

Expected Outcome

Related to

↓

Etiology (Related Factors)

Nursing Interventions**

As Manifested by

↓

**Signs and Symptoms
(Defining Characteristics)**

Evaluative Statement

*More than one patient goal may be appropriate. For the purposes of this exercise, develop the one patient
goal that demonstrates a direct resolution of the patient problem identified in the nursing diagnosis.
**Be sure you are able to list the scientific rationale for each nursing intervention you ordered.

UNIT VIII

Promoting Healthy Physiologic Reponses

CHAPTER 36

Hygiene

CHAPTER OVERVIEW

- Personal hygiene refers to measures of personal cleanliness and grooming that promote physical and psychologic well-being.

- People differ in personal hygiene practices, which may be affected by culture, socioeconomic class, religion, developmental level, knowledge level, health state, and personal preferences.

- A comprehensive assessment of the skin and mucous membranes includes the collection of data about usual hygiene practices (showering or bathing practices; skin, hair, and scalp care; eye, ear, nose, and mouth care; nail and foot care; and perineal care); an assessment of any sensory, cognitive, endurance, mobility, or motivational deficit that interferes with the individual's hygiene practices; the identification of any existing problems of the skin or mucous membranes and associated care and its effectiveness; and a physical examination of the skin and mucous membranes.

- Because lifestyle factors, changes in health state, illness, and certain diagnostic and therapeutic measures may adversely affect the skin, the nurse needs to identify high-risk populations and perform the appropriate skin assessment, teach the patient how to examine and care for the skin, and institute preventive skin care measures.

- Nursing diagnoses may be written that specifically address problems of deficient hygiene (Self Care Deficit: Bathing/Hygiene) or that identify the effects problems of the skin, hair, scalp, eye, ear, nose, mouth, nails, feet, or perineum have on other areas of human functioning (comfort, mobility, nutrition).

- The individual with cognitive, sensory, endurance, mobility, or motivation deficits may require nursing assistance with any or all aspects of personal hygiene. The nurse promotes independence in these measures consistently. Whenever possible, the nurse offers assistance compatible with the individual's preferences and usual routines. When indicated, the patient and family are taught necessary hygiene measures.

- Hospitalized patients receive scheduled hygienic care. This care includes careful attention to ensuring the safety and comfort of the patient's bedside unit. Because of the long hours many ill patients spend in bed, the condition of bed linens is checked periodically throughout the day.

- A pressure ulcer is caused by unrelieved pressure that results in damage to underlying tissue.

- Patients most at risk for developing a pressure ulcer include older adults, those who are immobile, and individuals living with chronic health problems.

- Family members who care for these individuals need information to effectively prevent pressure ulcers from developing.

■ Learning Checklist

Review the learning checklist at the end of the chapter in your textbook and be sure you can meet each objective.

■ Exercises

MATCHING

Match the oral diseases/conditions in Part A with their definitions listed in Part B.

PART A

a. stomatitis

b. gingivitis

c. pyorrhea

d. halitosis

e. plaque

f. tartar

g. glossitis

h. cheilosis

i. dry oral mucosa

j. oral malignancies

k. caries

l. *Candida albicans*

PART B

1. _____ A strong mouth odor.

2. _____ A marked inflammation of the gums involving the alveolar tissues.

3. _____ Ulceration of the lips, most often caused by vitamin B complex deficiencies.

4. _____ Lumps or ulcers.

5. _____ Inflammation of the oral mucosa with numerous causes (bacteria, virus, mechanical trauma, irritants, nutritional deficiencies, and systemic infection).

6. _____ May be related to dehydration or may be caused by mouth breathing, an alteration in salivary functioning, or certain medications.

7. _____ Hard deposits at the gum lines that attack the fibers that fasten teeth to the gums and eventually attack bone tissue.

8. _____ An inflammation of the tissue that surrounds the teeth.

9. _____ An invisible, destructive bacterial film that builds up on everyone's teeth and eventually leads to the destruction of tooth enamel.

10. _____ An inflammation of the tongue.

11. _____ The formation of cavities.

CORRECT THE FALSE STATEMENTS

Circle the word true or false that follows the statement. If the word false has been circled, change the underlined word/words to make the statement true. Place your answer in the space provided.

1. The integumentary system comprises <u>the skin, the subcutaneous layer directly under the skin, and the appendages of the skin</u>.

   True   False   _____

2. The <u>epidermis</u> consists of smooth, muscular tissue; nerves; hair follicles; certain glands and their ducts; arteries; veins and capillaries; and fibrous, elastic tissue.

   True   False   _____

3. The <u>sebaceous glands</u> secrete cerumen, which consists of a heavy oil and brown pigment, into the external ear canals.

   True   False   _____

4. Fluid loss through fever, vomiting, or diarrhea reduces the fluid volume of the body and is called <u>dehydration</u>.

   True   False   _____

5. Jaundice, a condition caused by excessive bile pigments in the skin, results in a <u>grayish</u> skin color.

   True   False   _____

6. The equipment for a <u>bag bath</u> consists of a plastic bag containing 10 wash cloths that have been moistened with a non-rinsable cleaner and water mixture warmed for a short time.

   True   False   _____

7. Antiembolism stockings are often used for patients with limited activity to help prevent <u>pressure ulcers</u>.

   True   False   _____

8. Before leaving the patient's bedside, the nurse should ensure that the bed is in <u>its highest position</u>.

   True   False   _____

9. The odor of perspiration occurs when <u>bacteria</u> act on the skin's normal secretions.

   True   False   _____

10. <u>Dry skin</u> is especially bothersome during adolescence.

    True   False   _____

11. Pressure ulcers are areas of cellular necrosis caused by <u>increased blood circulation</u> to the involved area.

    True   False   _____

12. Hard contact lenses should be removed before sleeping and should not be worn more than <u>12 to 16 hours</u>.

    True   False   _____

13. Another name for baldness is <u>alopecia</u>.

    True   False   _____

14. <u>Pediculus humanus capitis</u> infests the body.

    True   False   _____

15. A physician who treats foot disorders is known as a <u>pediatrician</u>.

    True   False   _____

16. When providing perineal care for an uncircumcised male patient, the foreskin <u>should be retracted</u> while washing the penis.

    True   False   _____

17. The second layer of the skin, which consists of smooth, muscular tissue; nerves; hair follicles; certain glands and their ducts; arteries, veins, and capillaries; and fibrous, elastic tissue is termed the <u>epidermis</u>.

    True   False   _____

18. Depending on the patient's self-care abilities, the nurse offers assistance with toileting, oral care, bathing, back massage, special skin care measures, cosmetics, dressing, and positioning for comfort during the <u>afternoon care</u> schedule.

    True   False   _____

MULTIPLE CHOICE

Circle the letter that corresponds to the best answer for each question.

1. When using antiembolism stockings on a patient, the nurse should be aware of which of the following facts?

    a. Embolism stockings are made "one size fits all."

    b. The stockings should be applied in the evening after the patient gets into bed.

    c. The legs should be massaged after removing the stockings in the evening.

    d. If the patient has been up and about, elevate the feet and legs 15 minutes before applying stockings.

2. Which of the following would be the appropriate treatment for acne?

    a. The infected areas should be gently squeezed to release the infection.

    b. A person with acne should wash his/her skin less frequently to avoid removing beneficial oils.

    c. Foods that are found to aggravate the condition should be eliminated.

    d. Cosmetics and emollients should be used to cover the condition.

3. When caring for a patient with dentures, which of the following should the nurse tell the patient?

    a. Keeping dentures out for long periods of time permits the gum line to change, affecting denture fit.

    b. Dentures should be wrapped in tissue or a disposable wipe when out of the mouth, and stored in a disposable cup.

    c. Dentures should never be stored in water because the plastic material may warp.

    d. A brush and nonabrasive powder should be used to clean the dentures, and hot water should be used to rinse them.

4. Which of the following techniques for cleaning a patient's eyes is appropriate?

    a. The eye should be cleaned from the outer canthus to the inner canthus.

    b. The eye should be wiped with a dry washcloth or cotton ball.

    c. Artificial tear solution should be used every 4 hours when the blink reflex is decreased or absent.

    d. The patient should be positioned on the opposite side of the eye being cleaned.

5. Which of the following is an appropriate measure when providing oral care for a patient?

    a. A firm brush should be used to brush the patient's teeth.

    b. Automatic toothbrushes are effective cleaning tools and may be used in a hospital setting.

    c. Salt and sodium bicarbonate are far less expensive than toothpastes on the market and may be used exclusively for hospital care.

    d. Mouthwashes should not be used on patients because they tend to mask odor, which must be assessed by the nurse.

6. When bathing your patient, you notice she has a rash on her arms. Which of the following would be an appropriate nursing intervention?

    a. Avoid washing the area as cleansing agents will only make the rash worse.

    b. Use a tepid bath to relieve inflammation and itching.

    c. Do not use over-the-counter products on unknown rashes.

    d. Use a moisturizing lotion on a wet rash to prevent itching.

7. When caring for the skin of patients of different age groups, which of the following should the nurse consider?

   a. An infant's skin and mucous membranes are protected from infection by a natural immunity.

   b. Secretions from skin glands are at their maximum from age 3 on.

   c. The skin becomes thicker and leathery with aging and is prone to wrinkles and dryness.

   d. An adolescent's skin ordinarily has enlarged sebaceous glands and increased glandular secretions.

COMPLETION

1. List six major functions of the skin.

   a. _____

   b. _____

   c. _____

   d. _____

   e. _____

   f. _____

2. Describe the general, normal condition of the skin in the following age groups:

   a. Children: _____

   b. Adolescents: _____

   c. Adults: _____

   d. Older adults: _____

3. Briefly describe how the following factors may influence personal hygiene behaviors.

   a. Culture: _____

   b. Socioeconomic class: _____

   c. Spiritual practices: _____

   d. Developmental level: _____

   e. Health state: _____

   f. Personal preference: _____

4. List four specific activities necessary to meet daily needs that may be addressed as self-care deficits.

   a. _____

   b. _____

   c. _____

   d. _____

5. A mother brings her 6-month-old baby to a well-baby clinic for immunizations. Upon examining the infant, you notice dirt accumulated in the skinfolds and a scaly scalp. Develop a nursing care plan for the infant and mother that includes teaching hygiene. Write a sample diagnosis for the infant's hygiene deficit: _____

6. Describe the activities the nurse would perform in the following scheduled care time periods.

   a. Early morning care: _____

   b. Morning care: _____

   c. Afternoon care: _____

d. Hour of sleep care: _____

_____

_____

e. As needed care: _____

_____

_____

7. List five benefits of bathing.

a. _____

b. _____

c. _____

d. _____

e. _____

8. Describe how you would prepare a bed bath for a patient who is able to wash himself: _____

_____

_____

_____

9. List four advantages of a towel bath.

a. _____

b. _____

c. _____

d. _____

10. List three benefits of a back rub.

a. _____

b. _____

c. _____

11. Describe how the following conditions should be controlled in order to provide a comfortable bedside unit for the patient.

a. Ventilation: _____

_____

_____

b. Odors: _____

_____

_____

c. Room temperature: _____

_____

_____

d. Lighting and noise: _____

_____

_____

12. You are visiting a patient at home who is recovering from heart surgery. When you prepare a bed bath for the patient, you notice her skin is dry and flaky. List four interventions you could use for this patient to prevent injury and irritation.

a. _____

b. _____

c. _____

d. _____

13. Describe the conditions you would look for when assessing the following areas:

a. Lips: _____

_____

_____

b. Buccal mucosa: _____

_____

_____

c. Gums: _____

_____

_____

d. Tongue: _____

_____

_____

e. Hard and soft palates: _____

_____

_____

f. Eye: _____

_____

_____

g. Ear: _____

_____

_____

h. Nose: _____

_____

_____

14. Describe how you would clean the following areas for a patient.

a. Eye: _____

_____

_____

b. Ear: _____

_____

_____

c. Nose: _____

_____

_____

15. Briefly describe the care necessary for the following corrective devices.

a. Contact lenses: _____

_____

_____

b. Artificial eye: _____

_____

_____

c. Hearing aids: _____

_____

_____

d. Dentures: _____

_____

_____

16. List four variables known to cause nail and foot problems.

a. _____

b. _____

c. _____

d. _____

GUIDE TO CRITICAL THINKING AND DEVELOPING BLENDED SKILLS

1. Think about nursing's responsibility to assist patients with daily hygiene. Then, reflect on how you would respond in the following situations. See if your classmates would respond as you do.

a. A same age, opposite sex patient requires total assistance with hygiene.

b. A patient confined to bed, but able to assist with hygiene, refuses to do so.

c. An elderly, incontinent patient refuses your offer to assist her with perineal care.

2. Interview patients of different backgrounds or cultures to find out how they perform their daily routine hygiene. Note how their routine is similar to or different from your personal routine. What would you do to assist these people if they were placed in your care in a healthcare setting?

PATIENT CARE STUDY

Read the following patient care study and use your nursing process skills to answer the questions below.

Dominic Gianmarco is a 78-year-old retired man with a history of Parkinson's disease, who lives alone in a small twin home. He was recently hospitalized for problems with cardiac rhythm, and a pacemaker was installed. The home healthcare nurse made a scheduled visit 1 week after the hospitalization to monitor his recovery and compliance with his medication regimen. The nurse observed that his appearance was disheveled and multiple stains were apparent on his clothing. Several food items were in various stages of preparation on the kitchen counter, and some appeared to have spoiled. Mr. Gianmarco had several days' growth of beard and a body odor was apparent. He was pleasant and oriented to place and person, but unable to identify the time or day of the week. "I lose track of what day it is. Time's not important when you're my age. The most important thing to me right now is to be able to take care of myself and stay in this house near my friends." A walker was visible in a corner of the living room, but Mr. Gianmarco ambulated slowly around the house with a minimum of difficulty and did not use the walker. He commented that he keeps busy "reading, watching old movies, and going to Senior Citizen activities with friends who stop by for me." His daughter, who lives several hours away, visits him every weekend and prepares his medications for the week in a plastic container that is easy for him to open. The nurse observed that all medications appeared to have been taken to date. "I don't mess around with my medicines. One helps my ticker and the others keep me from shaking so much."

1. Identify pertinent patient data by placing a single underline beneath the objective data in the case study and a double underline beneath the subjective data.

2. Complete the Nursing Process Worksheet on the next page to develop a three-part diagnostic statement and related plan of care for this patient.

3. Write down the patient and personal nursing strengths you hope to draw upon as you assist this patient to better health.

Patient strengths: _____

_____

_____

Personal strengths: _____

_____

_____

4. Pretend that you are performing a nursing assessment of this patient after the plan of care is implemented. Document your findings below.

_____

_____

_____

_____

NURSING PROCESS WORKSHEET

Health Problem (Title)	Expected Outcome
Related to ↓	
Etiology (Related Factors)	Nursing Interventions**
As Manifested by ↓	
Signs and Symptoms (Defining Characteristics)	Evaluative Statement

*More than one patient goal may be appropriate. For the purposes of this exercise, develop the one patient goal that demonstrates a direct resolution of the patient problem identified in the nursing diagnosis.
**Be sure you are able to list the scientific rationale for each nursing intervention you ordered.

CHAPTER 37

Skin Integrity and Wound Care

CHAPTER OVERVIEW

- A pressure ulcer is caused by unrelieved pressure that results in damage to underlying tissue.

- Patients most at risk for developing a pressure ulcer include older adults, those who are immobile, and individuals living with chronic health problems.

- Family members who care for these individuals need information to effectively prevent pressure ulcers from developing.

- The most susceptible areas for development of a pressure ulcer are the sacrum, coccyx, trochanter, and heels.

- The Agency for Health Care Policy and Research (AHCPR) and the National Pressure Ulcer Advisory Panel (NPUAP) have adopted a four-stage classification system for pressure ulcers.

- The Norton scale and the Braden scale are risk assessment tools that have been used and tested extensively and are recommended for use in any healthcare setting.

- Skin assessment for a pressure ulcer includes a thorough nursing history and physical assessment describing the location, dimensions, and stage of the ulcer; presence of abnormal pathways, necrotic tissue, exudate, or granulation tissue; and occurrence of epithelialization.

- The nursing diagnoses that specifically address the presence of a pressure ulcer are Impaired Skin Integrity and Risk for Impaired Skin Integrity for stage I and II ulcers, and Impaired Tissue Integrity and Risk for Impaired Tissue Integrity for stage III and IV ulcers.

- Normal saline is the agent recommended for cleansing and irrigation of a pressure ulcer because it does not cause damage to tissue.

- A moisture-retentive dressing creates a healing environment that allows epithelial cells to bridge the open surface of a pressure ulcer more easily.

■ Learning Checklist

Review the learning checklist at the end of the chapter in your textbook and be sure you can meet each objective.

■ Exercises

MATCHING

Match the term in Part A with the correct definition in Part B.

PART A

a. dehiscence

b. ischemia

c. eschar

d. wound

e. exudate

f. granulation tissue

g. epithelialization

h. scar

i. hemorrhage

j. evisceration

k. serous wound drainage

l. sanguineous wound drainage

m. purulent wound drainage

n. red wounds

o. yellow wounds

p. black wounds

q. dressing

PART B

1. _____ The partial or total disruption of wound layers.

2. _____ New tissue, pink-red in color, composed of fibroblasts and small blood vessels that fill an open wound when it starts to heal.

3. _____ Used as a protective cover over a wound.

4. _____ The protrusion of viscera through the incisional area.

5. __k__ Composed of fluid and cells that escape from the blood vessels and are deposited in or on tissue surfaces.

6. __D__ Wounds in the proliferative stage of healing that are the color of granulation tissue.

7. __L__ Wound drainage that is composed of the clear, serous portion of the blood and drainage from serous membranes.

8. __P__ Wounds that are covered with thick eschar, which is usually black but may be brown, gray, or tan.

9. _____ May occur from a slipped suture, a dislodged clot from stress at the suture line, infection, or the erosion of a blood vessel by a foreign body (such as a drain).

10. __K__ Wound drainage that is made up of white blood cells, liquefied dead tissue debris, and both dead and live bacteria.

11. _____ Wounds that are characterized by oozing from the tissue covering the wound, often accompanied by purulent drainage.

12. __h__ Necrotic tissue.

13. _____ A disruption in the normal integrity of the skin.

14. _____ Avascular collagen tissue that does not sweat, grow hair, or tan in sunlight.

15. _____ Wound drainage that consists of large numbers of red blood cells and looks like blood.

Match the wound care dressings and wraps in Part A with their definition/indication listed in Part B. Some answers may be used more than once.

PART A

a. Telfa

b. gauze dressings

c. Soft-Wick

d. ABDs, Surgipads

e. transparent dressings

f. bandages

g. binders

h. roller bandages

PART B

16. __F__ Strips of cloth, gauze, or elasticized material used to wrap a body part.

17. __A__ A special gauze that covers the incision line and allows drainage to pass through and be absorbed by the center absorbent layer.

18. __g__ Wraps that are designed for a specific body part.

19. __A__ Prevents outer dressings from adhering to the wound and causing further injury when removed.

20. __B__ Commonly used to cover wounds; they come in various sizes and are commercially packaged as single units or in packs.

21. __D__ Placed over the smaller gauzes to absorb drainage and protect the wound from contamination or injury.

22. __C__ Precut halfway to fit around drains or tubes.

23. __E__ Applied directly over a small wound or tube; these dressings are occlusive, decreasing the possibility of contamination while allowing visualization of the wound.

24. __g__ They may be made of cloth (flannel or muslin) or an elasticized material that fastens together with Velcro.

25. __E__ The type of dressing often used over intravenous sites, subclavian catheter insertion sites, and healing wounds.

Match the type of moisture-retentive dressings, listed in Part A, with their intended purpose, listed in Part B. Describe the type of wound care for which each dressing is used on the line provided.

PART A

a. transparent films

b. absorptive fillers

c. alginates

d. hydrocolloids

e. hydrogels

f. synthetic barrier dressings

g. VAC therapy

h. retention dressings

PART B

26. ___F___ These are pastes that dry to form transparent, semipermeable dressings. Pores in the dried paste allow drainage to move from the wound to an absorbent dressing.

_____

27. ___A___ These are semipermeable dressings that allow an exchange of oxygen between the wound and environment, protect against contamination, and maintain a moist wound environment.

_____

28. ___C___ These masses of fiber form a moisture-retentive gel on contact with exudate.

_____

29. ___G___ This is the application of negative pressure to pull the cells closer together. It allows the epithelial cells to multiply rapidly and form granulation tissue so healing can begin.

_____

30. ___B___ These dressings absorb drainage and maintain a moist surface by forming a gelatinous mass. They conform to the shape of the wound and can remain in place up to 24 hours.

_____

31. ___D___ These are wafer-shaped dressings that come in many shapes and thicknesses to absorb drainage, maintain a moist wound surface, and decrease the risk of infection.

_____

32. ___E___ These are oxygen-permeable and nonadhesive dressings that maintain moisture. They may consist of powders, pastes, or beads, and may remain in place for 8 to 48 hours.

_____

MULTIPLE CHOICE

Circle the letter that corresponds to the best answer for each question.

1. A patient who is being treated for self-inflicted wounds admits to the nurse that she is anorexic. Which of the following criteria would alert the healthcare worker to her nutritional risk?

    a. an albumin level of 3.5 mg/dL

    b. total lymphocyte count of 1500/mm^3

    c. body weight decrease of 5%

    d. arm muscle circumference 90% of standard

2. A patient with a pressure ulcer on his back should be treated by which of the following methods?

    a. A foam wedge should be used to keep body weight off his back.

    b. A ring cushion should be used to protect reddened areas from additional pressure.

    c. The amount of time the head of the bed is elevated should be increased.

    d. Positioning devices and techniques should be used to maintain posture and distribute weight evenly for patients in a chair.

3. When cleaning a wound, the nurse should adhere to which of the following protocols?

    a. The wound should be cleaned with each dressing change.

    b. Friction should be used with cleaning materials to loosen dead cells.

    c. Povidone-iodine or hydrogen peroxide should be used to fight infection in the wound.

    d. Irrigating devices should not be used on wounds because they damage cells needed for healing.

4. Which of the following recommendations for wound dressing is accurate?

   a. Use wet-to-dry dressings continuously.

   b. Keep the intact, healthy skin surrounding the ulcer moist because it is susceptible to breakdown.

   c. Select a dressing that absorbs exudate, if it is present, but still maintains a moist environment.

   d. Pack wound cavities tightly with dressing material.

5. You are giving a back rub to an older patient at home and notice a stage II pressure ulcer. Which of the following treatments would you suggest for this patient?

   a. Treat the ulcer by using pressure-relieving devices.

   b. Use a wet-to-dry dressing on the wound.

   c. Cover the wound with a nonadherent dressing and change every 8 to 12 hours.

   d. Maintain a moist healing environment, with a saline or occlusive dressing to promote natural healing.

6. Which of the following drains provides sinus tract and would be used after incision and drainage of an abscess, in abdominal surgery?

   a. T-tube

   b. Jackson-Pratt

   c. Penrose

   d. Hemovac

7. A patient's pressure ulcer is superficial and presents clinically as an abrasion, blister, or shallow crater. His ulcer would be categorized as which of the following stages?

   a. stage I

   b. stage II

   c. stage III

   d. stage IV

8. Which of the following is an effect of applying heat to a body part?

   a. constriction of peripheral blood vessels

   b. reduced blood flow to tissues

   c. increased venous congestion

   d. increased supply of oxygen and nutrients to the area

9. Which of the following is a recommended technique for administering an alcohol or cold water sponge bath?

   a. Prepare a water and alcohol solution at about 29.5°C to 32°C.

   b. Keep the patient uncovered to promote evaporation of the water.

   c. Sponge the body for a total of 5 to 10 minutes.

   d. Rub the patient dry after the bath to raise the body temperature gradually.

10. When irrigating a wound, the nurse should follow which of the following guidelines?

    a. For irrigation to clean a wound effectively, the pressure of the irrigation must measure between 2 to 5 pounds per square inch.

    b. Irrigation with a bulb syringe effectively cleans a wound.

    c. Irrigation pressure above 15 psi may cause trauma and force bacteria into the wound.

    d. A Water Pic set at the highest setting effectively and safely cleans a wound.

11. Which of the following patients would be at greatest risk for developing a pressure ulcer?

    a. a newborn infant

    b. a patient with cardiovascular disease

    c. an older patient with arthritis

    d. a critical care patient

12. Which of the following patients would most likely develop a pressure ulcer from shearing forces?

    a. a patient sitting in a chair who slides down

    b. a patient who lifts himself up on his elbows

    c. a patient who lies on wrinkled sheets

    d. a patient who must remain on his back for long periods

13. A large wound with considerable tissue loss allowed to heal naturally by formation of granulation tissue would be classified as which of the following categories of wound healing?

    a. primary intention

    b. secondary intention

    c. tertiary intention

    d. none of the above

14. Which of the following vitamins is needed for collagen synthesis, capillary formation, and resistance to infection?

   a. vitamin A

   b. vitamin B

   c. vitamin C

   d. vitamin K

COMPLETION

1. Describe how the following mechanisms contribute to pressure ulcer development.

   a. External pressure: *Compresses blood vessels and causes friction*

   b. Friction and shearing forces: *Tear and injure blood vessels*

2. Give an example of how the following factors affect predisposition to develop a pressure ulcer.

   a. Nutrition: *Vitamin C deficiency causes capillary to become fragile + poor circulation*

   b. Hydration: *dehydration can interfere E circulation + subsequent cell division*

   c. Moisture on the skin: *increases risk of skin damage*

   d. Mental status: _____

   e. Age: _____

3. When visiting a patient recovering from a stroke in her home, you notice a pressure ulcer developing on her coccyx. Develop a nursing care plan for this patient that involves the family in the treatment of the ulcer.

   _____

   _____

   _____

4. Briefly describe the three phases of wound healing.

   a. Inflammatory phase: _____

   b. Fibroplasia phase: _____

   c. Maturation phase: _____

5. List three goals for patients who are at risk for impaired skin integrity.

   a. _____

   b. _____

   c. _____

6. Give two examples of interview questions that could be asked to assess a patient's skin integrity in the following areas.

   a. Overall appearance of the skin: _____

   b. Recent changes in skin condition: _____

   c. Contributing factors: activity/mobility: _____

   d. Nutrition: _____

e. Pain: _____

_____

_____

f. Elimination: _____

_____

_____

7. Describe how you would assess the following aspects of wound healing.

a. Appearance: _____

_____

_____

b. Wound drainage: _____

_____

_____

c. Pain: _____

_____

_____

d. Sutures and staples: _____

_____

_____

e. Drains and tubes: _____

_____

_____

8. List the purposes for wound dressings.

_____

_____

_____

_____

9. Describe the RYB color classification and care of open wounds.

a. R = red = protect: _____

_____

_____

b. Y = yellow = cleanse: _____

_____

_____

c. B = black = debride: _____

_____

_____

10. Briefly describe the use of the following methods of applying heat and any advantages or disadvantages.

a. Hot water bags or bottles: _____

_____

_____

b. Electric heating pads: _____

_____

c. Aquathermia pads: _____

_____

d. Heat lamps: _____

_____

e. Heat cradles: _____

_____

f. Hot packs: _____

_____

g. Warm moist compresses: _____

_____

h. Sitz baths: _____

_____

i. Warm soaks: _____

_____

_____

GUIDE TO CRITICAL THINKING AND DEVELOPING BLENDED SKILLS

1. Develop a nursing plan to assist the following patients who are at high risk for pressure ulcers:

   a. A comatose 35-year-old man.

   b. A frail elderly man who is confined to bed.

   c. A 20-year-old woman who is in a lower body cast.

   d. A premature baby on life support.

   What knowledge and skills do you need to prevent pressure ulcers in these patients?

2. Follow the wound care for three patients with different types of wounds (for example, a gunshot wound, a wound from surgery, a pressure ulcer). Help the nurse assess the wound each day and apply the dressings. Interview the patients to see how the wound has affected their mobility, sensory perception, activity, nutrition and exposure to friction and shear. Keep a log of the daily changes in the wound.

PATIENT CARE STUDY

Read the following patient care study and use your nursing process skills to answer the questions below.

Mrs. Chijioke, an 88-year-old woman who lived alone for years, was brought to the hospital after neighbors found her lying at the bottom of her cellar steps. She had broken her hip and is now 3 days after hip repair surgery. The nurse assigned to care for Mrs. Chijioke noticed during the patient's bath that the skin of her coccyx, heels, and elbows was reddened. The skin did return to a normal color when pressure was relieved in these areas. There was no edema, nor was there induration or blistering. Although Mrs. Chijioke was able to be lifted out of bed into a chair, she spent most of the day in bed, lying on her back with an abductor pillow between her legs. At 5 feet 0 inches and 89 pounds, Mrs. Chijioke looked lost in the big hospital bed. Her eyes were bright and she usually attempted a warm smile, but she had little physical strength and would lie seemingly motionless for hours. Her skin was wrinkled and paper thin, and her arms were already bruised from unsuccessful attempts at intravenous therapy. Dehydrated on admission, since she had spent almost 48 hours crumpled at the bottom of her steps before being found by her neighbors, Mrs. Chijioke was clearly in need of nutritional, fluid, and electrolyte support. A long-time diabetic, Mrs. Chijioke is now spiking a temperature (39.0°C/102.2°F), which concerns her nurse.

1. Identify pertinent patient data by placing a single underline beneath the objective data in the patient care study and a double underline beneath the subjective data.

2. Complete the Nursing Process Worksheet on the next page to develop a three-part diagnostic statement and related plan of care for this patient.

3. Write down the patient and personal nursing strengths you hope to draw upon as you assist this patient to better health.

   Patient strengths: _____

   _____

   _____

   Personal strengths: _____

   _____

   _____

   _____

   _____

4. Pretend that you are performing a nursing assessment of this patient after the plan of care is implemented. Document your findings below.

   _____

   _____

   _____

   _____

NURSING PROCESS WORKSHEET

Health Problem (Title)	**Expected Outcome**
Related to ↓	
Etiology (Related Factors)	**Nursing Interventions****
As Manifested by ↓	
Signs and Symptoms (Defining Characteristics)	**Evaluative Statement**

*More than one patient goal may be appropriate. For the purposes of this exercise, develop the one patient goal that demonstrates a direct resolution of the patient problem identified in the nursing diagnosis.
**Be sure you are able to list the scientific rationale for each nursing intervention you ordered.

CHAPTER 38

Activity

CHAPTER OVERVIEW

- The fulfillment of most human needs depends, at least partially, on the body's ability to move. Purposeful, coordinated movement of the body requires the integrated functioning of the skeletal, muscular, and nervous systems of the body.

- Bones and joints provide form for the body and serve as the levers and fulcrums that make body movement possible. It is the contraction and relaxation of skeletal muscles, however, that actually produce movement by pulling on bones, and it is nerve impulses that stimulate the muscles to contract.

- Good body mechanics is the efficient use of the body as a machine and as means of locomotion. To role model healthy body mechanics, the nurse pays special attention to body alignment, balance, and coordinated body movement during work and leisure activities.

- Factors that influence body alignment and mobility include developmental considerations, physical health, mental health, lifestyle variables, attitudes and values, fatigue and stress level, and external factors.

- The active exertion of muscles involving the contraction and relaxation of muscle groups is termed exercise. Isotonic exercise involves muscle shortening and active movement, and its potential benefits include increased muscle mass, tone, and strength; improved joint mobility; increased cardiac and respiratory function; increased circulation; and increased osteoblastic activity. Isometric exercise involves contraction without movement, and potential benefits are increased muscle mass, tone, and strength; increased circulation to the exercised body part; and increased osteoblastic activity.

- Individuals who choose to live inactive lifestyles place themselves at high risk for serious health problems. Problems of immobility include increased cardiac workload, thrombus formation, orthostatic hypotension, ineffective breathing patterns, ineffective airway clearance, impaired gas exchange, activity intolerance, pathologic fractures, nutritional alterations, fluid volume excesses, constipation, alteration in urinary elimination, potential for urinary tract infection, impairment of skin integrity, disturbances in self-esteem, powerlessness, impaired social interaction, altered thought processes, ineffective coping, and sleep pattern disturbances.

- People beginning exercise programs should be familiar with the following guidelines: Begin program slowly and allow the body time to adjust to the new stress; know your body and respect its limitations; and follow the safety guidelines for specific exercises.

- When assessing mobility status, interview the patient regarding daily activity level, endurance, exercise and fitness goals, mobility problems, physical or mental problems that affect mobility, and external factors that affect mobility. The physical assessment of mobility status includes an assessment of general ease of movement and gait; alignment; joint structure and function; muscle mass, tone, and strength; and endurance.

- Nursing diagnoses for mobility problems include Activity Intolerance and Impaired Physical Mobility. Both problem statements have multiple etiologies. Because mobility influences so many other areas of human functioning, many nursing diagnoses have as their etiology a problem with mobility.

- The aim of nursing care for both well and ill patients is that the patient follow a program of regular physical exercise that improves cardiovascular function, endurance, flexibility, and strength.

- Nursing strategies that promote mobility for patients on bed rest include careful attention to positioning that maintains correct alignment and facilitates physiologic functioning, safe transfer of patient from bed to chair or stretcher, and the early and safe ambulation of patients. The nurse may also play a key role in teaching patients to use mechanical aids for walking.

- Patients require specialized nursing care if they have the following mobility diagnoses: Activity Intolerance, Impaired Physical Mobility, Risk for Injury related to complications for immobility, and Altered Health Maintenance related to lack of exercise program.

■ Learning Checklist

Review the learning checklist at the end of the chapter in your textbook and be sure you can meet each objective.

■ Exercises

MATCHING

Match the type of joint listed in Part A with the examples listed in Part B.

PART A

a. ball-and-socket joint
b. condyloid joint
c. gliding joint
d. hinge joint
e. pivot joint
f. saddle joint

PART B

1. _____ The joints between the axis and atlas and the proximal ends of the radius and ulna.

2. _____ Carpal bones of the wrist; tarsal bones of the feet.

3. _____ The joint between the trapezium and metacarpal of the thumb.

4. _____ Wrist joint.

5. _____ Shoulder and hip joint.

Match the bed position listed in Part A with its definition or purpose listed in Part B. Answers may be used more than once.

PART A

a. Fowler's position
b. protective supine position
c. protective side-lying or lateral position
d. protective Sims' position
e. protective Prone position
f. oblique position

PART B

6. _____ A semi-sitting position that calls for the head of the bed to be elevated 45 to 60 degrees.

7. _____ Recommended as an alternative to the side-lying position because it places significantly less pressure on the trochanter region.

8. _____ The patient lies on the side, but the lower arm is behind the patient and the upper arm is flexed at both the shoulder and the elbow.

9. _____ The patient lies flat on the back with the head and shoulders slightly elevated with a pillow, unless contraindicated.

10. _____ The patient lies on the side, and the main weight of the body is borne by the lateral aspect of the lower scapula and the lateral aspect of the lower ilium.

11. _____ When patients on bed rest use this position periodically, it helps to prevent flexion contractures of the hips and knees; however, it produces a marked forward curvature of the lumbar spine.

12. _____ This position is often used to promote cardiac and respiratory functioning because abdominal organs drop in this position and provide maximal space in the thoracic cavity.

13. _____ This position is comfortable for sleeping and relieves pressure on the scapulae, sacrum, and heels, and allows the legs and feet to be comfortably flexed.

14. _____ In this position the main body weight is borne by the anterior aspects of the humerus, clavicle, and ilium.

15. _____ The patient lies on the abdomen with the head turned to the side; the body is straightened out in this position because the shoulders, head, and neck are in an erect position with the arms placed in correct alignment with the shoulder girdle.

Match the term used to describe body positions and movements in Part A with its definition listed in Part B.

PART A

a. abduction

b. adduction

c. circumduction

d. flexion

e. extension

f. hyperextension

g. dorsiflexion

h. plantar flexion

i. rotation

j. internal rotation

k. external rotation

l. pronation

m. supination

n. inversion

o. eversion

PART B

16. _____ The assumption of a prone position.

17. _____ Lateral movement of a body part away from the midline of the body.

18. _____ Backward bending of the hand or foot.

19. _____ Movement of the sole or foot outward.

20. _____ The state of being bent.

21. _____ A body part turning on its axis away from the midline of the body.

22. _____ Lateral movement of a body part toward the midline of the body.

23. _____ Movement of the sole of the foot inward.

24. _____ Movement of the distal part of the limb to trace a complete circle while the proximal end of the bone remains fixed.

25. _____ The assumption of a supine position.

26. _____ A body part turning on its axis toward the midline of the body.

27. _____ Flexion of the foot.

28. _____ The state of being in a straight line.

29. _____ The turning point of a body part on the axis provided by its joint.

Match the condition related to muscle mass listed in Part A with its definition listed in Part B.

PART A

a. atrophy

b. hypertrophy

c. muscle tone

d. flaccidity

e. spasticity

f. paresis

g. hemiparesis

h. paraplegia

i. quadriplegia

PART B

30. _____ Increased muscle mass resulting from exercise or training.

31. _____ Increased tone that interferes with movement.

32. _____ Impaired muscle strength or weakness.

33. _____ Muscle mass that is decreased through disuse or neurologic impairment.

34. _____ Paralysis of the arms and legs.

35. _____ The slight residual tension that remains in a resting normal muscle with an intact nerve supply.

36. _____ Decreased tone that results from disuse or neurologic impairment.

37. _____ Weakness of one half of the body.

CORRECT THE FALSE STATEMENT

Circle the word true or false that follows the statement. If the word false has been circled, change the underlined word/words to make the statement true. Place your answer in the space provided.

1. The bones of the jaw and spinal column would be classified as <u>short bones</u>.

   True   False   _____

2. In a <u>gliding joint</u>, articular surfaces are flat; flexion-extension and abduction-adduction are permitted.

   True   False   _____

3. <u>Ligaments</u> are tough, fibrous bands that bind joints together and connect bones and cartilage.

   True   False   _____

4. It is a <u>nerve impulse</u> that stimulates muscles to contract.

   True   False   _____

5. <u>Body dynamics</u> is the efficient use of the body as a machine and as a means of locomotion.

   True   False   _____

6. <u>Tonus</u> is the term used to describe the state of slight contraction-the usual state of skeletal muscles.

   True   False   _____

7. The <u>narrower</u> a base of support, and the lower the center of gravity, the greater the stability of the object.

   True   False   _____

8. The <u>labyrinthine sense</u> informs the brain of the location of a limb or body part as a result of joint movements stimulating special nerve endings in muscles, tendons, and fascia.

   True   False   _____

9. The <u>cerebral motor cortex</u> integrates semivoluntary movements such as walking, swimming, and laughing.

   True   False   _____

10. Rehabilitative exercises for knee or elbow injuries are examples of <u>isokinetic exercises</u>.

    True   False   _____

11. <u>Atelectasis</u> is an incomplete expansion or collapse of lung tissue.

    True   False   _____

12. <u>Footdrop</u> is a complication of immobility in which the foot is unable to maintain itself in the perpendicular position, heel–toe gait is impossible, and the patient experiences extreme difficulty in walking.

    True   False   _____

13. Should a patient faint or begin to fall while walking, the nurse should stand with feet apart to create a wide base of support and rock the pelvis out on the side <u>opposite</u> the patient.

    True   False   _____

14. When a patient stands between the back legs of a walker, <u>the walker should extend</u> from the floor to the <u>patient's</u> hip joint; the patient's elbows should be flexed about 30 degrees.

    True   False   _____

15. A nurse should <u>lift</u> an object to be moved to reduce the energy needed to overcome the pull of gravity.

    True   False   _____

MULTIPLE CHOICE

Circle the letter that corresponds to the best answer for each question.

1. Joints are classified according to which of the following criteria?
   a. bone type they connect
   b. amount of movement they permit
   c. size of the joint
   d. amount of space between the bones

2. Which of the following terms describes the lateral movement of a body part toward the midline of the body?
   a. adduction
   b. abduction
   c. circumduction
   d. extension

3. An object has greater stability under which of the following conditions?
   a. a wide base of support and high center of gravity
   b. a narrow base of support and high center of gravity
   c. a wide base of support and low center of gravity
   d. a narrow base of support and low center of gravity

4. Which of the following postural reflexes informs the brain of the location of a limb or body part as a result of joint movements stimulating special nerve endings in muscles, tendons, and fascia?

    a. labyrinthine sense

    b. extensor reflexes

    c. optic reflexes

    d. proprioceptor sense

5. The CNS part that integrates semi-voluntary movements, such as walking, swimming, and laughing, is which of the following?

    a. basal ganglia

    b. cerebral motor cortex

    c. cerebellum

    d. pyramidal pathways

6. A patient who is bedridden may experience which of the following conditions?

    a. increase in the movement of secretions in the respiratory tract

    b. increase in circulating fibrinolysin

    c. predisposition to renal calculi

    d. an increased metabolic rate

7. Which of the following parts of the CNS assists the motor cortex and basal ganglia by making body movements smooth and coordinated?

    a. cerebral motor cortex

    b. cerebellum

    c. basal ganglia

    d. pyramidal pathways

8. On assessing an ambulatory patient, you observe that both arms swing freely in alternation with leg swings. You are assessing which of the following?

    a. alignment

    b. joint function

    c. gait

    d. muscle tone

9. Mr. Drennan will be ambulating for the first time since his cardiac surgery. Which of the following should the nurse consider when assisting Mr. Drennan?

    a. Patients who are fearful of walking should be told to look at their feet when walking to assure correct positioning.

    b. Patients who can lift their legs only 1 to 2 inches off the bed do not have sufficient muscle power to permit walking.

    c. Nurses should never assist patients with ambulation without a physical therapist present.

    d. If an ambulating patient a nurse is assisting begins to fall, she should slide the patient down her own body to the floor, carefully protecting the patient's head.

10. The ribs are an example of which of the following types of bones?

    a. long bones

    b. short bones

    c. flat bones

    d. irregular bones

11. Which of the following traumas to the musculoskeletal system is a break in the continuity of the structure of a bone or cartilage?

    a. fracture

    b. sprain

    c. strain

    d. dislocation

12. Swimming, jogging, and bicycling are examples of which of the following types of exercises?

    a. isotonic exercises

    b. isometric exercises

    c. isokinetic exercises

    d. stretching exercises

13. Mr. Bellas is a 40-year-old man in a sedentary job who is beginning an exercise program. Which of the following effects will exercise have on his cardiovascular system?

    a. decreased efficiency of the heart

    b. decreased heart rate and blood pressure

    c. decreased blood flow to all body parts

    d. decreased circulating fibrinolysin

14. The joint between the trapezium and metacarpal of the thumb is an example of which of the following types of joints?

    a. gliding joint

    b. condyloid joint

    c. pivot joint

    d. saddle joint

15. A body that is in correct alignment when standing maintains which of the following positions?

    a. The chest is held upward and backward.

    b. The abdominal muscles are held downward and the buttocks upward.

    c. The knees are slightly bent.

    d. The base of support is on the soles of the feet.

16. In which of the following crutch gaits is weight-bearing permitted on both feet?

    a. 2-point gait

    b. 3-point gait

    c. 4-point gait

    d. swing-to gait

COMPLETION

1. Briefly explain the effects of exercise and immobility on the body systems listed on the chart below. Place your answers in the space provided on the chart.

Body System	Effects of Exercise	Effects of Immobility
Cardiovascular		
Respiratory		
Gastrointestinal		
Urinary		
Musculoskeletal		
Metabolic		
Integumentary		
Psychological well-being		

2. List three functions performed by the muscles through contraction.

   a. _____

   b. _____

   c. _____

3. Describe the following points of attachment of muscle to bone.

   a. Point of origin: _____

   _____

   _____

   b. Point of insertion: _____

   _____

   _____

4. Describe the four steps the nervous system completes to stimulate muscles to contract.

   a. _____

   _____

   _____

   b. _____

   _____

   _____

   c. _____

   _____

   _____

   d. _____

   _____

   _____

5. Briefly describe the following concepts of body mechanics.

   a. Body alignment or posture: _____

   _____

   _____

   b. Balance: _____

   _____

   _____

   c. Coordinated body movement: _____

   _____

   _____

6. List four guidelines for the use of body mechanics when a person is at work.

   a. _____

   _____

   _____

   b. _____

   _____

   _____

   c. _____

   _____

   _____

   d. _____

   _____

   _____

7. Briefly describe how the following types of exercise provide health benefits to patients, and give an example of each.

   a. Aerobic exercises: _____

   _____

   _____

   b. Stretching exercises: _____

   _____

   _____

   c. Strength and endurance exercises: ____

   _____

   _____

   d. Activities of daily living: _____

   _____

   _____

8. List four psychologic benefits of regular exercise.

   a. _____

   b. _____

   c. _____

   d. _____

9. Briefly describe how the following devices are used to promote correct alignment or alleviate discomfort on body parts.

   a. Pillows: _____

   _____

   _____

   b. Mattresses: _____

   _____

   _____

   c. Adjustable bed: _____

   _____

   _____

   d. Bed side rails: _____

   _____

   _____

   e. Trapeze bar: _____

   _____

   f. Cradle: _____

   _____

   g. Sandbags: _____

   _____

   h. Trochanter rolls: _____

   _____

   i. Hand-wrist splints or rolls: _____

   _____

   _____

10. Describe how you would teach a patient the following exercises.

    a. Quadriceps drills: _____

    _____

    _____

    b. Push-ups: _____

    _____

    _____

c. Dangling: _____

_____

_____

11. Mrs. Mulherin is a 60-year-old female patient admitted to a healthcare facility for degenerative joint disease. Explain how you would assess, diagnose, and plan an exercise program for this patient.

    a. Physical assessment: _____

    _____

    _____

    b. Diagnosis: _____

    _____

    _____

    c. Exercise program: _____

    _____

    _____

12. Give two examples of normal and abnormal findings when assessing mobility status for a patient in the following areas:

    a. General ease of movement:

    Normal: _____

    Abnormal: _____

    b. Gait and posture:

    Normal: _____

    Abnormal: _____

    c. Alignment:

    Normal: _____

    Abnormal: _____

    d. Joint structure and function:

    Normal: _____

    Abnormal: _____

    e. Muscle mass, tone, and strength:

    Normal: _____

    Abnormal: _____

    f. Endurance:

    Normal: _____

    Abnormal: _____

GUIDE TO CRITICAL THINKING AND DEVELOPING BLENDED SKILLS

1. Visit a center for rehabilitative medicine and observe how the physical therapists assist patients to become mobile. Interview several patients to find out how the lack of mobility has affected their lives. See if you can help with some of the exercise routines, and try out some of the exercises yourself. Develop a nursing care plan to incorporate what you learned about mobility and exercise into your own patient care routine.

2. Using a partner, practice putting each other into the following positions: Fowler's, supine, prone, lateral side-lying, and Sims'. What did this teach you about the experience of being positioned that will be helpful in your practice? Assess each position for health risks that may arise from the following factors: comfort level, body alignment, and pressure points. Write down the advantages and disadvantages of each position.

3. Try maneuvering on a busy street on crutches or in a wheelchair. How does impaired mobility affect your ability to perform everyday chores? How did the public react to your impaired mobility? What effects might a permanent disability have on patients, and how can you best promote their coping?

PATIENT CARE STUDY

Read the following patient care study and use your nursing process skills to answer the questions below.

Robert Witherspoon, a 42-year-old university professor, presented for his first "physical" shortly after his father's death. His father died of complications of coronary artery disease. Mr. Witherspoon is 5 feet, 9 inches, weighs 235 pounds, has a decided "paunch," and reports that until now he has made no time for exercise because he preferred to use his free time reading or listening to classical music. He enjoys French cuisine, including rich desserts, and has a cholesterol level of 310 mg/dL (normal is 150 to 250 mg/dL). He admits being frightened by his father's death, and is appropriately concerned about his elevated cholesterol level. "I guess I've never given much thought to my health before, but my dad's death changed all that. I know coronary artery disease runs in families and I can tell you that I'm not ready to pack it all in yet. Tell me what I have to do to fight this thing." He admits that he used to tease a colleague—who lowered his own cholesterol from 290 to 200 mg/dL by diet and exercise alone—by accusing him of being a fitness freak. "Now I'm recognizing the wisdom of his health behaviors and wondering if diet and exercise won't do the trick for me. Can you help me design an exercise program that will work?"

1. Identify pertinent patient data by placing a single underline beneath the objective data in the patient care study and a double underline beneath the subjective data.

2. Complete the Nursing Process Worksheet on the opposite page to develop a three-part diagnostic statement and related plan of care for this patient.

3. Write down the patient and personal nursing strengths you hope to draw on as you assist this patient to better health.

Patient strengths: _____

_____

Personal strengths: _____

_____

4. Pretend that you are performing a nursing assessment of this patient after the plan of care has been implemented. Document your findings below.

_____

_____

_____

NURSING PROCESS WORKSHEET

Health Problem (Title)

Expected Outcome

Related to

↓

Etiology (Related Factors)

Nursing Interventions**

As Manifested by

↓

**Signs and Symptoms
(Defining Characteristics)**

Evaluative Statement

*More than one patient goal may be appropriate. For the purposes of this exercise, develop the one patient
goal that demonstrates a direct resolution of the patient problem identified in the nursing diagnosis.
**Be sure you are able to list the scientific rationale for each nursing intervention you ordered.

CHAPTER 39

Rest and Sleep

CHAPTER OVERVIEW

- Most people spend about one third of their lives asleep; sleep of some quality and duration is an essential component of well-being.

- Sleep is a state of altered consciousness throughout which varying degrees of stimuli produce wakefulness. It is an active and complex rhythmic state, a progression of repeated cycles.

- The cyclic nature of sleep is controlled by the reticular activating system and bulbar synchronizing region in the brain stem. Biochemical changes and hormones also influence the sleep process.

- Circadian synchronization occurs when an individual's sleep–wake patterns follow the inner biologic clock. Shift work, traveling across time zones, and irregular sleep–wake patterns can easily lead to desynchronization, poor quality sleep, and decreased work performance.

- There is both NREM sleep and REM sleep. During a sleep cycle, a person passes through the four stages of NREM sleep and through REM sleep. The average person has four or five complete sleep cycles each night.

- Factors affecting sleep include age, physical activity, psychologic stress, motivation, diet, alcohol intake, caffeine intake, nicotine use, environment, lifestyle, illness, and medications. Most people with sleep disturbances can initiate lifestyle changes that will improve sleep.

- Nurses should explore parents' perceptions about the amount of sleep their infant or child needs and the schedule the parent uses for sleep and rest times. Development variations and the need for consistent sleep–wake patterns and bedtime rituals may need to be taught.

- For the young adult, the sleep–wakefulness cycle is the most important of all the rhythmic patterns and the one most likely to be abused. Multiple stressors can interfere with the young adult obtaining sufficient rest and sleep and can encourage the use of alcohol or sleep medications. Teaching needs to include the importance of developing good sleep habits to promote long-term wellness.

- The nurse who wishes to be an effective role model in promoting rest and sleep uses appearance and energy level to communicate to patients the value of proper rest and sleep self-care behaviors.

- A comprehensive sleep history includes data on sleep–wakefulness pattern, the effect of the sleep pattern on everyday functioning, sleep aids, sleep disturbance, and contributing factors.

- When a sleep disturbance exists, the assessment attempts to identify the nature of the problem, its cause, related signs and symptoms, onset and frequency, effect on everyday living, severity, whether the problem can be treated independently by nursing, and the coping means the patient has used and their success. A sleep diary and information from a bed partner may be needed to establish a diagnosis.

- Common sleep problems include insomnia, narcolepsy, sleep apnea, parasomnias (sleep walking, sleep talking, enuresis), and sleep deprivation.

- Nursing diagnoses may be written to address sleep pattern disturbances specifically (insomnia: difficulty falling asleep, difficulty remaining asleep, or premature awakening); or to identify the effect sleep pattern disturbances have on other areas of human functioning (anxiety, comfort, coping, alteration in thought process).

- Nursing interventions to promote rest and sleep include establishing a trusting relationship, preparing a restful sleep environment, attending to bedtime rituals, offering appropriate bedtime snacks, promoting relaxation and comfort, respecting normal sleep–wake patterns, scheduling nursing care to avoid disturbances, using medications to promote sleep, and teaching the patient about rest and sleep.

■ Learning Checklist

Review the learning checklist at the end of the chapter in your textbook and be sure you can meet each objective.

■ Exercises

MATCHING

Match the sleep disorder listed in Part A with its appropriate definition listed in Part B.

PART A

a. insomnia

b. hypersomnia

c. narcolepsy

d. sleep apnea

e. parasomnia

f. somnambulism

g. enuresis

h. bruxism

i. sleep deprivation

j. nocturnal myoclonus

PART B

1. _____ Bedwetting during sleep.

2. _____ Difficulty in falling asleep, intermittent sleep, or early awakening from sleep.

3. _____ A condition characterized by an uncontrollable desire to sleep.

4. _____ Grinding teeth during sleep.

5. _____ A condition characterized by excessive sleep, particularly during the day.

6. _____ Periods of no breathing between snoring intervals.

7. _____ Sleepwalking.

8. _____ Decrease in the amount, consistency, and quality of sleep.

9. _____ Marked muscle contraction that results in the jerking of one or both legs during sleep.

Match the stage of NREM sleep listed in Part A with the characteristics of that stage, listed in Part B. Some answers may be used more than once.

PART A

a. stage I

b. stage II

c. stage III

d. stage IV

PART B

10. _____ The depth of sleep increases and arousal becomes increasingly difficult.

11. _____ It is a transitional stage between wakefulness and sleep.

12. _____ Involuntary muscle jerking may occur and waken the person.

13. _____ The person reaches the greatest depth of sleep, called delta sleep.

14. _____ The person falls into a deep sleep from which he/she cannot be aroused with ease.

15. _____ Constitutes about 10% of sleep.

16. _____ Constitutes 50% to 55% of sleep.

17. _____ Metabolism slows and the body temperature is low.

18. _____ Constitutes about 5% of sleep.

CORRECT THE FALSE STATEMENT

Circle the word true or false that follows the statement. If the word false has been circled, change the underlined word/words to make the statement true. Place your answer in the space provided.

1. During sleep, stimuli from the cortex are <u>minimal</u>.

   True   False   _____

2. <u>Sleep stages III and IV</u> are deep-sleep states termed delta sleep, or slow-wave sleep.

   True   False   _____

3. If a person is awakened from sleep at any time, he/she will return to sleep again by starting <u>at the point in the cycle where he/she was when disturbed</u>.

   True   False   _____

4. Most people go through <u>8 to 10</u> cycles of sleep each night.

   True   False   _____

5. On the average, infants sleep from <u>10 to 14</u> hours each day.

   True   False   _____

6. During times of stress REM sleep <u>decreases</u> in amount, which tends to add to anxiety and stress.

   True   False   _____

7. A <u>small protein snack</u> before bedtime is recommended for patients with insomnia.

   True   False   _____

8. Exercise that occurs within a 2-hour interval before normal bedtime <u>stimulates</u> sleep.

   True   False   _____

9. The administration of a <u>larger mid-afternoon dose</u> of asthma medication may more effectively prevent attacks that commonly occur at night during sleep.

   True   False   _____

10. <u>Parasomnias</u> are patterns of waking behavior that appear during sleep.

    True   False   _____

11. <u>Narcolepsy</u> refers to periods of no breathing between snoring intervals.

    True   False   _____

MULTIPLE CHOICE

Circle the letter that corresponds to the best answer for each question.

1. You notice that a patient admitted to your unit sleeps for an abnormally long time. This patient may have suffered damage to which of the following areas of the brain?

   a. cerebral cortex

   b. hypothalamus

   c. medulla

   d. midbrain

2. Wakefulness occurs when which of the following is activated with stimuli from the cerebral cortex and peripheral sensory organs?

   a. reticular activating system

   b. bulbar synchronizing region

   c. circadian rhythm

   d. medulla

3. Which of the following is a characteristic of REM sleep?

   a. Small muscles are immobile, as in paralysis.

   b. Pulse is slow and regular.

   c. Body temperature decreases.

   d. Eyes dart back and forth quickly.

4. When an individual's sleep–wake patterns follow the inner biologic clock, which of the following conditions exist?

   a. circadian rhythm

   b. circadian synchronization

   c. bulbar synchronization

   d. sleep cycle

5. Which of the following instruments receives and records electrical currents from the brain?

   a. electroencephalograph

   b. electrooculogram

   c. electromyograph

   d. electrocardiogram

6. The arousal threshold is usually greatest in which of the following stages of NREM sleep?

   a. stage I

   b. stage II

   c. stage III

   d. stage IV

7. In normal adults, the REM state consumes what percentage of nightly sleep?

   a. 5% to 10%

   b. 10% to 20%

   c. 20% to 25%

   d. 25% to 35%

8. On which of the following patients should a sleep history be obtained?

   a. Only patients who have been suffering from a sleep disorder.

   b. Patients who suffer from a sleep disorder or have been unconscious.

   c. Patients who suffer from a sleep disorder or who are spending time in CCU.

   d. All patients admitted to a healthcare agency.

9. A patient who has been diagnosed with hypothyroidism is admitted to a nursing home. On performing a sleep history on this patient, you find out that the patient is suffering from fatigue, lethargy, depression, and difficulty executing the tasks of everyday living. This patient is probably experiencing which of the following types of sleep deprivation?

   a. REM deprivation

   b. NREM deprivation

   c. total sleep deprivation

   d. Insomnia

10. Most authorities agree that an individual's sleep–wake cycle is fully developed by what age?

    a. 9 months to 1 year

    b. 1 year to 18 months

    c. 2 to 3 years

    d. 4 to 6 years

11. Which of the following interventions would be recommended for a patient with insomnia?

    a. Nap frequently during the day to make up for the lost sleep of night.

    b. Eliminate caffeine and alcohol in the evening because both are associated with disturbances in the normal sleep cycle.

    c. Exercise vigorously before bedtime to promote drowsiness.

    d. Avoid food high in carbohydrates before bedtime.

12. Mrs. Leister, a new admit to the medical–surgical unit, complains of difficulty sleeping. She is scheduled for an exploratory laparotomy in the morning. Your diagnosis is Sleep Pattern Disturbance: Insomnia related to fear of impending surgery. Which one of the following steps is the most appropriate in planning care designed for this diagnosis?

    a. Help her maintain her normal bedtime routine and time for sleep.

    b. Provide opportunity for her to talk about her concerns.

    c. Use tactile relaxation techniques, such as a back massage.

    d. Bring her a warm glass of milk at bedtime.

COMPLETION

1. List three benefits of sleep.

   a. _____

   b. _____

   c. _____

2. List the average amount of sleep required for the following age groups.

   a. Infants: _____

   b. Growing children: _____

   c. Adults: _____

   d. Older adults: _____

3. Briefly describe how the following factors influence sleep.

   a. Physical activity: _____

   _____

   _____

   b. Psychologic stress: _____

   _____

   _____

   c. Motivation: _____

   _____

   _____

   d. Culture: _____

   _____

   _____

e. Diet: _____

_____

_____

f. Alcohol and caffeine: _____

_____

_____

g. Smoking: _____

_____

_____

h. Environmental factors: _____

_____

_____

i. Lifestyle: _____

_____

_____

j. Exercise: _____

_____

_____

k. Illness: _____

_____

_____

l. Medications: _____

_____

_____

4. List the information that should be determined in a sleep history when a sleep disturbance is noted:

_____

_____

_____

5. Describe four physical findings that either confirm that a patient is getting sufficient rest to provide energy for the day's activities, or validate the existence of a sleep disturbance that is decreasing the quantity or quality of sleep.

a. _____

b. _____

c. _____

d. _____

6. Describe how you would prepare a restful environment for a home healthcare patient who is experiencing a sleep disorder: _____

_____

_____

_____

7. Write a sample nursing diagnosis for the following sleep problems:

a. Mr. Smith is admitted to the hospital for surgery. He normally has no problem falling asleep, but the noise of the hospital and need for periodic treatments keep him awake at night:

_____

b. Mr. Loper, a 74-year-old patient in a long-term healthcare facility, is bored during the day and admits taking a nap in the afternoon and early evening. He is not able to sleep at night:

_____

c. Dr. Harris, a resident working varying shifts in the emergency room, complains that he is sleepy all the time, but cannot sleep when he lies down after work: _____

_____

d. Mrs. Maher, age 28, consumes four alcoholic drinks when watching television at night before bedtime. After eliminating the alcohol from her diet, she complains of waking after a short period and not being able to fall back to sleep:

_____

e. Mrs. Eichorn, age 45, has two teenage sons who are often out late at night. She is unable to sleep until they are both home safely, and even then continues to worry about their future:

_____

8. Describe how each of the following is affected by REM sleep.

a. Eyes: _____

b. Muscles: _____

c. Respirations: _____

d. Pulse: _____

e. Blood pressure: _____

f. Gastric secretions: _____

g. Metabolism: _____

h. Sleep–wake cycle: _____

9. List three measures a nurse can take to help alleviate a patient's sleep problem.

   a. _____

   b. _____

   c. _____

10. Give an example of a question you would ask a patient to assess for the following sleep factors.

    a. Usual sleeping and waking times: _____

    _____

    _____

    b. Number of hours of undisturbed sleep: _____

    _____

    _____

    c. Quality of sleep: _____

    _____

    _____

    d. Number and duration of naps: _____

    _____

    _____

    e. Energy level: _____

    _____

    _____

    f. Means of relaxing before bedtime: _____

    _____

    _____

    g. Bedtime rituals: _____

    _____

    _____

    h. Sleep environment: _____

    _____

    _____

    i. Pharmacologic aids: _____

    _____

    _____

    j. Nature of a sleep disturbance: _____

    _____

    _____

    k. Onset of a disturbance: _____

    _____

    _____

    l. Causes of a disturbance: _____

    _____

    _____

    m. Severity of a disturbance: _____

    _____

    _____

    n. Symptoms of a disturbance: _____

    _____

    _____

    o. Interventions attempted and results: _____

    _____

    _____

GUIDE TO CRITICAL THINKING AND DEVELOPING BLENDED SKILLS

1. Visit a busy hospital unit at night. Assess the factors on the ward that would contribute to a patient's sleep deficit. What could be done to change the hospital environment to promote healthy sleeping patterns in the occupants?

2. Develop a sleep teaching tool that explains the typical sleep patterns and requirements for patients of all ages: infancy to older adult. Be sure to include common factors that disrupt sleep patterns, total amount of sleep required, and possible interventions to minimize sleep pattern disturbances. Interview individuals who have tried your interventions and evaluate the likelihood that your teaching tool will successfully resolve sleep problems.

3. Interview several friends or relatives to find out what they do to prepare for a restful night's sleep. Do they have any bedtime routines that are different from yours? What are some methods they use when they are unable to fall asleep? Discuss the effect of lack of sleep on their work performance the following day.

PATIENT CARE STUDY

Read the following patient care study and use your nursing process skills to answer the questions below.

Gina Cioffi, a 23-year-old graduate nurse, has been in her new position as a critical care staff nurse in a large tertiary care medical center for 3 months. "I was so excited about working three 12-hour shifts a week when I started this job, thinking I'd have lots of time for other things I want to do, but I'm not so sure anymore. I've been doing extra shifts when we're shortstaffed because the money is so good, and right now it seems I'm always tired and all I think about all day long is how soon I can get back to bed. Worst of all, when I do finally get into bed, I often can't fall asleep, especially if things have been busy at work and someone 'went bad.' Does everyone else feel like me?" Looking at Gina, you notice dark circles under her eyes and are suddenly struck by the change in her appearance from when she first started working. At that time, she "bounced into work" looking fresh each morning, and her features were always animated. Now her skin color is pale, her hair and clothes look rumpled, and the "brightness" that was so characteristic of her earlier is strikingly absent. With some gentle questioning, you discover that she frequently goes out with new friends she has made at the hospital when her shift is over, and sometimes goes for 48 hours without sleep. "I know I've gotten myself into a rut. How do I get out of it? I used to think my sleep habits were bad at school, but this is a hundred times worse, because there never seems to be time to crash. I have to just keep on going."

1. Identify pertinent patient data by placing a single underline beneath the objective data in the case study and a double underline beneath the subjective data.

2. Complete the Nursing Process Worksheet on the next page to develop a three-part diagnostic statement and related plan of care for this patient.

3. Write down the patient and personal nursing strengths you hope to draw on as you assist this patient to better health.

   Patient strengths: _____

   _____

   _____

   Personal strengths: _____

   _____

   _____

NURSING PROCESS WORKSHEET

Health Problem (Title)

Expected Outcome

Related to

↓

Etiology (Related Factors)

Nursing Interventions**

As Manifested by

↓

**Signs and Symptoms
(Defining Characteristics)**

Evaluative Statement

*More than one patient goal may be appropriate. For the purposes of this exercise, develop the one patient
goal that demonstrates a direct resolution of the patient problem identified in the nursing diagnosis.

**Be sure you are able to list the scientific rationale for each nursing intervention you ordered.

CHAPTER 40

Comfort

CHAPTER OVERVIEW

- Pain is a universal human experience, yet no two individuals experience and respond to pain exactly the same way. The most important services nurses offer a patient experiencing pain are belief that the patient's pain is real, willingness to become involved in the patient's pain experience, and competence in developing effective pain management regimens.

- Pain may originate from physical (cutaneous, somatic, or visceral) causes or mental or emotional (psychogenic) causes. Most often pain is a blend of both. There is no direct and constant relation between a stimulus for pain and its perception. Little is understood about what causes individuals to perceive pain differently.

- The transmission of pain stimuli is a complex process involving the release of potent chemicals that sensitize the nerve endings, help transmit the pain message, and set the stage for healing; transmission of the pain signal as an electrochemical impulse along the length of the nerve to the dorsal horn of the spinal cord; and relay of the pain signal to the thalamus and eventually to the cortex.

- The gate control theory of pain transmission postulates that only a limited amount of sensory information can be processed by the nervous system at any given moment. The effectiveness of many nursing measures to relieve pain (cutaneous stimulation, imagery) may result from their overstimulation of nerve fibers and the "closing of the gate" to pain stimuli.

- Pain is a mixed sensation and occurs in varying degrees. Pain characteristics include duration, severity, quality, and periodicity. Pain responses may be physiologic, behavioral, or affective.

- Many factors influence the pain experience. Among these are culture, religion, environment, support people, anxiety and other stressors, and past experience with pain.

- Numerous misconceptions about pain by both patients and healthcare professionals interfere with the patient's communication of pain and relief needs and with pain assessment and management.

- It is helpful for nurses to assume that all patients are experiencing some degree of discomfort or pain and to initiate a pain assessment rather than waiting for the patient to indicate experiencing pain.

- Pain flow sheets clearly demonstrate the effectiveness of treatment modalities and the development of undesirable side effects.

- Multiple nursing diagnoses may be written that specifically address pain problems or identify the effect of pain problems on other areas of human functioning. Nursing diagnoses developed for pain problems should identify type of pain; etiologic factors; patient responses; and other factors affecting pain stimulus and transmission, perception, and response.

- Expected patient outcomes regarding pain are directed toward the reduction and elimination of discomfort and pain and, whenever possible, to the patient's management of a pain-relief program that allows the patient to resume his or her normal lifestyle pattern.

- Nurses are often reluctant to become involved in pain management because of a natural tendency to avoid pain and because pain in the past has evoked in them feelings of fear, frustration, inadequacy, uselessness, and incompetence.

- The unique relationship that can be developed between a patient, the family, and the nurse makes the nurse a critical member of the pain management team. Nursing skills are ideal for developing in the patient and family the needed self-care behavior to direct an effective pain management program.

- Nursing interventions for pain relief include education, empowerment, manipulating factors that affect the pain experience, initiation of nonpharmacologic treatment modalities (distraction, relaxation, cutaneous stimulation), safe and effective administration of analgesics, and participation in alternate methods of administering analgesics.

- Cancer pain requires specialized nursing skills. The chief objective with severe cancer pain is to prevent rather than treat the pain and this most often involves regular doses of opioid analgesics. Until the patient with cancer pain trusts that the pain can be effectively managed, he or she has little psychic energy for other life activities. The nurse's vigilant control of newly developing symptoms can contribute greatly to the patient's comfort.

• Evaluation of the plan of care necessitates the nurse's ongoing attention to the patient's pain experience and the continual modification of pain therapies as needed. Integral to evaluation is feedback from the patient and family regarding their feelings about themselves and their current ability to deal with pain.

■ Learning Checklist

Review the learning checklist at the end of the chapter in your textbook and be sure you can meet each objective.

■ Exercises

MATCHING

Match the type of pain listed in Part A with its definition listed in Part B.

PART A

a. nociceptive pain

b. cutaneous pain

c. somatic pain

d. visceral pain

e. neuropathic pain

f. allodynia pain

g. psychogenic pain

h. referred pain

i. acute pain

j. chronic pain

k. intractable pain

PART B

1. _____ Pain that results from an injury to or abnormal functioning of peripheral nerves or the central nervous system.

2. _____ Pain that is resistant to therapy and persists despite a variety of interventions.

3. _____ Pain that occurs following a normally weak or nonpainful stimuli, such as a light touch or a cold drink.

4. _____ Pain that may be limited, intermittent, or persistent, but that lasts for 6 months or longer and interferes with normal functioning.

5. _____ Pain that is usually acute and transmitted following normal processing of noxious stimuli.

6. _____ Pain that is diffuse or scattered and originates in tendons, ligaments, bones, blood vessels, and nerves.

7. _____ Pain for which a physical cause cannot be found.

8. _____ Superficial pain that usually involves the skin or subcutaneous tissue.

9. _____ Pain that is poorly localized and originates in body organs, the thorax, cranium, and abdomen.

10. _____ Pain that is perceived in an area that is distant from its point of origin.

Match the pain syndrome in Part A with its origin listed in Part B.

PART A

a. causalgia

b. postherpetic neuralgia

c. phantom limb pain

d. thalamic syndrome

e. trigeminal neuralgia

f. arthritis

g. diabetic neuropathy

PART B

11. _____ Syndrome characterized by severe, spontaneous, and often continuous pain, often accompanied by a myriad of symptoms that may result from damage caused by a cerebrovascular accident or brain attack.

12. _____ Pain occurs in the area of a partially injured peripheral nerve and occurs most commonly on the palms of the hands, soles of the feet, and in the digits.

13. _____ Metabolic and vascular changes result in damage to peripheral and autonomic nerves. Symptoms include sensations of numbness, prickling, or tingling.

14. _____ Pain syndrome that follows an acute central nervous system infection such as shingles.

15. _____ May occur in a person who has had a body part amputated either surgically or traumatically.

16. _____ Paroxysms of lightening-like stabs of intense pain in the distribution of one or more divisions of the trigeminal nerve, the fifth cranial nerve.

Match the examples in Part B with the type of pain listed in Part A. Answers may be used more than once.

PART A

a. cutaneous pain

b. deep somatic pain

c. visceral pain

d. referred pain

PART B

17. _____ Pain associated with cancer of the uterus.

18. _____ Pain associated with a myocardial infarction.

19. _____ Pain associated with a knee injury.

20. _____ Pain associated with burns.

21. _____ Pain associated with a brain tumor.

22. _____ Pain associated with a gash in the skin.

23. _____ Pain associated with a broken leg.

24. _____ Pain associated with ulcers.

Match the term for nonpharmacologic pain relief listed in Part A with its definition listed in Part B.

PART A

a. imagery

b. relaxation techniques

c. TENS

d. cutaneous stimulation

e. placebo

f. hypnosis

g. acupuncture

h. biofeedback

i. acupressure

j. therapeutic touch

k. distraction

PART B

25. _____ Involves using one's hands to consciously direct an energy exchange from the practitioner to the patient.

26. _____ Involves four elements: assuming a comfortable position with the body in good alignment, being in quiet surroundings, repeating certain words, and adopting a passive attitude when distracting thoughts enter the individual's consciousness.

27. _____ Involves stimulating the skin's surface to relieve pain; can be explained by the gate control theory.

28. _____ Requires the patient to focus attention on something other than the pain.

29. _____ An example of mind–body interaction being used to decrease pain sensation that involves one or all of the senses, and focus on a mental picture.

30. _____ Involves the application of pressure or massage or both to usual acupuncture sites.

31. _____ A noninvasive alternative technique that involves electrical stimulation of large diameter fibers to inhibit transmission of painful impulses carried over small diameter fibers.

32. _____ A technique that produces a subconscious condition by means of suggestion.

33. _____ A technique that uses a teaching machine with a signal to help the patient learn by trial and error to control the supposedly involuntary body mechanisms that may cause pain.

34. _____ A technique that uses needles of various lengths to prick specific parts of the body to produce insensitivity to pain.

MULTIPLE CHOICE

Circle the letter that corresponds to the best answer for each question.

1. Pain that is poorly localized and originates in body organs is known as which of the following?

   a. cutaneous pain

   b. somatic pain

   c. visceral pain

   d. perceived pain

2. You are visiting a patient at home who is recovering from a bowel resection. She complains of constant pain and discomfort, and displays symptoms of depression. When assessing this patient for pain, you should be aware of which of the following facts about pain?

    a. As her primary healthcare giver, you are the authority about the existence and nature of your patient's pain sensation.

    b. The pain your patient is experiencing is probably an emotional or psychologic problem due to depression.

    c. A placebo should be administered to the patient to see if the pain is manufactured or psychogenic before starting drug therapy.

    d. The patient is the only authority about the existence and nature of her pain, and pain management therapy should be reviewed and revised if necessary.

3. Which of the following is a powerful vasodilator that increases capillary permeability and constricts smooth muscles, playing a role in the chemistry of pain at the injury site?

    a. bradykinin

    b. prostaglandins

    c. substance P

    d. serotonin

4. Pain receptors consisting of free nerve endings that are involved in fast-conducting, acute, well-localized pain include which of the following?

    a. C fibers

    b. gamma fibers

    c. B fibers

    d. A-delta fibers

5. The highest level of integration of sensory impulses of pain occurs in which of the following regions?

    a. cortex

    b. medulla

    c. CNS

    d. spinal cord

6. A patient with a recently amputated limb complains of pain in the amputated part. The nurse should explain to the patient which of the following?

    a. The pain cannot exist because the leg has been amputated.

    b. The pain is a phenomenon known as "ghost pain."

    c. The pain is a real experience for the patient.

    d. The patient is experiencing central pain syndrome.

7. The fact that a person can tolerate a higher temperature as water is gradually heated to the pain level than if the hand had been plunged into hot water without any preparation can be explained by which of the following theories?

    a. threshold of pain theory

    b. adaptation theory

    c. gate control theory

    d. regulation by neuromodulators

8. Which of the following means of pain control can be generally explained on the basis of the gate control theory?

    a. biofeedback

    b. distraction

    c. hypnosis

    d. acupuncture

9. Aspirin, acetaminophen, and ibuprofen are examples of which of the following types of pharmaceutical agents that relieve pain?

    a. NSAIDs

    b. opioids

    c. nonopioid analgesics

    d. adjuvant drugs

10. A patient complains of severe pain following a mastectomy. A good choice for an analgesic for this patient would be which of the following?

    a. acetaminophen

    b. aspirin

    c. morphine

    d. methadone

11. A prn drug regimen is an effective means of administering pain medication in which of the following cases?

    a. A patient experiencing acute pain

    b. A patient in the early postoperative period

    c. A patient experiencing chronic pain

    d. A patient in the postoperative stage with occasional pain

12. Your patient is experiencing acute pain following the amputation of a limb. Which of the following nursing interventions should you keep in mind when treating this patient?

    a. Treat the pain as it occurs to prevent drug addiction.

    b. Encourage the use of non-drug complementary therapies as adjuncts to the medical regime.

    c. Increase and decrease the serum level of the analgesic as needed.

    d. Do not provide analgesia if there is any doubt about the likelihood of pain occurring.

13. Which of the following groups of opioids are produced at neural synapses at various points in the CNS pathway and are powerful pain-blocking chemicals?

    a. dymorphins

    b. endorphins

    c. enkephalins

    d. bradykinins

14. When assessing a patient for pain, the nurse should consider which of the following facts about pain?

    a. Patients frequently complain about pain that is not there to get attention.

    b. People with pain should be taught to have a high tolerance for pain.

    c. All real pain has an identifiable, physical cause.

    d. Having an emotional reaction to pain does not mean the pain is a result of an emotional problem.

15. Three days postsurgery, Mrs. Dodds continues to have moderate to severe incisional pain. According to the gate control theory, the nurse should do which of the following?

    a. Administer pain medications in smaller doses, but more frequently.

    b. Decrease external stimuli in the room during painful episodes.

    c. Reposition Mrs. Dodds and gently massage her back.

    d. Advise Mrs. Dodds that she should try to sleep following administration of pain medication.

16. When treating a child who is in pain and cannot vocalize this pain, which of the following measures should the nurse employ?

    a. Ignore the child's pain if he is not complaining about it.

    b. Ask the child to draw a cartoon about the color or shape of his pain.

    c. Medicate the child with analgesics to reduce the anxiety of experiencing pain.

    d. Distract the child so he does not notice his pain.

17. After sedating a patient, you assess that he is frequently drowsy and drifts off during conversations. What number on the sedation scale would best describe your patient's sedation level?

    a. 1

    b. 2

    c. 3

    d. 4

COMPLETION

1. Read each of the situations below and use the accompanying chart to describe behavioral, physiologic, and affective responses to pain that you might observe in these patients:

   Situation A: Mrs. Novinger tells you that she frequently gets migraine headaches and feels one coming on.

   Situation B: Ryan Goode, age 3, reached out to pet a stray cat who hissed and scratched his forearm.

Situation C: Mrs. Carol Chung is 2 days post-cesarean section and using her call light to request something for incisional pain.

Situation D: Joseph Miles, age 79, has a long history of degenerative joint disease and tells you this is a "bad morning" for his joints. He states: "I think the weather must be affecting my arthritis."

Write a three-part diagnosis statement for each of the above patients, using the assessment data in the above chart.

Situation	Behavioral	Physiological	Affective
A			
B			
C			
D			

Situation A: _____

_____

_____

Situation B: _____

_____

_____

Situation C: _____

_____

_____

Situation D: _____

_____

_____

2. Briefly describe the events that occur when the threshold of pain has been reached and there is injured tissue.

_____

_____

_____

_____

3. Explain why referred pain can be transmitted to a cutaneous (skin) site different from its origin.

_____

_____

_____

4. Explain the mechanics of the gate control theory and how it is believed to control pain.

_____

_____

_____

5. Describe the following types of pain and give an example of each from your own experience with patients.

a. Acute pain: _____

_____

_____

b. Chronic pain: _____

_____

_____

c. Intractable pain: _____

_____

_____

6. Give an example of how the following factors may influence a patient's pain experience.

a. Culture: _____

_____

_____

b. Ethnicity: _____

_____

_____

c. Family, gender, or age: _____

_____

_____

d. Religious beliefs: _____

_____

_____

e. Environment and support people: _____

_____

_____

f. Anxiety and other stressors: _____

_____

_____

g. Past pain experiences: _____

_____

_____

7. List two experiences you have had with pain management for patients. Note your response to their pain and the effectiveness of your pain management techniques. Which pain control measures were most effective, and what could you have done differently to provide better pain control?

a. _____

_____

_____

_____

b. _____

_____

_____

8. Describe how you would respond to a patient who tells you the following about their pain experience.

a. "I know you will know when I am in pain and will do something to relieve it."

_____

_____

b. "If I ask for something for pain, I'm afraid I may become addicted."

_____

_____

c. "It's natural to have pain when you get older. It's just something I've learned to live with."

_____

_____

9. Give an example of an interview question you could use to assess a patient for the following characteristics of pain.

a. Duration of the pain: _____

_____

_____

b. Quantity and intensity of the pain: _____

_____

_____

c. Quality of the pain: _____

_____

_____

d. Physiologic indicators of the pain: _____

_____

_____

10. State your opinion of the use of placebos to satisfy a person's demand for a drug. Is lying to the patient ever justifiable? How could this action affect the nurse–patient relationship? What, if anything, would you say to a physician who prescribed a placebo for your patient?

_____

_____

_____

11. How would you modify your means of assessing for pain in the following patients?

a. A patient with a cognitive impairment: _____

_____

_____

b. A 5-year-old patient: _____

_____

_____

c. An elderly patient: _____

_____

_____

GUIDE TO CRITICAL THINKING AND DEVELOPING BLENDED SKILLS

1. Think back to the last time you experienced acute pain (for example, a toothache, headache, backache). If you were in a work environment, were you able to concentrate on anything but the pain? How did the people around you respond to your pain? What measures did you take to relieve the pain, and how successful were they? Interview several patients who are experiencing acute pain. How are they coping psychologically and physically with the pain? What comfort measures work best for them? How has medication helped to control their pain? How can you use this knowledge to improve your care?

2. Find a tool to assess pain. Be sure it includes physical assessment, pain scales, location and duration of the pain, coping measures, pain management, and the effect of pain on daily living. Use this tool to assess the pain of individuals with similar problems (for example, migraine, cramps, arthritis) and look for factors to explain their different experiences.

3. You notice a young woman who is experiencing intense pain. When you ask the nurses about this patient, they tell you she is in end stage cancer and has received all the pain medication she has been prescribed. They could not administer more medication without a doctor's order. How would you react to this patient? What would you do to provide alternative comfort measures? Would you be an advocate for this patient and attempt to have more medication prescribed? How might who you are and your competence in pain management affect this woman's last days?

PATIENT CARE STUDY

Read the following case study and use your nursing process skills to answer the questions below.

Tabitha Wilson is a 24-month-old infant with AIDS who is hospitalized, this admission, with infectious diarrhea. She is well known to the pediatric staff, and there is real concern that she might not pull through this admission. She has suffered many of the complications of AIDS and is no stranger to pain. At the present time, the skin on her buttocks is raw and excoriated, and tears stream down her face whenever she is moved. Her blood pressure also shoots up when she is touched. The severity of her illness has left her extremely weak and listless, and her foster mother reports that she no longer recognizes her child. When alone in her crib, she seldom moves, and moans softly. Several nurses have expressed great frustration caring for Tabitha because they find it hard to perform even simple nursing measures like turning, diapering, and weighing her when they see how much pain these procedures cause.

1. Identify pertinent patient data by placing a single underline beneath the objective data in the case study and a double underline beneath the subjective data.

2. Complete the Nursing Process Worksheet on the opposite page to develop a three-part diagnostic statement and related plan of care for this patient.

3. Write down the patient and personal nursing strengths you hope to draw on as you assist this patient to better health.

    Patient strengths: _____

    _____

    _____

    Personal strengths: _____

    _____

    _____

    _____

4. Pretend that you are performing a nursing assessment of this patient after the plan of care is implemented. Document your findings below.

    _____

    _____

    _____

    _____

NURSING PROCESS WORKSHEET

Health Problem (Title)	Expected Outcome
Related to ↓	
Etiology (Related Factors)	Nursing Interventions**
As Manifested by ↓	
Signs and Symptoms (Defining Characteristics)	Evaluative Statement

*More than one patient goal may be appropriate. For the purposes of this exercise, develop the one patient goal that demonstrates a direct resolution of the patient problem identified in the nursing diagnosis.

**Be sure you are able to list the scientific rationale for each nursing intervention you ordered.

CHAPTER 41

Nutrition

CHAPTER OVERVIEW

- A person's state of energy balance can be determined by comparing caloric intake with caloric expenditure, which is the sum of calories used during physical activity, for basal metabolism, and for specific dynamic action.

- The six classes of nutrients needed by the body are carbohydrates, protein, fats, vitamins, minerals, and water.

- Carbohydrates provide most of the calories in the diet. Glucose, the only carbohydrate present in systemic circulation, may be burned for energy, stored as glycogen, or converted to fat and stored as adipose.

- Protein is broken down by the body into amino acids, which are then recombined to form proteins. Eight or nine amino acids are considered essential because they cannot be made in the body and must be supplied in the diet. Protein is used in the body for tissue growth and repair, and for the production of enzymes, hormones, antibodies, blood and other substances, and secretions; it also may be oxidized for energy. Excess protein is converted to fat and stored as adipose.

- Lipids provide more than twice the calories per unit of either carbohydrates or protein. Essential fatty acids cannot be made by the body, and therefore must be supplied through the diet. Dietary fat not used for immediate energy is stored as adipose.

- Vitamins and minerals do not provide calories but are needed for the metabolism of energy.

- Water provides the medium for all chemical reactions within the body; it is more vital to life than food.

- Tools used to evaluate a diet for adequacy include food groups and RDAs or RNIs. Dietary guidelines issued by health and governmental agencies focus on avoiding excesses rather than on obtaining sufficient quantities of nutrients. Most experts recommend that Americans eat a variety of food; maintain their ideal weight; reduce their intake of fat, saturated fat, cholesterol, salt, and alcohol; and eat more complex carbohydrates and fiber.

- A person's food habits are a product of many variables, such as physical factors (geographic location, food technology, income), physiologic factors (state of health, hunger, stage of development), and psychosocial factors (culture, religion, tradition, education, politics, social status, food ideology).

- Factors that influence nutrient requirements include age, sex, state of health, alcohol abuse, the use of medications, and megadoses of nutrient supplements. Nutrient intake can be affected by numerous physiologic and psychologic factors.

- A systematic approach is used to identify the patient's actual or potential needs, formulate a plan to meet those needs, initiate the plan or assign others to implement it, and evaluate the effectiveness of the plan.

- Nutritional assessment data can be collected through history taking (dietary data and medical–socioeconomic data), physical examination (anthropometric data and clinical data), and laboratory data.

- Nursing diagnoses may be written to address nutritional problems specifically (Altered Nutrition: Less Than Body Requirements, More Than Body Requirements, Risk for More Than Body Requirements) or to identify the effect nutritional problems have on other areas of human functioning (Activity Intolerance, Anxiety, Constipation, Diarrhea).

- Implementing a plan of care may involve nursing actions that are concerned with stimulating appetite, providing special diets, assisting with eating, withholding food, feeding by tube, feeding by vein, and conducting diet instructions.

- A nasogastric or nasointestinal tube is used to provide enteral nutrition for short-term use (less than 6 weeks) while a gastrostomy or jejunostomy tube can be used to supply nutrients via the enteral route for long-term use.

- Total parenteral nutrition (TPN) is a hypertonic, nutrient-rich solution that is administered intravenously through a central vein. Partial or peripheral parenteral nutrition (PPN) is an intravenous supplement for patients who have inadequate intake of oral nutrition and is delivered through a peripheral vein.

■ Learning Checklist

Review the learning checklist at the end of the chapter in your textbook and be sure you can meet each objective.

■ Exercises

MATCHING

Match the nutrient in Part A with the type of function it performs listed in Part B. Answers will be used more than once.

PART A

a. carbohydrates
b. protein
c. fat

PART B

1. _____ Spares protein so it can be used for other functions.
2. __C__ Insulates the body.
3. __D__ Stimulates tissue growth and repair.
4. _____ Prevents ketosis from inefficient fat metabolism.
5. _____ Helps regulate fluid balance through oncotic pressure.
6. __C__ Cushions internal organs.
7. _____ Delays glucose absorption.
8. __C__ Is necessary for absorption of fat-soluble vitamins.
9. _____ Detoxifies harmful substances.
10. _____ Forms antibodies.

Match the vitamins and minerals listed in Part A with the signs/symptoms of their deficiency listed in Part B.

PART A

a. vitamin C
b. vitamin B complex
c. riboflavin
d. niacin
e. B-6
f. folate
g. B-12
h. vitamin A
i. vitamin D
j. vitamin K
k. calcium
l. sodium
m. potassium
n. iron
o. fluoride

PART B

11. _____ Pellagra, dermatitis
12. __a__ Scurvy, hemorrhaging, delayed wound healing
13. _____ Hemorrhagic disease of newborn, delayed blood clotting
14. __m__ Hypokalemia, muscle cramps and weakness, irregular heartbeat
15. _____ Microcytic anemia, pallor, decreased work capacity, fatigue, weakness
16. _____ Beriberi, mental confusion, fatigue
17. __e__ Anemia, CNS problems
18. _____ Pernicious anemia
19. _____ Night blindness, rough skin
20. __l__ Hyponatremia; muscle cramps, cold and clammy skin
21. _____ Tooth decay; risk of osteoporosis
22. __i__ Retarded bone growth, bone malformation
23. __K__ Tetany, osteoporosis
24. _____ Ariboflavinosis, symptoms related to inflammation and poor wound healing

Match the function in Part B with the mineral listed in Part A. List one food source for each mineral on the line provided at the end of the sentence.

PART A

a. calcium

b. phosphorus

c. magnesium

d. sulfur

e. sodium

f. selenium

g. chlorine

h. iron

i. iodine

j. zinc

k. copper

l. manganese

m. fluoride

n. chromium

o. molybdenum

PART B

25. _____ Promotes certain enzyme reactions and detoxification reactions _____.

26. _____ Bone and tooth formation, blood clotting, nerve transmission, muscle contraction _____.

27. _____ Component of HCl in stomach; fluid balance; acid-base balance _____.

28. _____ Component of thyroid hormones _____.

29. _____ Major ion of extracellular fluid; fluid balance; acid-base balance _____.

30. _____ Aids in iron metabolism and activity of enzymes _____.

31. _____ Tooth formation and integrity; bone formation and integrity _____.

32. _____ Antioxidant _____.

33. _____ Oxidizes sulfur and products of sulfur metabolism _____.

34. _____ Bone and tooth formation; acid–base balance; energy metabolism _____.

35. _____ Oxygen transported by way of hemoglobin; constituent of enzyme systems _____.

36. _____ Tissue growth; sexual maturation; immune response _____.

37. _____ Part of enzyme system needed for protein and energy metabolism _____.

38. _____ Cofactor for insulin; proper glucose metabolism _____.

Match the terms listed in Part A with their definition, listed in Part B.

PART A

a. nutrition

b. nutrients

c. macronutrients

d. micronutrients

e. calories

f. basal metabolism

g. RDA

h. cholesterol

i. Food Guide Pyramid

PART B

39. _____ The measurement of energy in the diet.

40. _____ The study of nutrients and how they are handled by the body.

41. _____ The recommendation for average daily amounts that healthy population groups should consume over time.

42. _____ Specific biochemical substances used by the body for growth, development, activity, reproduction, lactation, health maintenance, and recovery from injury or illness.

43. _____ A graphic device designed to represent a total diet and provide a firm foundation for health.

44. _____ Essential nutrients that supply energy and build tissue.

45. _____ The amount of energy required to carry on the involuntary activities of the body at rest.

46. _____ Vitamins and minerals that are required in much smaller amounts to regulate and control body processes.

MULTIPLE CHOICE

Circle the letter that corresponds to the best answer for each question.

1. When assessing the nutritional requirements of an adult, which of the following facts about nutrition should be considered?

    a. Most nutrients work better alone than they do together.

    b. Nutrient needs remain the same throughout the life cycle.

    c. All nutrients are synthesized in the body.

    d. Nonessential nutrients do not have to be supplied though exogenous sources.

2. Which of the following nutrients supplies energy to the body?

    a. proteins

    b. vitamins

    c. minerals

    d. water

3. Of the following factors, which increases BMR?

    a. aging

    b. fever

    c. fasting

    d. sleep

4. What would be the approximate BMI for a 220-pound man who is 6 feet, 3 inches tall?

    a. 26.5

    b. 27.5

    c. 28.5

    d. 29.5

5. According to the U.S. guidelines, which of the following would be the daily caloric requirement for a sedentary male whose IBW is 165?

    a. 2640

    b. 2740

    c. 2800

    d. 2850

6. Approximately what range in grams of carbohydrates is needed daily to prevent ketosis?

    a. 25 to 50 grams

    b. 50 to 100 grams

    c. 100 to 150 grams

    d. 150 to 200 grams

7. Most healthcare experts recommend that protein intake should contribute what percentage of total caloric intake?

    a. 0% to 10%

    b. 10% to 20%

    c. 20% to 30%

    d. 30% to 40%

8. What percentage of an adult's total body weight is water?

    a. 20% to 30%

    b. 30% to 40%

    c. 40% to 50%

    d. 50% to 60%

9. Mrs. Blase is an obese patient who visits a weight control clinic. When considering a weight reduction plan for this patient, the nurse should consider which of the following guidelines?

    a. To lose 1 pound/week, the daily intake should be decreased by 200 calories.

    b. One pound of body fat equals approximately 5000 calories.

    c. Psychologic reasons for overeating should be explored, such as eating as a release for boredom.

    d. Obesity is very treatable, and 50% of obese people who lose weight maintain the weight loss for 7 years.

10. Which of the following is the most abundant and least expensive source of calories in the world?

    a. carbohydrates

    b. fats

    c. proteins

    d. milk

11. Which of the following sugars must be broken down by enzymes in the intestinal tract before they can be absorbed?

    a. glucose

    b. fructose

    c. galactose

    d. lactose

12. Which of the following is the primary function of carbohydrates?
    a. to supply energy
    b. to form antibodies
    c. to maintain body tissues
    d. to provide the blood-clotting factor

13. Which of the following foods provides a complete protein?
    a. vegetables
    b. meats
    c. grains
    d. legumes

14. Which of the following vitamins is water soluble?
    a. vitamin A
    b. vitamin B
    c. vitamin E
    d. vitamin C

15. Men have a higher need than women for which of the following nutrients, due to their larger muscle mass?
    a. carbohydrates
    b. minerals
    c. proteins
    d. vitamins

16. Which of the following procedures is appropriate when aspirating fluid from small-bore feeding tubes?
    a. Use a small syringe and insert 10 mL of air.
    b. If fluid is obtained when aspirating, measure its volume and pH and flush the tube with water.
    c. Continue to instill air until fluid is aspirated.
    d. Place the patient in the Trendelenburg position to facilitate the fluid aspiration process.

17. Checking placement of a gastrostomy or jejunostomy tube requires regular comparisons of which of the following?
    a. tube length
    b. gastric fluid
    c. pH
    d. air pressure

18. If a patient is able to attempt eating regular meals during the day and is prepared to ambulate and resume activities, supplemental feedings should be provided by which of the following methods?
    a. continuous feeding
    b. intermittent feeding
    c. cyclic feeding
    d. ambulatory feeding

19. When performing nursing actions associated with successful tube feedings, the nurse should do which of the following?
    a. Check tube placement by adding food dye to the tube feed as a means of detecting aspirated fluid.
    b. Check residual before each feeding or every 4 to 8 hours during a continuous feeding.
    c. Assess for bowel sounds at least four times per shift to ensure presence of peristalsis and a functional intestinal tract.
    d. Prevent contamination during enteral feedings by using an open system.

20. A nutritional therapy for patients who have nonfunctional gastrointestinal tracts or who are comatose would most likely be accomplished by which of the following?
    a. enteral feeding pump
    b. PEG
    c. nasointestinal tube
    d. TPN

21. Which of the following is the best indicator of a patient who is in need of TPN?
    a. a serum albumin level 2.5 g/dL or less
    b. a residual of more than 100 mL
    c. absence of bowel sounds
    d. presence of dumping syndrome

COMPLETION

1. Briefly explain the body's state of nitrogen balance.

   _____

   _____

   _____

   _____

2. Explain the difference between the following fatty acids and give an example of each. Note which of the two lowers serum cholesterol levels.

   a. Saturated fatty acids: _____

   _____

   _____

   b. Unsaturated fatty acids: _____

   _____

   _____

3. List four conditions that may predispose a person to mild or subclinical deficiencies of vitamin A, vitamin C, folate, and vitamin B-6.

   a. _____

   b. _____

   c. _____

   d. _____

4. Briefly describe the nutritional needs of the following age groups:

   a. Infants: _____

   b. Toddlers and preschoolers: _____

   c. School age: _____

   d. Adolescents: _____

   e. Adults: _____

   f. Pregnant women: _____

   g. Older adults: _____

5. Complete the chart at the bottom of the page that depicts the function and recommended percentage of the diet for the energy nutrients.

6. List four interventions to increase fiber in a patient's diet.

   a. _____

   b. _____

   c. _____

   d. _____

7. Briefly describe the following eating disorders and the typical characteristics of individuals affected by them.

   a. Anorexia nervosa: _____

   _____

   _____

   b. Bulimia: _____

   _____

   _____

8. Give an example of how the following variables may affect a patient's nutritional needs:

   a. Sex: _____

   b. State of health: _____

   c. Alcohol abuse: _____

   d. Medications: _____

   e. Megadoses of nutrient supplements: _____

   f. Religion: _____

   g. Economics: _____

Nutrient	Function	Recommended %
a. carbohydrates		
b. proteins		
c. fats		
d. vitamins		
e. minerals		
f. water		

9. Describe the following methods of collecting dietary data.

   a. Food diaries: _____

   b. Diet history: _____

10. Describe how you would assess a patient you are caring for at home for adequate nourishment:

    _____

    _____

    _____

11. List three teaching strategies a nurse may employ to achieve compliance with diet instructions.

    a. _____

    b. _____

    c. _____

12. Describe the following types of diets, noting their nutritional value, and give an example of the types of food provided in each.

    a. Clear liquid diet: _____

    _____

    _____

    b. Full liquid diet: _____

    _____

    _____

    c. Soft diet: _____

    _____

    _____

13. Briefly describe the following types of enteral feedings, noting their advantages and disadvantages.

    a. Nasogastric feeding tube: _____

    _____

    _____

    b. Nasointestinal feeding tube: _____

    _____

    _____

14. List five areas that need to be evaluated for a patient at home on TPN.

    a. _____

    b. _____

    c. _____

    d. _____

    e. _____

15. Devise a diet plan for a patient who is moderately to morbidly obese: _____

    _____

    _____

    _____

GUIDE TO CRITICAL THINKING AND DEVELOPING BLENDED SKILLS

1. Develop a nutritional assessment for the following patients. What developmental factors influence their nutritional needs?

   a. An 18-month-old healthy infant.

   b. A 5-year-old child who is extremely active.

   c. A 12-year-old child who is 50 pounds overweight.

   d. A teenager who is concerned about body image and borders on being anorexic.

   e. A middle-aged adult with high blood pressure.

   f. A senior citizen who is anemic.

2. Keep a diary of all the foods you eat in a week. Does your diet follow the USDA's dietary guidelines for a healthy diet? Does your diet include the recommended number of servings of foods from the food pyramid? Is your diet high or low in fat? Perform a nutritional nursing assessment of your dietary habits. Develop a plan of care to improve your nutritional intake, if necessary. What personal factors might interfere with your making the necessary changes? How might this self-knowledge influence your nursing care?

PATIENT CARE STUDY

Read the following case study and use your nursing process skills to answer the questions below.

Mr. Church, a 74-year-old white male, is being admitted to the geriatric unit of the hospital for a diagnostic work-up. He was diagnosed as having Alzheimer's disease 4 years ago, and just 1 year ago was admitted to a long-term care facility. His wife of 49 years is extremely devoted, and informed the nurse taking the admission history that she instigated his admission to the hospital because she was alarmed with the amount of weight he was losing. Assessment revealed a 6 feet, 1 inch, emaciated male, who weighed 149 pounds. His wife reported he lost 20 pounds in the last 2 months. The staff at the long-term care facility report that he was eating his meals, and his wife validated that this was the case. No one seemed sure, however, of the caloric content of his diet. His wife nodded her head vigorously when asked if her husband seemed more agitated and hyperactive recently. Mr. Church has dull, sparse hair, pale, dry skin, and dry mucous membranes.

1. Identify pertinent patient data by placing a single underline beneath the objective data in the case study and a double underline beneath the subjective data.

2. Complete the Nursing Process Worksheet on the opposite page to develop a three-part diagnostic statement and related plan of care for this patient.

3. Write down the patient and personal nursing strengths you hope to draw on as you assist this patient to better health.

   Patient strengths: _____

   _____

   _____

   Personal strengths: _____

   _____

   _____

4. Pretend that you are performing a nursing assessment of this patient after the plan of care is implemented. Document your findings below.

   _____

   _____

   _____

   _____

NURSING PROCESS WORKSHEET

Health Problem (Title)	Expected Outcome
Related to ↓	
Etiology (Related Factors)	**Nursing Interventions****
As Manifested by ↓	
Signs and Symptoms (Defining Characteristics)	**Evaluative Statement**

*More than one patient goal may be appropriate. For the purposes of this exercise, develop the one patient goal that demonstrates a direct resolution of the patient problem identified in the nursing diagnosis.

**Be sure you are able to list the scientific rationale for each nursing intervention you ordered.

CHAPTER 42

Urinary Elimination

CHAPTER OVERVIEW

- Urinary elimination, a natural process in which the body excretes waste products and materials that exceed bodily needs, usually is taken for granted. When urinary problems arise, the nurse realizes that many patients consider urination a private act and may become embarrassed when they need to discuss urination or require assistance with elimination. The nurse implements nursing interventions accordingly.

- Healthy urinary elimination presupposes well-functioning kidneys, ureters, urinary bladder, and urethra. Problems in any of these areas can affect both the amount and the quality of the urine formed and the manner in which it is expelled from the body.

- Other factors that affect urination include growth and development, food and fluid intake, lifestyle variables, psychologic variables, activity and muscle tone, pathologic conditions, and medications.

- A comprehensive assessment of the urinary system includes the collection of data about voiding patterns and urinary problems and the physical assessment of the kidneys, bladder, urethral meatus, skin integrity, and urine. These findings may need to be correlated with the results of diagnostic tests and procedures for examining urine and the urinary tract.

- Identification of patient health problems often is aided by the nurse's careful monitoring of fluid intake and output, collection of urine specimens, and testing of urine specimens for abnormalities.

- Nursing diagnoses may be written specifically addressing problems in urinary functioning (incontinence, pattern alteration, and retention) and identifying the effect urinary problems have on other areas of human functioning (anxiety, comfort, skin integrity).

- Nursing attention to the patient's usual voiding schedule, need for privacy, natural position while voiding, and hygiene habits will help ensure the patient's comfort and satisfactory urine output. Other measures facilitating normal urination include promoting an optimal fluid intake, strengthening tone in the perineal and abdominal muscles, and using specific measures (running tap water) to initiate voiding.

- The patient with cognitive, sensory, motor, neurologic, or endurance deficits may need nursing assistance with the toilet, bedpan, commode, or urinal. Family members also may need to be taught how to assist the patient with elimination needs.

- Urinary catheterization may be indicated to relieve urinary retention, obtain select urine specimens, measure residual urine, or empty the bladder before and during surgery and before certain diagnostic procedures. Catheterization is considered the most prominent cause of nosocomial infections, and should be avoided whenever possible.

- Obstructions or tumors in the urinary tract may require surgical diversion of the urinary flow. In the ileal conduit, the ureters are connected to the ileum, and a stoma is created on the abdominal wall. Nursing care is directed toward patient education and the achievement of optimal self-care.

■ Learning Checklist

Review the learning checklist at the end of the chapter in your textbook and be sure you can meet each objective.

■ Exercises

MATCHING

Match the body part listed in Part A with the appropriate area on the diagrams pictured in Part B. Answers may be used more than once.

PART A

a. urethra

b. ureter

c. bladder

d. kidney

PART B

1. _____

2. _____

3. _____

4. _____

5. _____

6. _____

7. _____

8. _____

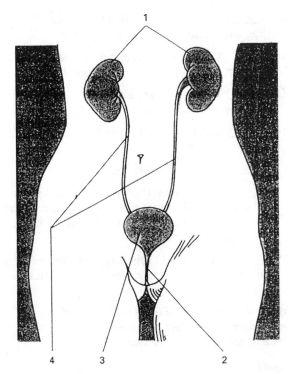

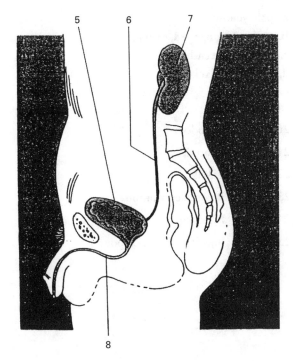

Match the terms associated with micturition in Part A, with their definitions, listed in Part B.

PART A

a. micturition

b. frequency

c. urinary retention

d. enuresis

e. autonomic bladder

f. hesitancy

g. stress incontinence

h. urge incontinence

i. mixed incontinence

j. overflow incontinence

k. functional incontinence

l. unconscious incontinence

PART B

9. _____ A delay or difficulty in initiating voiding.

10. _____ The involuntary loss of urine associated with an abrupt and strong desire to void.

11. _____ Urine loss caused by factors outside the lower urinary tract, such as chronic impairments of physical or cognitive functioning.

12. _____ The process of emptying the bladder.

13. _____ Involuntary urination that occurs after an age when continence should be present.

14. _____ Occurs when urine is produced normally but not appropriately excreted from the bladder.

15. _____ The involuntary loss of urine associated with overdistention and overflow of the bladder.

16. _____ Common in paraplegics and patients with multisystem failure.

17. _____ Voiding by reflex only.

18. _____ Occurs when there is an involuntary loss of urine related to an increase in intra-abdominal pressure during coughing, sneezing, laughing, or other physical activities.

19. _____ Symptoms of urge and stress incontinence are present although one type may predominate.

Match the color of urine listed in Part A with the medication that produces that color listed in Part B. Answers may be used more than once.

PART A

a. pale yellow

b. orange, orange-red, or pink

c. green or green-blue

d. brown or black

PART B

20. _____ Levodopa

21. _____ Diuretics

22. _____ Elavil

23. _____ B complex vitamins

24. _____ Pyridium

25. _____ Injectable iron compounds

MULTIPLE CHOICE

Circle the letter that corresponds to the best answer for each question.

1. Which of the following statements about kidney function is accurate?

   a. It is estimated that the total blood volume passes through the kidneys for waste removal about every two hours.

   b. One of the most significant functions of the kidneys is to maintain the composition and volume of body fluids.

   c. Because of varying kinds and amounts of food and fluids ingested, body fluids are relatively inconsistent in their amount and composition.

   d. There are about 1000 nephrons in each kidney.

2. When collecting a urine specimen for urinalysis, the nurse should be aware of which of the following facts?

   a. A sterile urine specimen is required for a routine urinalysis.

   b. If a woman is menstruating, a urine specimen cannot be obtained for urinalysis.

   c. Strict aseptic technique must be used when collecting and handling urine specimens.

   d. Urine should be left standing at room temperature for a 24-hour period before being sent to the laboratory.

3. A woman who notices an involuntary loss of urine following a coughing episode is most likely experiencing which of the following types of incontinence?

   a. stress incontinence

   b. urge incontinence

   c. overflow incontinence

   d. functional incontinence

4. Measurement of residual urine by catheterization after voiding verifies which of the following conditions?

   a. urinary tract infection

   b. urinary retention

   c. urinary incontinence

   d. urinary suppression

5. Which of the following catheters should be used to drain a patient's bladder for short periods (5 to 10 minutes)?

a. Foley catheter

b. suprapubic catheter

c. indwelling urethral catheter

d. straight catheter

6. Which of the following facts about the lower urinary tract system should be kept in mind when considering catheterization?

a. The bladder normally is a sterile cavity.

b. The external opening to the urethra should always be sterilized.

c. Pathogens introduced into the bladder remain in the bladder.

d. A normal bladder is as susceptible to infection as an injured one.

7. Which of the following events occurs when micturition is initiated?

a. The detrusor muscle expands.

b. The internal sphincter contracts.

c. Urine enters the posterior urethra.

d. The muscles of the perineum and external sphincter contract.

8. Which of the following collection devices is a nurse's best option when collecting urine from a nonambulatory male patient?

a. specimen hat

b. large urine collection bag

c. bedpan

d. urinal

9. You are preparing a patient for catheterization. Which of the following is an appropriate step for this procedure?

a. Place patient in the dorsal recumbent position.

b. Explain to the patient that the procedure is painless and should cause no discomfort.

c. Place the patient on a soft surface, preferably a soft mattress or pillow.

d. Place the patient in a prone position.

10. Mr. Gonos is being transferred to the hospital from a nursing home with a diagnosis of dehydration and urinary bladder infection. His skin is also excoriated from urinary incontinence. Which of the following is the most appropriate nursing diagnosis for Mr. Gonos?

a. Impaired skin integrity related to functional incontinence

b. Urinary incontinence related to urinary tract infection

c. Impaired skin integrity related to urinary tract infection and dehydration

d. Risk for urinary tract infection related to dehydration

11. Which of the following nursing interventions would be *least* effective when trying to maintain safety for the patient with an indwelling catheter?

a. Maintain a closed drainage system.

b. Restrict fluid intake

c. Apply a topical antibiotic ointment to urinary meatus.

d. Report signs of infection immediately.

12. A nurse determines that her patient has costovertebral tenderness. Which of the following conditions is indicated by this physical finding?

a. a bladder infection

b. a bladder obstruction

c. an inflamed kidney

d. the presence of a kidney stone

13. Mrs. Babb has had four urinary tract infections in the past year. Which physiologic change of aging is likely causing Mrs. Babb's problem?

a. decreased bladder contractility

b. diminished ability to concentrate urine

c. decreased bladder muscle tone

d. neurologic weakness

14. The doctor has ordered the collection of a fresh urine sample for a particular examination. Which urine sample would the nurse discard?

a. the sample collected immediately after lunch

b. the bedtime voiding

c. the voiding collected at 4:00 PM

d. the first voiding of the day

15. Mr. Morris has a urinary obstruction and is not a candidate for surgery. Which of the following devices would be an appropriate intervention for this patient?

 a. insertion of an indwelling urethral catheter

 b. insertion of a suprapubic catheter

 c. insertion of a straight catheter

 d. insertion of a urologic stent

COMPLETION

1. Describe how the following factors affect micturition.

 a. Developmental considerations: _____

 _____

 _____

 b. Food and fluid: _____ /____

 _____

 _____

 c. Psychologic variables: _____

 _____

 _____

 d. Activity and muscle tone: _____

 _____

 _____

 e. Pathologic conditions: _____

 _____

 _____

 f. Medications: _____

 _____

 _____

2. List three factors that indicate a child is ready for toilet training.

 a. _____

 b. _____

 c. _____

3. Describe special urinary considerations that should be included in the nursing history for the following patients.

 a. Infants and young children: _____

 _____

 _____

 b. Older adults: _____

 _____

 _____

 c. Patients with limited or no bladder control or urinary diversions: _____

 _____

 _____

4. Describe how you would examine the following areas of the urinary system when performing a physical assessment.

 a. Kidneys: _____

 _____

 _____

 b. Bladder: _____

 _____

 c. Urethral orifice: _____

 _____

 _____

 d. Skin integrity and hydration: _____

 _____

 _____

 e. Urine: _____

 _____

 _____

5. Briefly describe the procedure for determining the specific gravity of urine with a urinometer or hydrometer: _____

 _____

 _____

 _____

6. List four expected outcomes that denote normal voiding in a patient.

   a. _____

   b. _____

   c. _____

   d. _____

7. Explain how the following factors influence a patient's voiding patterns.

   a. Schedule:

   _____

   _____

   b. Privacy:

   _____

   _____

   c. Position:

   _____

   _____

   d. Hygiene:

   _____

   _____

8. List three reasons for catheterization.

   a. _____

   b. _____

   c. _____

9. List two expected outcomes for a patient with a urinary appliance.

   a. _____

   b. _____

GUIDE TO CRITICAL THINKING AND DEVELOPING BLENDED SKILLS

1. Develop a teaching plan to teach a postsurgical patient and his wife how to insert and care for a Foley catheter in a home setting. What factors are likely to influence the success of your teaching plan?

2. Keep a record of your fluid intake and output for 3 days. Note how your intake influenced urinary elimination. Write down the factors that could affect urine elimination. Are you at risk for urinary problems? If possible, perform routine tests on a sample of your urine and record the results.

PATIENT CARE STUDY

Read the following case study and use your nursing process skills to answer the questions below.

Mr. Eisenberg, age 84, was hurriedly admitted to a nursing home when his wife of 62 years died. He has two adult children, neither of whom feels prepared to care for him the way his wife did. "We don't know how mom did it year after year. After he retired from his law practice, he was terribly demanding, and it just seemed nothing she did for him pleased him. His Parkinson's disease does make it a bit difficult for him to get around, but he's able to do a whole lot more than he is letting on. He's always been this way." You are talking with his son and daughter because the aides have reported to you that he is frequently incontinent of both urine and stool during the day as well as during the night. He is alert and appears capable of recognizing the need to void or defecate and signaling for any assistance. His son and daughter report that this was never a problem at home, that he was able to go into the bathroom with assistance. He has been depressed about his admission to the home and seldom speaks, even when directly approached. He has refused to participate in any of the floor social events since his arrival.

1. Identify pertinent patient data by placing a single underline beneath the objective data in the case study and a double underline beneath the subjective data.

2. Complete the Nursing Process Worksheet on the next page to develop a three-part diagnostic statement and related plan of care for this patient.

3. Write down the patient and personal nursing strengths you hope to draw on as you assist this patient to better health.

Patient strengths: _____

_____

_____

Personal strengths: _____

_____

_____

_____

4. Pretend that you are performing a nursing assessment of this patient after the plan of care is implemented. Document your findings below.

_____

_____

_____

_____

NURSING PROCESS WORKSHEET

Health Problem (Title)	**Expected Outcome**
Related to ↓	
Etiology (Related Factors)	**Nursing Interventions****
As Manifested by ↓	
Signs and Symptoms (Defining Characteristics)	**Evaluative Statement**

*More than one patient goal may be appropriate. For the purposes of this exercise, develop the one patient goal that demonstrates a direct resolution of the patient problem identified in the nursing diagnosis.

**Be sure you are able to list the scientific rationale for each nursing intervention you ordered.

CHAPTER 43

Bowel Elimination

CHAPTER OVERVIEW

- Bowel elimination, a natural process in which the body excretes the waste products of digestion, is an essential component of healthy body functioning.

- Problems with bowel elimination may affect fluid and electrolyte balance, nutritional status, skin integrity, and self-concept.

- Healthy bowel elimination presupposes a well-functioning gastrointestinal tract. The large intestine is the primary organ of bowel elimination.

- Defecation and bowel movement are the terms used to describe the emptying of the intestines. People vary in the frequency of their bowel movements. The aim is to have the bowels move regularly and for the stools to be formed, soft, and passed without discomfort.

- Factors that affect bowel elimination include growth and development, daily patterns, food and fluid intake, activity and muscle tone, lifestyle variables, psychologic variables, pathologic conditions, medications, diagnostic tests, surgery, and anesthesia.

- A comprehensive assessment of bowel elimination includes the collection of data about usual patterns of elimination; recent changes in these patterns; aids to elimination; elimination problems; physical assessment of the abdomen, anus, and rectum; and stool characteristics. These findings may need to be correlated with the results of diagnostic studies of the stool and gastrointestinal tract.

- When caring for a debilitated, confused, or unconscious patient, the nurse needs to monitor bowel status daily to identify and treat bowel elimination problems early. Nursing care is directed to the prevention of bowel problems.

- Endoscopic examinations using a lighted tube allow the direct visualization of the gastrointestinal tract and are helpful in the diagnosis of inflammatory, ulcerative, and infectious diseases; neoplastic diseases; and lesions of the esophageal, gastric, and intestinal mucosa.

- Indirect visualization of the gastrointestinal tract is achieved through radiography. Important nursing responsibilities are assisting the patient to complete a safe and effective dietary and bowel preparation program and ensuring that the patient eliminates the contrast medium (barium sulfate) used in the study. Standard bowel preparation agents may be contraindicated for some patients.

- Nursing diagnoses may be written to address specific problems in bowel elimination (constipation, diarrhea, bowel incontinence) and to identify the effect bowel elimination problems have on other areas of human functioning (anxiety, comfort, self-concept, skin integrity).

- Regular bowel elimination may be promoted in both well and ill patients by attention to timing, positioning, privacy, nutrition, and exercise. Patients need to understand the importance of heeding the urge to defecate and the relation between bowel elimination and nutrition and exercise.

- Specific nursing strategies for bowel elimination include use of cathartics, laxatives, and antidiarrheals; techniques for emptying the colon of feces (enemas, rectal suppositories, oral intestinal lavage, and digital removal of stool); bowel training programs; and comfort measures.

- Although laxatives have valid uses, they frequently are abused. Many people who take laxatives for what they think is constipation do not realize that the habitual use of laxatives is the most common cause of chronic constipation.

- A physician's order may be needed before the nurse digitally removes a fecal impaction because this may result in irritation of the rectal mucosa and bleeding, and because vagal stimulation can decrease the heart rate.

- The purpose of a bowel training program is to manipulate factors within the person's control (food and fluid intake, exercise, time of defecation) and to achieve the elimination of a soft, formed stool at regular intervals without laxative support.

- The patient with a bowel diversion needs physical and psychologic support both preoperatively and postoperatively. The nurse works collaboratively with the physician and enterostomal therapist to ensure that the patient and family can manage the care of the bowel diversion after discharge.

- Patients with acute or chronic constipation, impaction, diarrhea, incontinence, or flatulence require special nursing care. These problems, if uncorrected, may seriously affect the patient's comfort, self-concept, and other areas of physical functioning.

■ Learning Checklist

Review the learning checklist at the end of the chapter in your textbook and be sure you can meet each objective.

■ Exercises

MATCHING

Match the bowel studies listed in Part A with their definition, listed in Part B.

PART A

a. endoscopy

b. esophagogastroduodenoscopy

c. colonoscopy

d. sigmoidoscopy

e. upper gastrointestinal examination

f. lower gastrointestinal examination

g. fecal occult blood test

h. timed specimens

i. pinworm test

PART B

1. __H__ The collection of a specimen of every stool passed within a designated time period.

2. __A__ The direct visualization of the lining of a hollow body organ using a long flexible tube containing glass fibers that transmits light into the organ and returns an image that can be viewed.

3. __D__ The visual examination of the lining of the distal sigmoid colon, the rectum, and the anal canal using either a flexible or rigid instrument.

4. __F__ Barium sulfate is instilled into the large intestine through a rectal tube inserted through the anus. Fluoroscopy projects consecutive x-ray images onto a screen for continuous observation of the flow of the barium.

5. __C__ Visual examination of the lining of the large intestine with a flexible, fiberoptic endoscope.

6. __E__ The patient drinks barium sulfate, which coats the esophagus, stomach, and small intestine to be better visualized.

7. __B__ Visual examination of the lining of the esophagus, the stomach, and the upper duodenum with a flexible, fiberoptic endoscope.

8. __G__ Use of a commercial tape, dipstick, or solution to test for pH or blood in the stool.

Match the type of enema in Part A with its use listed in Part B.

PART A

a. oil-retention enemas

b. carminative enemas

c. medicated enemas

d. anthelmintic enemas

e. nutritive enemas

f. return flow or Harris flush enemas

PART B

9. _____ Used to lubricate the stool and intestinal mucosa, making defecation easier.

10. _____ Administered to destroy intestinal parasites.

11. _____ Used to administer medications that are absorbed through the rectal mucosa.

12. _____ Used to administer fluids and nutrition rectally.

13. _____ Used to help expel flatus from the rectum and provide relief from gaseous distention.

Match the term in Part A with its definition listed in Part B.

PART A

a. chyme

b. feces

c. stool

d. flatus

e. bowel movement

f. hemorrhoids

g. constipation

h. diarrhea

i. incontinence

j. Valsalva maneuver

k. peristalsis

PART B

14. ___G___ The passage of dry, hard stools.

15. ___A___ Waste product of digestion.

16. ___H___ The passage of excessively liquid and unformed stools.

17. ___B___ Waste product that reaches the distal end of the colon.

18. ___D___ Intestinal gas.

19. ___i___ The inability of the anal sphincter to control the discharge of fecal and gaseous material.

20. ___C___ Excreted feces.

21. ___E___ The emptying of the intestines.

22. ___K___ The contraction of the circular and longitudinal muscles of the intestine.

Match the organs of the gastrointestinal system listed in Part A with the illustration in Part B.

PART A

a. splenic flexure

b. sigmoid colon

c. cecum

d. hepatic flexure

e. common bile duct

f. stomach

g. esophagus

h. descending colon

i. ileum

j. hepatic duct

k. gallbladder

l. duodenum

m. jejunum

n. rectum

o. ascending colon

p. pancreatic duct

q. ileocecal junction

r. transverse colon

PART B

23. _____

24. _____

25. _____

26. _____

27. _____

28. _____

29. _____

30. _____

31. _____

32. _____

33. _____

34. _____

35. _____

36. _____

37. _____

38. _____

39. _____

40. _____

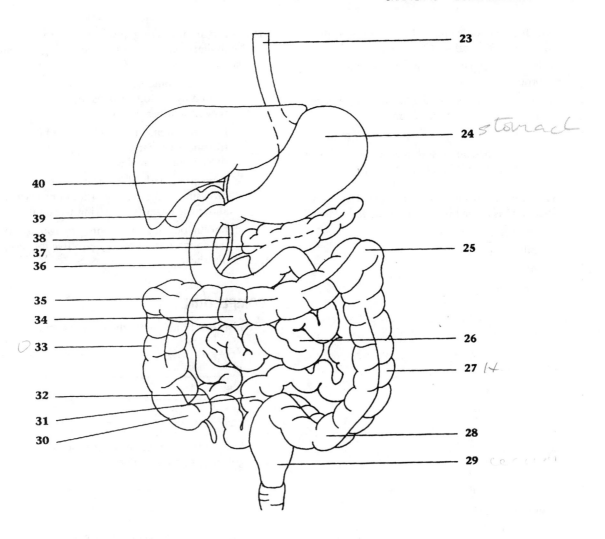

23

24 *storach*

40

39

38
37
36

35

34

33

32

31
30

25

26

27 *It*

28

29 *cecum*

MULTIPLE CHOICE

Circle the letter that corresponds to the best answer for each question.

1. Which of the following statements concerning peristalsis is accurate?

   a. The sympathetic nervous system inhibits movement.

   b. Peristalsis occurs every 25 to 30 minutes.

   c. One half to three quarters of ingested food waste products normally is excreted in the stool within 24 hours.

   d. Mass peristaltic sweeps occur one to four times every 24 hours in most people.

2. A patient who is experiencing constipation should avoid which of the following foods?

   a. beans

   b. chocolate

   c. cheese

   d. onions

3. The acronym BRAT stands for which of the following combinations of foods?

   a. beans, rice, applesauce, tea

   b. bananas, rice, applesauce, tomato juice

   c. bananas, rice, applesauce, tea

   d. bran, rice, applesauce, tea

4. Which of the following is the correct procedure when using a rectal tube?

   a. Position the patient on his/her back and drape properly.

   b. Introduce the rectal tube beyond the anal canal into the rectum about 10 cm.

   c. Leave the tube in place for 45 to 60 minutes.

   d. Have the patient lie still in a side-lying position when the tube is in place.

5. Tympany, the normal sound percussed over the abdomen, is caused by which of the following?

   a. excess flatus

   b. hollow organs

   c. intestinal fluid

   d. fecal contents

6. Which of the following is the barrier between the large intestine and the ileum of the small intestine?

   a. ileocecal junction

   b. sphincter

   c. splenic flexure

   d. hepatic flexure

7. Approximately how much water is absorbed daily by the intestinal tract?

   a. 300 to 400 mL

   b. 400 to 600 mL

   c. 600 to 800 mL

   d. 800 to 1000 mL

8. Which of the following indicates the most logical sequence of tests to ensure an accurate diagnosis?

   a. barium studies, endoscopic examination, fecal occult blood test

   b. fecal occult blood test, barium studies, endoscopic examination

   c. barium studies, fecal occult blood test, endoscopic examination

   d. endoscopic examination, barium studies, fecal occult blood test

9. Which of the following drugs acts by increasing intestinal bulk to enhance mechanical stimulation of the intestine?

   a. Cascara

   b. Bisacodyl

   c. magnesium sulfate

   d. phenolphthalein

10. When administering antidiarrheals to a patient with diarrhea, which of the following guidelines should be considered?

   a. Opiates should be used to treat diarrhea that is caused by poisons, toxins, or infections because they hasten peristalsis.

   b. Dose requirements of opiates used for treatment of diarrhea usually are larger than those used for analgesia.

   c. Some antidiarrheal medications may cause drowsiness, and patients should be warned about the hazards of driving when taking them.

   d. Kaolin–pectin preparations are available over the counter and are very effective for severe diarrhea.

COMPLETION

1. List four functions of the large intestine.

   a. _____

   b. _____

   c. _____

   d. _____

2. List the two centers of the nervous system that govern the reflex to defecate.

   a. _____

   b. _____

3. Describe two effects the following surgical procedures may have on peristalsis.

   a. Direct manipulation of the bowel: _____

   _____

   _____

   b. Inhalation of general anesthetic agents: _____

   _____

   _____

4. List the characteristics of the abdomen the nurse would assess by the following methods.

   a. Inspection: _____

   _____

   _____

b. Auscultation: _____

_____

_____

c. Percussion: _____

_____

_____

d. Palpation: _____

_____

_____

5. Give an example of how the following factors might affect the bowel elimination of a patient.

a. Developmental considerations: _____

_____

_____

b. Daily patterns: _____

_____

_____

c. Food and fluid: _____

_____

_____

d. Activity and muscle tone: _____

_____

_____

e. Lifestyle: _____

_____

_____

f. Psychologic variables: _____

_____

_____

g. Medications: _____

_____

_____

h. Diagnostic studies: _____

_____

_____

6. Mrs. Manganello is a 52-year-old patient presenting with acute stomach pain related to diverticular disease. Prepare an interview to assess Mrs. Manganello for bowel elimination:

_____

_____

_____

7. List four factors that promote healthy elimination patterns.

a. _____

b. _____

c. _____

d. _____

8. Give three examples of foods that have the following effects on elimination:

a. Constipating: _____

b. Laxative effect: _____

c. Gas producing: _____

9. Mrs. Azhner is a 65-year-old postsurgical patient complaining of painful defecation due to hard, dry stools. List three expected outcomes for this patient.

a. _____

b. _____

c. _____

10. Specify dietary measures to alleviate the following gastrointestinal problems.

a. Constipation: _____

b. Diarrhea: _____

c. Flatulence: _____

d. Ostomies: _____

11. Describe the following exercises designed for patients with weak abdominal and perineal muscles who are using a bedpan.

a. Abdominal settings: _____

_____

_____

b. Thigh strengthening: _____

_____

_____

12. List four reasons for prescribing cleansing enemas.

   a. _____

   b. _____

   c. _____

   d. _____

13. Briefly describe the following types of ostomies.

   a. Ileostomy: _____

   _____

   _____

   b. Colostomy: _____

   _____

   _____

14. Describe how the following factors help promote healthy bowel habits in patients:

   a. Timing: _____

   b. Positioning: _____

   c. Privacy: _____

   d. Nutrition: _____

   e. Exercise: _____

GUIDE TO CRITICAL THINKING AND DEVELOPING BLENDED SKILLS

1. Develop a list of preferred foods to ensure healthy bowel elimination for the following patients:

   a. A woman complains of constipation following a C-section.

   b. A 40-year-old man who is under stress in his job complains of frequent diarrhea.

   c. A toddler's stools are hard and dry and he complains of frequent stomach aches.

   What other factors are likely to promote healthy bowel elimination in these patients?

2. Perform a physical assessment and write a nursing diagnosis for a patient who has just had a colostomy performed. What types of changes in his life will this patient face, and what can be done to help him cope with them? How can you best learn this? Be sure to assess this patient's physical and psychologic factors, body image, coping mechanisms and support system. Develop a nursing care plan to provide postoperative care, hospital care, and follow-up care for this patient.

PATIENT CARE STUDY

Read the following patient care study and use your nursing process skills to answer the questions below.

Ms. Elgaresta, age 54, a single, Hispanic woman, is being followed by a cardiologist who monitors her heart arrhythmia. Last month, she was started on a new heart medication. At this visit, she complains to the nurse practitioner who works with the cardiologist: "Right after I started taking that medication, I got terribly constipated and nothing seems to help. I'm desperate and about ready to try dynamite unless you can think of something else!" She reports a change in her bowel movements from one soft stool daily to one to two hard stools weekly, stools that cause much straining. The nurse practitioner realizes that regulating Ms. Elgaresta's heart is difficult and that her best cardiac response to date has been with the medication that is now causing constipation. Reluctant to suggest substituting another medication too quickly, she asks more questions and discovers the following: "I've never been much of a drinker. Two cups of coffee in the morning and maybe a glass of wine at night. Water? Almost never. And I don't drink juices or soft drinks." Analysis of her diet reveals a diet low in fiber: "I never was one much for vegetables, and they can just keep all this bran stuff that's out on the market! Coffee and a cigarette. That's for me!" Ms. Elgaresta is a workaholic computer programmer who has little leisure time and spends what little spare time she has watching TV. She reports tiring after walking one flight of stairs, and states that she avoids all forms of vigorous exercise.

1. Identify pertinent patient data by placing a single underline beneath the objective data in the case study and a double underline beneath the subjective data.

2. Complete the Nursing Process Worksheet on the opposite page to develop a three-part diagnostic statement and related plan of care for this patient.

3. Write down the patient and personal nursing strengths you hope to draw upon as you assist this patient to better health.

Patient strengths: _____

_____

_____

Personal strengths: _____

_____

_____

_____

4. Pretend that you are performing a nursing assessment of this patient after the plan of care is implemented. Document your findings below.

_____

_____

_____

_____

NURSING PROCESS WORKSHEET

Health Problem (Title)

Expected Outcome

Related to

↓

Etiology (Related Factors)

Nursing Interventions**

As Manifested by

↓

**Signs and Symptoms
(Defining Characteristics)**

Evaluative Statement

*More than one patient goal may be appropriate. For the purposes of this exercise, develop the one patient goal that demonstrates a direct resolution of the patient problem identified in the nursing diagnosis.
**Be sure you are able to list the scientific rationale for each nursing intervention you ordered.

CHAPTER 44

Oxygenation

CHAPTER OVERVIEW

- The functioning units of the respiratory system are the alveoli, where the actual exchange of oxygen and carbon dioxide between the lung and circulation occurs. Airways conduct available gases during inspiratory and expiratory phases of ventilation.

- There are normal variations in respiratory functioning unique to specific ages that allow appropriate oxygenation to meet cellular needs. These differences involve chest shape, breath sounds, and presence of landmarks. In addition to age, other factors affect adequate respiratory functioning: level of health, growth and development, environment, and psychologic health. Persons with health deviations in respiratory functioning can initiate changes to improve the work of breathing.

- The health history is an essential component of respiratory function assessment. The patient's physical examination and laboratory findings can provide information to identify the nature of the problem, its course, related signs and symptoms, onset and frequency, and effect on everyday living.

- Nursing diagnoses can be written to address inadequate breathing patterns, ineffective airway clearance, and impaired gas exchange. Nursing diagnoses also can be written to address how altered respiratory functioning has an effect on other areas of human functioning (e.g., anxiety).

- Nursing interventions to promote adequate respiratory functioning include educating patients to maintain a pollution-free environment, promoting effective breathing and coughing exercises, maintaining adequate fluid intake, maintaining good nutrition, promoting comfort by positioning, providing supplemental oxygen, and using medications to promote adequate respiratory functioning.

- Evaluation is ongoing. The health care team and the patient examine progress toward achieving the established outcomes. The plan is modified based on the patient's response to nursing actions.

■ Learning Checklist

Review the learning checklist at the end of the chapter in your textbook and be sure you can meet each objective.

■ Exercises

MATCHING

Match the definition in Part B with the term listed in Part A.

PART A

a. ventilation

b. inspiration

c. expiration

d. lung compliance

e. airway resistance

f. diffusion

g. perfusion

h. hypoventilation

i. atelectasis

j. hyperventilation

k. hypoxia

PART B

1. _____ Movement of muscles and thorax to bring air into the lungs.

2. _____ The movement of oxygen and carbon dioxide between the air and the blood.

3. _____ Incomplete lung expansion or lung collapse.

4. _____ An inadequate amount of oxygen in the cells.

5. _____ The movement of air in and out of the lungs.

6. _____ Any impediment or obstruction that air meets as it moves through the airway.

7. _____ The stretchability of the lungs or the ease with which the lungs can be inflated.

8. _____ The process in which the oxygenated capillary blood passes through tissue.

9. _____ A decreased rate of air movement into the lungs.

10. _____ An increased rate and depth of ventilation above the body's normal metabolic requirements.

Match the organs of the respiratory tract listed in Part A with the illustration in Part B.

PART A

a. right main bronchus

b. epiglottis

c. terminal bronchioles

d. esophagus

e. pleura

f. left main bronchus

g. nasal cavity

h. thyroid cartilage

i. trachea

j. oral cavity

PART B

11. _____

12. _____

13. _____

14. _____

15. _____

16. _____

17. _____

18. _____

19. _____

20. _____

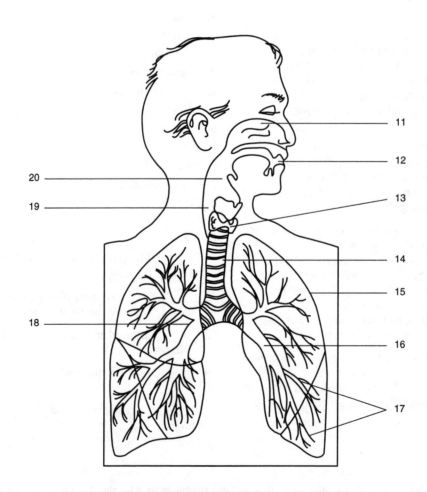

Match the type of medication used to improve respiratory functioning listed in Part A with its activity listed in Part B.

PART A

a. epinephrine

b. isoproterenol

c. theophylline

d. corticosteroids

e. antihistamines

f. cromolyn sodium

PART B

21. _____ Reduces inflammation.

22. _____ Relaxes muscles that line bronchi and bronchioles.

23. _____ Blocks histamine and relieves congestion of an allergic origin.

24. _____ Bronchodilator (inhaler).

25. _____ Prevents the release of histamines, serotonin, and prostaglandin by the mast cell in an antigen–antibody reaction in asthma.

Match the type of oxygen delivery system listed in Part A with its description listed in Part B.

PART A

a. nasal cannula

b. nasal catheter

c. simple oxygen mask

d. partial rebreather mask

e. nonrebreather mask

f. Venturi mask

g. oxygen tent

h. transtracheal oxygen delivery

PART B

26. _____ Connects to oxygen tubing, a humidifier, and flowmeter, and delivers 35% to 60% oxygen; should cover nose and mouth; has vents in sides to allow room air to leak in at many places, diluting the source oxygen.

27. _____ Produces the highest concentration of oxygen with a mask; contains two one-way valves that prevent conservation of exhaled air, which escapes through side vents.

28. _____ A tube is inserted into the throat through one nostril and must be changed to the other nostril every 9 hours. Gastric distention often occurs.

29. _____ This mask delivers the most precise concentrations of oxygen, and has a large tube with an oxygen inlet. As tube narrows, pressure drops, causing air to be sucked in through side ports.

30. _____ Probably the most commonly used respiratory aid, consisting of a disposable, plastic device with two protruding prongs for insertion into nostrils; connected to oxygen source with humidifier and flowmeter.

31. _____ A small catheter is inserted into the trachea under local anesthesia.

32. _____ This mask is equipped with a reservoir bag for the collection of the first parts of the patient's exhaled air. The air is mixed with 100% oxygen for next inhalation.

Match the lung values and capacities listed in Part A with their description, listed in Part B.

PART A

a. tidal volume

b. inspiratory reserve volume

c. expiratory reserve volume

d. residual volume

e. vital capacity

f. inspiratory capacity

g. functional residual volume

h. total lung capacity

PART B

33. _____ The amount of air inspired and expired in a normal respiration. Normal is 500 mL.

34. _____ The largest amount of air that can be inhaled following a normal quiet exhalation. Normal is 3600 mL.

35. _____ The amount of air that can be exhaled beyond tidal volume. Normal is 1200 mL.

36. _____ The amount of air that can be inspired beyond tidal volume. Normal is 3100 mL.

37. _____ The sum of the TV + IRV + ERV + RV. Normal is 6000 mL.

38. _____ The amount of air remaining in the lungs after a maximal expiration. Normal is 1200 mL.

39. _____ The maximal amount of air that can be exhaled following a maximal inhalation. Normal is 4800 mL.

MULTIPLE CHOICE

Circle the letter that corresponds to the best answer for each question.

1. Which of the following is the primary purpose of surfactant?
   a. to propel sheets of mucus toward the upper airway
   b. to warm inspired air
   c. to produce watery mucus
   d. to reduce surface tension of the fluid lining the alveoli

2. The small air sacs at the end of the terminal bronchioles that are the sites of gas exchange are known as which of the following?
   a. alveoli
   b. pleurae
   c. labules
   d. bronchioles

3. A patient who has difficulty breathing, increased respiratory and pulse rates, and pale skin color with regions of cyanosis may be suffering from which of the following?
   a. hyperventilation
   b. hypoxia
   c. perfusion
   d. atelectasis

4. When a nurse inspects a patient's chest to assess respiratory status, she should be aware of which of the following normal findings?
   a. The contour of the intercostal spaces should be rounded.
   b. The skin at the thorax should be cool and moist.
   c. The anteroposterior diameter should be greater than the transverse diameter.
   d. The chest should be slightly convex with no sternal depression.

5. When percussing a normal lung, which of the following sounds should be heard?
   a. tympany
   b. resonance
   c. dullness
   d. hyperresonance

6. Which of the following normal breath sounds should be heard over the trachea?
   a. vesicular
   b. bronchovesicular
   c. bronchial
   d. tympanic

7. A patient who develops air in the pleural space is experiencing which of the following conditions?
   a. pleural effusion
   b. hemothorax
   c. pneumothorax
   d. pleurathorax

8. When caring for a patient with a chest tube, it is the nurse's responsibility to do which of the following?
   a. Maintain the drainage unit above the patient's chest level.
   b. Assess drainage every hour postoperatively for 24 hours.
   c. After the first 24 hours postsurgery, perform subsequent checks every 12 hours.
   d. Notify the physician if drainage exceeds 200 mL/hr.

9. Which of the following cough suppressants is generally preferred, despite its addictive quality?
   a. cough syrup with codeine
   b. Benylin
   c. Balminil DM
   d. Benadryl

10. A patient who complains of difficulty breathing should be placed in which of the following positions?
    a. prone position
    b. lateral position
    c. supine position
    d. Fowler's position

11. Which of the following guidelines should be used to help a coughing patient maintain adequate fluid intake?

   a. Secretions should be kept thin by having the patient drink 1 to 1.5 quarts of clear fluids daily.

   b. If the patient has right-sided heart failure, fluid intake should exceed 1.5 to 2 quarts daily.

   c. Milk products should be used to thin secretions and congestion.

   d. The patient's fluid intake should be increased to the maximum that his/her health can tolerate.

12. To drain the apical sections of the upper lobes of the lungs, the nurse should place the patient in which of the following positions?

   a. left side with a pillow under the chest wall

   b. side-lying position, half on the abdomen and half on the side

   c. high Fowler's position

   d. Trendelenburg's position

13. Which of the following inhalers is used to liquefy or loosen thick secretions?

   a. bronchodilators

   b. mucolytic agents

   c. corticosteroids

   d. metered dose inhalers

14. The brain is sensitive to hypoxia and will sustain irreversible brain damage after how many minutes?

   a. 2 to 4 minutes

   b. 4 to 6 minutes

   c. 6 to 8 minutes

   d. 8 to 10 minutes

15. Mr. Parks has chronic obstructive pulmonary disease. His nurse has taught him pursed-lip breathing, which helps him in which of the following ways?

   a. Increases carbon dioxide, which stimulates breathing.

   b. Teaches him to prolong inspiration and shorten expiration.

   c. Helps liquefy his secretions.

   d. Decreases the amount of air trapping and resistance.

16. A nurse suctioning his patient through a tracheostomy tube should be careful not to occlude the Y-port when inserting the suction catheter, because it would cause which of the following to occur?

   a. trauma to the tracheal mucosa

   b. prevention of suctioning

   c. loss of sterile field

   d. suctioning of carbon dioxide

17. When caring for a tracheotomized patient, the nurse should be aware of which of the following?

   a. The wound around the tube and inner cannula, if one is present, should be cleaned at least every 24 hours.

   b. The tracheotomized patient has no impaired speaking function.

   c. A newly inserted tracheostomy tube requires no immediate attention.

   d. Suctioning of the tracheostomy tube must be done using sterile technique.

18. When percussing the lungs of a patient with emphysema, the nurse would probably hear which of the following sounds?

   a. resonance

   b. hyperresonance

   c. tympany

   d. dullness

19. Which of the following is a function of the upper airway?

   a. conduction of air

   b. mucociliary clearance

   c. production of pulmonary surfactant

   d. purification of inspired air

COMPLETION

1. List three factors on which normal respiratory functioning depends.

   a. _____

   b. _____

   c. _____

2. Briefly describe the functions of the upper and lower airway, listing their main components.

   a. Upper airway: _____

   _____

   _____

   b. Lower airway: _____

   _____

   _____

3. Define Boyle's law: _____

   _____

   _____

4. List four factors that influence the diffusion of gas in the lungs.

   a. _____

   b. _____

   c. _____

   d. _____

5. Describe the two ways that oxygen is carried in the body.

   a. _____

   b. _____

6. Briefly describe the variations in respiration experienced by the following age groups.

   a. Infant: _____

   _____

   _____

   b. Preschool and school-age child: _____

   _____

   _____

   c. Older adult: _____

   _____

   _____

7. Explain how you would assess a patient for the following respiratory conditions.

   a. Respiratory excursion: _____

   _____

   _____

b. Tactile fremitus: _____

   _____

   _____

8. Describe nursing responsibilities before, during, and after a thoracentesis: _____

   _____

   _____

   _____

9. How would you describe the effects of smoking on the lungs to a patient who smokes a pack of cigarettes a day?

   _____

   _____

   _____

10. Briefly describe the following techniques designed to promote proper breathing.

    a. Deep breathing: _____

    _____

    _____

    b. Using incentive spirometry: _____

    _____

    _____

    c. Abdominal or diaphragmatic breathing: _____

    _____

    _____

11. You are the visiting nurse for a patient with emphysema who is receiving oxygen therapy. List five precautions you would take to prevent fire and injury to this patient.

    a. _____

    b. _____

    c. _____

    d. _____

    e. _____

12. Briefly describe the following types of airways and their uses.

    a. Oropharyngeal or nasopharyngeal airway: ____

    _____

    _____

    b. Endotracheal tube: _____

    _____

    _____

    c. Tracheostomy tube: _____

    _____

    _____

13. Describe the ABCs of basic life support:

    A: _____

    B: _____

    C: _____

14. What is the nurse's responsibility when aspirating a patient's pleural cavity?

    _____

    _____

15. Describe seven comfort measures for patients with impaired respiratory functioning.

    a. _____

    b. _____

    c. _____

    d. _____

    e. _____

    f. _____

    g. _____

GUIDE TO CRITICAL THINKING AND DEVELOPING BLENDED SKILLS

1. Develop a set of nursing strategies to promote adequate respiratory functioning in the following patients:

    a. A patient with lung cancer presents with blood in his sputum.

    b. A child with cystic fibrosis is having difficulty breathing.

    c. A young woman with asthma develops pneumonia.

    d. A 48-year-old man who smokes a pack of cigarettes a day presents with emphysema.

    What is it that makes the strategies you selected appropriate/effective?

2. Interview young people who are smokers to find out their opinions about the health risks associated with smoking. See if they would be willing to quit with your help. Is the knowledge of health risk sufficient to motivate lifestyle modifications? What are the implications for your practice?

PATIENT CARE STUDY

Read the following case study and use your nursing process skills to answer the questions below.

Toni is a 14-year-old girl who is in the adolescent mental health unit following a suicide attempt. Her chart reveals that on several occasions when her mother was visiting, she began hyperventilating (respiratory rate of 42 and increased depth). Gasping for breath on these occasions, she nevertheless pushed away all who approached her to assist. Her mother confided that she and her husband are in the midst of a divorce and that it hasn't been easy for Toni at home. "I know she's been having a rough time at school, and I guess I've been too caught up in my own troubles to be there for her." When you attempt to discuss this with Toni and mention her mother's concern, she begins hyperventilating again.

1. Identify pertinent patient data by placing a single underline beneath the objective data in the case study and a double underline beneath the subjective data.

2. Complete the Nursing Process Worksheet on the next page to develop a three-part diagnostic statement and related plan of care for this patient.

3. Write down the patient and personal nursing strengths you hope to draw on as you assist this patient to better health.

   Patient strengths: _____

   _____

   _____

   Personal strengths: _____

   _____

   _____

4. Pretend that you are performing a nursing assessment of this patient after the plan of care is implemented. Document your findings below.

   _____

   _____

   _____

   _____

NURSING PROCESS WORKSHEET

Health Problem (Title)	Expected Outcome
Related to ↓ **Etiology (Related Factors)**	**Nursing Interventions****
As Manifested by ↓ **Signs and Symptoms** **(Defining Characteristics)**	**Evaluative Statement**

*More than one patient goal may be appropriate. For the purposes of this exercise, develop the one patient goal that demonstrates a direct resolution of the patient problem identified in the nursing diagnosis.

**Be sure you are able to list the scientific rationale for each nursing intervention you ordered.

CHAPTER 45

Fluid, Electrolyte, and Acid–Base Balance

CHAPTER OVERVIEW

- Whereas life can be sustained for many days without food, it can be sustained for only a few days without water.

- There are two major compartments for body fluids: (1) intracellular fluid (ICF), which is the fluid within cells, and (2) extracellular fluid (ECF), located outside of body cells, which includes intravascular fluid (plasma) and interstitial fluid (fluid in which tissue cells are bathed).

- A person's age, lean body mass, and sex can all influence the distribution of body fluids in the different compartments. Because lean tissue has higher water content than fat, thin people, males, and younger people tend to have higher percentages of total body water in relation to body weight than obese, female, and older people because of their increased lean body mass.

- Sodium and chloride are the principal ions of ECF; potassium and phosphate are principal ions of ICF.

- The most common routes for transporting fluid and electrolytes among the body compartments are osmosis, diffusion, active transport, and filtration.

- In a healthy adult, fluid intake and loss should average about 2500 mL over 2 to 3 days. The output of urine generally approximates the ingestion of liquids; water from food and oxidation is balanced by water loss through the feces, the skin, and the respiratory process.

- Deficiencies in the amount of both water and electrolytes in ECF in near-normal proportions are termed fluid volume deficits. Excessive retention of water and electrolytes in ECF is termed fluid volume excess.

- To prevent the serious complications that can result from untreated electrolyte imbalances, nurses must be familiar with the causes, defining characteristics, and treatment of imbalances of sodium, potassium, calcium, magnesium, and phosphate.

- Normal blood plasma is slightly alkaline and has a normal pH range from 7.35 to 7.45. Slight deviations in either direction (acid–base imbalances), if untreated, may result in death.

- The narrow range of normal pH is achieved by complex buffer systems (bicarbonate, phosphate, protein) and specific respiratory and renal mechanisms.

- Failure of acid–base regulating mechanisms may result in respiratory or metabolic disturbances, which can be acidosis or alkalosis.

- Risk factors for fluid, electrolyte, and acid-base imbalances include pathologies involving homeostatic regulators of fluid balance (e.g., diabetes mellitus, congestive heart failure, renal failure); abnormal losses of body fluids; burns and trauma; and therapies with the potential to disrupt fluid and electrolyte balance (e.g., medications such as diuretics and steroids, IV therapy, TPN).

- Pertinent assessment measures include maintaining accurate intake and output records, recording daily weights, observing for the signs and symptoms that characterize specific imbalances, and monitoring results of laboratory studies.

- Nursing diagnoses may be developed in which the fluid imbalance is the problem statement (Fluid Volume Deficit or Fluid Volume Excess), or the etiology (Pain related to edema, Impaired Oral Mucous Membrane related to dehydration).

- Nursing interventions are directed to maintaining a patient's fluid, electrolyte, and acid–base balance; preventing disturbances; and correcting imbalances.

- When fluids are being encouraged or restricted, it is important that both the nursing staff and patient understand the target amount of fluid to be taken each shift and that the patient's fluid preferences be respected.

- Nurses administering IV fluids should accurately prepare the prescribed solution; understand the desired effect of treatment and possible adverse responses; and assume responsibility for initiating, monitoring, and, when ordered, discontinuing the therapy.

- Complications associated with IV infusions include infiltration, phlebitis, thrombus, speed shock, fluid overload, embolus, and infection.

- Administering blood transfusions requires a careful pretransfusion assessment of the patient, accurate identification and matching of the blood to be transfused with its intended recipient, and ongoing monitoring of the patient throughout the transfusion for transfusion reactions. These include hemolytic, febrile, allergic, and hypervolemic reactions.

- In TPN, hypertonic solutions of dextrose, amino acids, and select electrolytes and minerals—capable of reestablishing positive nitrogen balance and weight gain—are infused using a central vein.

■ Learning Checklist

Review the learning checklist at the end of the chapter in your textbook and be sure you can meet each objective.

■ Exercises

MATCHING

Match the cation in Part A with its function listed in Part B. Some answers may be used more than once.

PART A

a. sodium

b. potassium

c. calcium

d. magnesium

PART B

1. _____ It is the chief regulator of cellular enzyme activity and cellular water content.

2. _____ It is necessary for nerve-impulse transmission and blood clotting.

3. _____ It controls and regulates the volume of body fluids.

4. _____ It is the primary regulator of ECF volume.

5. _____ It is important for the metabolism of carbohydrates and proteins.

6. _____ It is a catalyst for muscle contraction.

7. _____ It assists in the regulation of acid–base balance by cellular exchange with H^+.

8. _____ It is necessary for protein and DNA synthesis, DNA and RNA transcription, and translation of RNA.

Match the anion in Part A with its function listed in Part B. Some answers may be used more than once.

PART A

a. chloride

b. bicarbonate

c. phosphate

d. sulfate

PART B

9. _____ It acts with sodium to maintain the osmotic pressure of the blood.

10. _____ It is important for cell division and for the transmission of hereditary traits.

11. _____ It is important in the buffering system that is activated by the exchange of oxygen and carbon dioxide between body tissues and red blood cells.

12. _____ It is found primarily within cells and is associated with intracellular protein.

13. _____ It is essential for acid–base balance and, in combination with carbonic acid, constitutes the body's primary buffer system.

14. _____ It participates in many important chemical reactions in the body; for example, it is necessary for many B vitamins to be effective and plays a role in carbohydrate metabolism.

15. _____ It is essential for the production of hydrochloric acid in gastric cells.

Match the organ function in Part B with the primary organ of homeostasis listed in Part A.

PART A

a. kidneys

b. cardiovascular system

c. lungs

d. adrenal glands

e. pituitary gland

f. thyroid gland

g. parathyroid glands

h. gastrointestinal tract

i. nervous system

PART B

16. _____ Secretes parathormone, which regulates the level of calcium in extracellular fluid.

17. _____ Responsible for pumping and carrying nutrients and water throughout the body.

18. _____ Normally filters 179 L plasma daily in the adult while excreting only 1.5 L urine.

19. _____ Acts as a switchboard that inhibits and stimulates mechanisms that influence fluid balance.

20. _____ Absorbs water and nutrients that enter the body through the intestines.

21. _____ Regulates oxygen and carbon dioxide levels of the blood.

22. _____ Stores antidiuretic hormone, which is manufactured in the hypothalamus.

23. _____ Secretes aldosterone, which is known as the great sodium conserver of the body.

Match the equations in Part B with the type of imbalance listed in Part A.

PART A

a. respiratory acidosis

b. metabolic acidosis

c. respiratory alkalosis

d. metabolic alkalosis

PART B

24. _____ Low pH, normal $PaCO_2$, low HCO_3

25. _____ Low pH, high $PaCO_2$, normal HCO_3

26. _____ High pH, normal $PaCO_2$, high HCO_3

27. _____ High pH, low $PaCO_2$, normal HCO_3

Match the infusion sites listed in Part A with their appropriate place on the diagram shown in Part B on the next page. Some answers will be used more than once.

PART A

a. basilic vein

b. radial vein

c. cephalic vein

d. median cubital vein

e. dorsal metacarpal veins

f. accessory cephalic veins

g. medial antebrachial vein

PART B

28. _____

29. _____

30. _____

31. _____

32. _____

33. _____

34. _____

35. _____

36. _____

Match the term in Part A with its definition listed in Part B.

PART A

a. ion

b. electrolyte

c. cation

d. anion

e. solvents

f. solutes

g. osmolarity

h. filtration

i. oncotic pressure

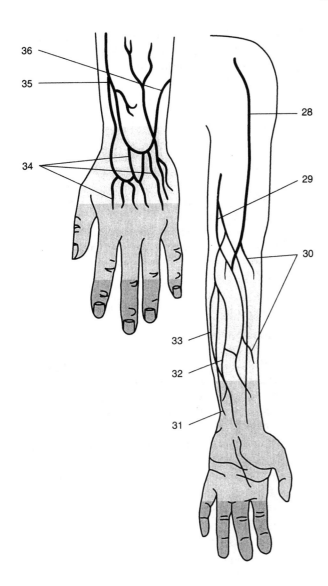

j. hydrostatic pressure
k. diffusion
l. active transport
m. filtration pressure
n. buffer
o. intravascular fluid
p. interstitial fluid

PART B

37. _____ Ions that develop a positive charge.

38. _____ Substances that are dissolved in a solution.

39. _____ Fluid that surrounds tissue cells and includes lymph.

40. _____ Measured in terms of their chemical combining power, or chemical activity.

41. _____ The liquid constituent of blood.

42. _____ A process that requires energy for the movement of substances through a cell membrane from an area of lesser concentration to an area of higher concentration.

43. _____ The passage of a fluid through a permeable membrane.

44. _____ An atom or molecule carrying an electric charge.

45. _____ An ion with a negative charge.

46. _____ Liquids that hold a substance in solution.

47. _____ A force exerted by a fluid against the container wall.

48. _____ The difference between colloid osmotic pressure and blood hydrostatic pressure.

49. _____ A substance that prevents body fluids from becoming overly acidic or alkaline.

50. _____ The concentration of particles in a solution, or its pulling power.

51. _____ The tendency of solutes to move freely throughout a solvent.

CORRECT THE FALSE STATEMENTS

Circle the word true or false that follows the statement. If the word false has been circled, change the underlined word/words to make the statement true. Place your answer in the space provided.

1. The human body is composed of anywhere from <u>50% to 60%</u> water by weight.

   True   False   _____

2. Substances capable of breaking into electrically charged ions when dissolved in a solution are called <u>solutes</u>.

   True   False   _____

3. A <u>hypertonic solution</u> has less osmolarity than plasma.

   True   False   _____

4. <u>Ingested liquids</u> make up the largest amount of water normally taken into the body.

   True   False   _____

5. Acidity or alkalinity of a solution is determined by its concentration of <u>oxygen ions</u>.

   True   False   _____

6. An <u>acid</u> is a substance that can accept or trap hydrogen ions.

   True   False   _____

7. Normal blood plasma is slightly <u>acidic</u> and has a normal pH range of 7.35 to 7.45.

   True   False   _____

8. The <u>kidneys</u> are the primary controller of the body's carbonic acid supply.

   True   False   _____

9. Excessive retention of water and sodium in ECF results in a condition termed fluid volume excess or <u>hypervolemia</u>.

   True   False   _____

10. <u>Hypokalemia</u> refers to a surplus of sodium in ECF that can result from excess water loss or an overall excess of sodium.

    True   False   _____

11. Acid–base imbalances occur when the ECF and ICF carbonic acid or bicarbonate levels become <u>equal</u>.

    True   False   _____

12. <u>Arterial blood gases</u> are most commonly used to assess and treat acid–base imbalances.

    True   False   _____

MULTIPLE CHOICE

Circle the letter that corresponds to the best answer for each question.

1. Which of the following short- or long-term venous access devices is usually introduced into the subclavian or internal jugular veins and passed to the superior vena cava just above the right atrium?
   a. peripherally inserted central catheters
   b. implanted port
   c. central venous catheter
   d. electronic infusion devices

2. When teaching a patient about foods that affect his fluid balance, the nurse will keep in mind that the electrolyte that primarily controls water distribution throughout the body is which of the following?
   a. Na^+
   b. K^+
   c. Ca^{++}
   d. Mg^{++}

3. A healthy patient eats a regular, balanced diet and drinks 3000 mL of liquids during a 24-hour period. In evaluating his urine output for the same 24-hour period, the nurse realizes that it should total approximately how many mL?
   a. 3750
   b. 3000
   c. 1000
   d. 500

4. For the patient with "hyperkalemia related to decreased renal excretion secondary to potassium-conserving diuretic therapy," an appropriate expected outcome would be which of the following?
   a. Bowel motility will be restored within 24 hours after beginning supplemental K^+.
   b. ECG will show no cardiac arrhythmias within 48 hours after removing salt substitutes, coffee, tea, and other K^+-rich foods from diet.
   c. ECG will show no cardiac arrhythmias within 24 hours after beginning supplemental K^+.
   d. Bowel motility will be restored within 24 hours after eliminating salt substitutes, coffee, tea, and other K^+-rich foods from the diet.

5. Which of the following nursing diagnoses would you expect to be based on the effects of fluid and electrolyte imbalance on human functioning?
   a. Constipation related to immobility.
   b. Pain related to surgical incision.
   c. Altered thought processes related to cerebral edema, including mental confusion and disorientation.
   d. Health risk for infection related to inadequate personal hygiene.

6. Which of the following is the liquid constituent of blood?

    a. intracellular fluid

    b. extracellular fluid

    c. interstitial fluid

    d. intravascular fluid

7. The body eliminates excess sodium through which of the following organs?

    a. kidneys

    b. bowels

    c. skin

    d. heart

8. Which of the following food items is a leading source of potassium?

    a. canned vegetables

    b. cheese

    c. bread

    d. bananas

9. Which of the following is the most abundant electrolyte in the body?

    a. sodium

    b. calcium

    c. potassium

    d. magnesium

10. "Pumping uphill" would describe which of the following means of transporting materials to and from intracellular compartments?

    a. osmosis

    b. diffusion

    c. filtration

    d. active transport

11. The desirable amount of fluid intake and loss in adults should average approximately which of the following amounts?

    a. 1000 mL/day

    b. 1500 mL/day

    c. 2500 mL/day

    d. 3500 mL/day

12. When considering a site for an IV infusion, the nurse should consider which of the following guidelines?

    a. Scalp veins should be selected for infants because of their accessibility.

b. Antecubital veins should be used for long-term infusions.

    c. Veins in the leg should be used to keep arms free for patient's use.

    d. Veins in surgical areas should be used to increase potency of medication.

13. Individuals with which of the following blood types are often called universal donors?

    a. type A

    b. type O

    c. type B

    d. type AB

14. A nurse who has diagnosed a patient as having "fluid volume excess" related to compromised regulatory mechanism (kidneys) may have been alerted by which of the following symptoms?

    a. muscular twitching

    b. distended neck veins

    c. fingerprinting over sternum

    d. nausea and vomiting

COMPLETION

1. List six functions of water in the body.

    a. _____

    b. _____

    c. _____

    d. _____

    e. _____

    f. _____

2. Briefly describe how the following processes transport materials to and from intracellular compartments.

    a. Osmosis: _____

    _____

    _____

    b. Diffusion: _____

    _____

    _____

    c. Active transport: _____

    _____

    _____

3. Give an example of how water is derived from the following sources.

   a. Ingested liquids: _____

   b. Food: _____

   c. Metabolic oxidation: _____

4. List three mechanisms for water loss in the body.

   a. _____

   b. _____

   c. _____

5. Explain how the following organs/systems of the body maintain fluid homeostasis.

   a. Kidneys: _____

   _____

   _____

   b. Cardiovascular system: _____

   _____

   _____

   c. Lungs: _____

   _____

   _____

   d. Thyroid: _____

   _____

   _____

   e. Parathyroid: _____

   _____

   _____

   f. Gastrointestinal system: _____

   _____

   _____

   g. Nervous system: _____

   _____

   _____

6. Give a brief description of the following conditions.

   a. Acidosis: _____

   _____

   _____

   b. Alkalosis: _____

   _____

   _____

7. Describe the following acid–base imbalances and their effect on the body.

   a. Respiratory acidosis: _____

   _____

   _____

   b. Respiratory alkalosis: _____

   _____

   _____

   c. Metabolic acidosis: _____

   _____

   _____

   d. Metabolic alkalosis: _____

   _____

   _____

8. Describe the causes of the following changes in hemoglobin and/or hematocrit.

   a. Increased hematocrit: _____

   b. Decreased hematocrit: _____

   c. Increased hemoglobin: _____

   d. Decreased hemoglobin: _____

9. Briefly describe the following screening tests.

   a. Urine pH and specific gravity: _____

   b. Serum electrolytes: _____

   _____

   c. Arterial blood gases: _____

10. You are the visiting nurse for an elderly patient with diabetes. List four factors you should consider to prevent fluid imbalance for this patient.

    a. _____

    b. _____

    c. _____

    d. _____

11. List four guidelines for selecting a vein for an IV.

    a. _____

    b. _____

    c. _____

    d. _____

12. List the important points a home healthcare nurse should address when caring for a patient on home infusion therapy.

    _____

    _____

    _____

In the following cases, determine the acid–base imbalance. Refer to the chart below entitled Rules of ABG Interpretation for your answers.

13. Mr. W. is a 90-year-old man who had a successful cardiopulmonary resuscitation a few hours ago. He received bicarbonate during that resuscitation.

    ABGs: pH = 7.55; $PaCO_2$ = 43; HCO_3 = 36

    _____

    _____

14. Mr. F. is a 56-year-old man with a known history of COPD.

    ABGs: pH = 7.36; $PaCO_2$ = 60; HCO_3 = 35

    _____

    _____

15. A 55-year-old woman is admitted with chronic renal failure. She is weak and tired.

    ABGs: pH = 7.24; $PaCO_2$ = 30; HCO_3 = 12

    _____

16. Mrs. S. is a 55-year-old woman with heart failure and dyspnea. She complains of pleuritic pain.

    ABGs: pH = 7.56; $PaCO_2$ = 22; HCO_3 = 24

    _____

17. Ms. S. is a 21-year-old woman who has been found by her friends on the floor of her room. She is "out of it."

    ABGs: pH = 7.18; $PaCO_2$ = 79; HCO_3 = 26

    _____

18. Indicate in the chart on page 300 the nature of the acid–base disturbance, whether compensation is present or not; and if present, whether compensation is renal or respiratory, and partial or complete.

Rules of Interpretation		
pH	**PaCO$_2$**	**HCO$_3$**
<7.35 = acidosis	>45 mm Hg = respiratory acidosis	<22 mEq/L = metabolic acidosis
>7.45 = alkalosis	<35 mm Hg = respiratory alkalosis	>26 mEq/L = metabolic alkalosis

- It is <u>OK</u> to use what you know about your patient.
- The body usually does the smart thing to compensate: metabolic disorders—compensated by the lung; respiratory disorders—compensated by the kidney.
- Any pH below 7.35—state of acidosis; Any pH greater than 7.45—state of alkalosis; CO_2 is an acid—HCO_3 is a base. Any change in CO_2 reflects a respiratory change. Any change in HCO_3 reflects a metabolic change.
- Usually, the initiating abnormality is the predominate abnormality.

- If the pH has returned to <u>normal</u>, compensation has taken place.
- If the primary event is a fall in pH—whether respiratory or metabolic in origin—the arterial pH stays on the <u>acid</u> side after compensation. If the primary event is an increase in pH—whether respiratory or metabolic in origin—the arterial pH stays on the <u>base</u> side after compensation.

pH	PaCO$_2$	HCO$_3$	Nature of Disturbance	Comp. Present?		Renal	Respiratory	Partial	Complete
				If Yes			If Yes		
				Yes	No				
7.28	63	25							
7.20	40	14							
7.52	40	35							
7.48	30	31							
7.16	82	30							
7.36	68	35							
7.56	23	26							
7.40	40	26							
7.56	23	26							
7.26	70	25							
7.52	44	38							
7.32	30	18							
7.49	34	26							
6.98	84	18							

GUIDE TO CRITICAL THINKING AND DEVELOPING BLENDED SKILLS

1. Assess the following patients for fluid, electrolyte, and acid–base balance. What knowledge of the factors that influence fluid and electrolyte and acid–base balance would you draw on to develop a plan to prevent recurrence of these patient problems?

   a. A long-distance runner who is practicing on a hot day experiences dizziness and shows signs of dehydration.

   b. A older male adult with persistent heartburn ingests a large amount of sodium bicarbonate in one day.

   c. An infant is brought to the ER severely dehydrated after an extended bout of diarrhea.

2. Plan a low-salt diet for a patient who has high blood pressure. List healthy foods that are low in salt, and foods that are high in salt and that should be avoided. Check the sodium content of fast food in restaurants to see if any of these foods could be included on the diet.

PATIENT CARE STUDY

Read the following patient care study and use your nursing process skills to answer the questions below.

Rebecca is a college freshman who, on the night she had her wisdom teeth removed, had an oral temperature of 39.5°C (103.1°F). She had a sore throat several days before the extraction, but neglected to mention this to the oral surgeon. Because of the soreness in her throat, she reported having greatly decreased both her food and fluid intake. Friends that night gave her some Tylenol, which brought her temperature down, and encouraged her to drink more fluids. When they checked on her in the morning, her temperature was elevated again and she said she had felt too weak during the night to drink. She was brought to the student health service, where the admitting nurse noticed her dry mucous membranes, decreased skin turgor, and rapid pulse. At 5 feet, 2 inches and 98 pounds, Rebecca was petite, but she had lost 4 pounds in the last week.

1. Identify pertinent patient data by placing a single underline beneath the objective data in the case study and a double underline beneath the subjective data.

2. Complete the Nursing Process Worksheet on the next page to develop a three-part diagnostic statement and related plan of care for this patient.

3. Write down the patient and personal nursing strengths you hope to draw on as you assist this patient to better health.

   Patient strengths: _____

   _____

   _____

   Personal strengths: _____

   _____

   _____

   _____

4. Pretend that you are performing a nursing assessment of this patient after the plan of care has been implemented. Document your findings below.

   _____

   _____

   _____

   _____

NURSING PROCESS WORKSHEET

Health Problem (Title)	**Expected Outcome**
Related to ↓ **Etiology (Related Factors)**	**Nursing Interventions****
As Manifested by ↓ **Signs and Symptoms (Defining Characteristics)**	**Evaluative Statement**

*More than one patient goal may be appropriate. For the purposes of this exercise, develop the one patient
goal that demonstrates a direct resolution of the patient problem identified in the nursing diagnosis.
**Be sure you are able to list the scientific rationale for each nursing intervention you ordered.

Answer Key

Chapter 1

MATCHING

1. a	2. c	3. a	4. b	5. d	6. b
7. c	8. d	9. d	10. a	11. c	12. d

CORRECT THE FALSE STATEMENT

1. True
2. True
3. False—licensure
4. False—registered nurse
5. False—distinct and separate
6. False—ICN
7. False—the patient
8. True
9. False—The nurse facilitates coping with disability or death.
10. False—person-centered process

MULTIPLE CHOICE

1. b	2. d	3. c	4. b	5. a	6. a
7. b	8. c	9. b	10. d		

COMPLETION

1. Nursing is the demonstration of nonpossessive caring for and about others.
2. Nursing is sharing self with patients, other health-team members, and other nurses.
3. Nursing is touching to provide comfort and give care.
4. Nursing is sharing with patients in the human feelings of sorrow, joy, frustration, and satisfaction.
5. Nursing is listening attentively to the verbal and nonverbal communication signals of others.
6. Nursing is accepting self in order to accept others.
7. Nursing is respecting individual differences through unconditional acceptance, ensuring confidences and privacy, and individualizing care.
8. a. Promoting wellness: The nurse caringly prepares the patient for tests, explaining each test thoroughly to the patient, focusing on any questions the patient may have. The nurse also identifies patient's strengths—e.g., healthy diet, daily exercise routine—and weaknesses, e.g., inability to quit smoking.
   b. Preventing illness: The nurse refers the patient to a smoking-cessation program and, if necessary, educates the patient about the nature and treatment of lung cancer.
   c. Restoring health: The nurse provides direct care for the patient, administers medications, and carries out procedures and treatments for the patient.
   d. Facilitating coping: The nurse facilitates patient and family coping by helping the patient to live with altered functioning or prepare for death.

Title	Education/Preparation	Role Description
EXAMPLE		
Nurse Researcher	Advanced degree	Conducts research relevant to nursing practice and education
9. Nurse Midwife	Certificate or advanced degree	Provides pre/postnatal care; delivers babies in uncomplicated pregnancies.
10. Nurse Practitioner	Advanced degree, certification	Works in a variety of settings, providing health assessment and primary care
11. Nurse Anesthetist	Advanced degree	Administers and monitors anesthesia
12. Nurse Administrator	Advanced degree	Functions at various levels of management in health care settings
13. Nurse Entrepreneur	Advanced degree	Manages a clinic or health related business, conducts research, provides education, or serves as an advisor or consultant to institutions, political agencies or businesses

Timeline	Role of Medicine in Society	Role of Nurse in Society
14. Precivilization (Theory of Animism)	Belief in good and evil spirits bringing health or illness; medicine man as physician.	Nurse portrayed as mother caring for family with physical care and health remedies; nurturing, caring role of nurse continues to present day.
15. Beginning of civilization	Temples were centers of medical care; belief that illness is caused by sin and gods' displeasure; priest as physician.	Nurse viewed as slave carrying out menial tasks based on orders of priest.
16. Beginning of 16th century	Focus on religion replaced by focus on warfare, exploration and expansion of knowledge.	Shortage of nurses; criminals recruited nursing viewed as disreputable.
17. 18th–19th century	Hospital schools organized; female nurses under control of male hospital administrators and physicians; male dominance of health care.	Florence Nightingale elevated nursing to a respected occupation; founded modern methods in nursing education.
18. World War II	Explosion of knowledge in medicine and technology.	Efforts made to upgrade nursing education; women are more assertive and independent.
19. 1950s to present	Varied healthcare settings developed.	Nursing broadened in all areas; practiced in wide variety of settings; growth of nursing as a profession.

20. a. Profession: A well-defined body of knowledge, strong service orientation, recognized authority as a professional group, code of ethics, professional organization that sets standards, ongoing research, autonomy.
   b. Discipline: An impressive body of lasting works, suitable techniques, concerns that are relevant to human activities, relevant traditions that inspire future knowledge development, considerable scholarly recognition and achievement.
21. a. Rapid advances in technology require nurses to update their knowledge and skills to use the technology to give safe, individualized care.
   b. Nursing autonomy has increased the need for nurses to use critical thinking based on knowledge to provide safe care.

Chapter 2

MATCHING

1. c	2. e	3. b	4. a	5. d	6. c
7. e	8. a	9. d	10. a	11. b	12. b
13. c	14. b	15. a	16. c	17. d	18. b
19. a	20. d				

MULTIPLE CHOICE

1. d	2. a	3. d	4. c	5. a

COMPLETION

1. a. Physical: A family lives in a comfortable home located in a safe neighborhood. This meets the family needs of safety and comfort and enhances growth and development of the children.
   b. Economic: A family is able to afford adequate housing, food, clothing and community demands. This meets the family's need for nourishment, shelter, and acceptance in society.
   c. Reproductive: A family seeks family planning to limit their offspring to three children. This provides the society's need for more members without putting too heavy a demand on the family to provide and care for their children.
   d. Affective and coping: Parents counsel their children to avoid drinking alcohol, smoking cigarettes and using drugs. This meets the children's needs to be productive members of society and avoid the pitfalls surrounding adolescence.
   e. Socialization: Parents seek expert counseling for a kindergarten child who is having difficulty adjusting to school and relating to other children. This meets the child's need to "fit in" with other schoolmates and helps correct a problem before it gets out of hand.
2. a. The nurse helps to prepare the mother for her C-section and administers any medications prescribed.
   b. The nurse monitors the mother's and baby's blood pressure during the procedure.
   c. The nurse helps the husband to cope with his fears and gets him ready to participate in the birth of his child.
   d. The nurse reassures the mother that having a C-section is a common procedure and she should not feel that she is responsible for not being able to have the baby vaginally.
   e. The nurse helps the mother post-surgery to continue with her original plan to breast-feed her infant.
3. a. More and more families are becoming two-income families in order to keep up with society's economic demands.
   b. There are more career opportunities available to women and many women prefer a career to staying home and raising children in the traditional manner.
4. Answers will vary with student's experiences.

Chapter 3

MATCHING

1. e	2. j	3. d	4. a	5. f	6. b
7. g	8. i	9. c	10. h	11. l	12. g
13. d	14. e	15. a	16. c	17. f	18. b
19. h	20. a	21. a,e,f	22. a,c	23. d	24. a
25. a,c,e	26. a	27. f,g	28. h	29. a	30. j
31. c	32. b	33. i	34. d	35. f	36. e

MULTIPLE CHOICE

1. c	2. d	3. d	4. a	5. b	6. b
7. c	8. a	9. d			

COMPLETION

1. (Sample Answers)
   a. Investigate bus routes from patient's home; check if medical services are available within walking distance of patient; see if insurance will cover transportation to and from medical services.
   b. Boil water before using it; Check with social services to see if they can provide any necessary services for patient.
   c. Refer patient to drug and alcohol counseling service.
2. (Sample Answers).
   a. Reassure the patient that the "granny" woman is an important key to her recovery and attempt to contact this person. Include the "granny" woman's assessment in medical history of patient.
   b. Ask family to allow patient to answer questions and reassure them that their input is also important and that they can add any information they feel is necessary at the end of the interview.
   c. Find out what herb patient has been taking and its efficacy and check with physician if patient can still take this herb. Explain the prescribed medications to the patient and how they will alleviate her symptoms.
3. Answers will vary with student's experiences.
4. Sample Answers
   a. Does the patient need an interpreter?
   b. What are the cultural characteristics of the patient's communication with others?
   c. How does the patient speak and write in English?
   d. What cultural values and beliefs of the patient may change your techniques of communication and care?
5. Sample Answers
   a. The number of female-headed households is increasing as a result of divorce, abandonment, unmarried motherhood, and changes in abortion laws. Many households depend on two incomes for economic survival and a single woman supporting a household is at a financial disadvantage.
   b. Most older adults live on fixed incomes which often do not keep up with inflation and many, particularly widows are on the borderline of poverty or have already slipped into poverty.

   c. In many cases poverty is passed from generation to generation. This is true in such groups as migrant farm workers, families living on welfare, and people who live in isolated areas of Appalachia.
6. Answers will vary with student's experiences.

Chapter 4

MATCHING

1. f	2. a	3. e	4. b	5. c	6. d
7. b	8. d	9. a	10. c	11. b	12. a
13. c	14. d	15. a	16. b	17. e	

MULTIPLE CHOICE

1. a	2. c	3. c	4. d	5. a	6. b

COMPLETION

1. Answers will vary with student's experiences.
2. a. Acute: A temporary condition of illness in which patient goes through four stages: 1. symptoms, 2. assuming sick role, 3. dependent role—accepting diagnosis and following the treatment plan, and 4. recovery and rehabilitation—person gives up dependent role and resumes normal activities and responsibilities.
   b. Chronic: A permanent change; caused by irreversible alterations in normal anatomy and physiology; requires patient education for rehabilitation; requires long period of care or support. Characteristics: slow onset, periods of remission.
3. a. Physical dimension: A woman with severe arthritis must learn to live with condition and control pain.
   b. Emotional dimension: Worried about work, a 35-year-old executive exacerbates his ulcer.
   c. Intellectual dimension: The mother of a toddler must learn to childproof her house.
   d. Environmental dimension: An older woman has hand rails installed on her bathtub.
   e. Sociocultural dimension: A homeless man does not seek treatment for chest pain.
   f. Spiritual dimension: A Catholic woman refuses treatment for cancer and arranges a pilgrimage to a " holy site" where miraculous cures have been recorded by her religious leaders.
4. Answers will vary with student's experiences.
5. a. Primary: giving immunizations, providing dental care teaching
   b. Secondary: providing physical therapy, giving medications
   c. Tertiary: facilitating a support system, doing diabetic teaching
6. a. Being: recognizing self as separate and individual
   b. Belonging: being part of a whole
   c. Becoming: growing and developing
   d. Making personal choices to befit the self for the future

Chapter 5

MATCHING

1. f	2. c	3. i	4. h	5. d	6. e
7. b	8. a	9. g	10. f	11. a	12. i
13. b	14. j	15. c	16. h	17. d	18. e

MULTIPLE CHOICE

1. d	2. a	3. c	4. b	5. a	6. d
7. c	8. b	9. a	10. c		

COMPLETION

1. a. General systems theory: This theory explains break-ing whole things into parts and then learning how these parts work together in "systems." It includes the relationship between the whole and the parts and defines concepts about how the parts will function and behave.
    b. Stress/adaptation theory: This theory defines adapta-tion as the adjustment of living matter to other living things and to environmental conditions. Adaptation is a dynamic or continuously changing process that effects change and involves interaction and response. Human adaptation occurs on three levels—internal, social and physical.
    c. Developmental theory: Outlines the process of growth and development of humans as orderly and predictable, beginning with conception and ending with death. The growth and development of an indi-vidual are influenced by heredity, temperament, emo-tional and physical environment, life experiences, and health status.

2. a. Nursing theories identify and define interrelated con-cepts specific to nursing and clearly state the relation between these concepts.
    b. Nursing theories must be logical in nature and use orderly reasoning and identify relations that are developed using a logical sequence.
    c. Nursing theories must be consistent with the basic assumptions used in their development. They should be simple and general.
    d. Nursing theories should increase the nursing profes-sion's body of knowledge by generating research and should guide and improve practice.

3. a. Florence Nightingale identified the role of the nurse in meeting the patient's personal needs; recognizing the importance of environmental influences on the care of sick people.
    b. She elevated the standards and acceptance of nursing by developing sound principles of nursing education.
    c. She also demonstrated efficient and knowledgeable nursing care, defining nursing practice as separate and distinct from medical practice, and differentiated between health nursing and illness nursing.

4. a. Cultural influences on nursing: Until the last two decades, nursing essentially had been considered "women's work," and women were considered inferi-or to men. After Nightingale established an accept-able occupation for educated women and facilitated improved attitudes toward nursing, the role of the woman as nurse became more favorably accepted.

b. Educational influences on nursing: The service orien-tation of nursing was the strongest influence on nurs-ing practice until the 1950s. After World War II, women increasingly entered the work force, became more independent and sought higher education. Nursing education began to focus on education instead of training. In the 1960s college and university based baccalaureate programs in nursing increased in number and enrollment and master's and doctoral programs in nursing were established.

c. Research and publishing in nursing: Beginning in the 1950s great advances were made in technology and medical research; nursing leaders realized that research about the practice of nursing was necessary to meet the health needs of modern society.

d. Improved communication in nursing: Nursing is based on communication with others—patients, other healthcare team members, community members as well as with nurses practicing in a variety of specialty settings. Nurses need a knowledge base and common terminology to use in communicating with other pro-fessionals.

e. Improved autonomy of nursing: Nursing is in the process of defining its own independent functions and contributions to healthcare. The development and use of nursing theory provide autonomy in the practice of nursing.

5. Sample Answers
    a. Johnson's behavioral systems model: Mark would be treated as a human with two major systems; biologic and behavioral. Balance would be fostered in Mark between his behavior (drinking) and the effects of his drinking upon his system.
    b. King's theory of goal attainment: Mark would be treated as a human with an open system who is social, rational, perceiving, controlling, purposeful and action and time-oriented. The nurse would com-municate to Mark the seriousness of his drinking and work with him to change his behavior and achieve personal goals.
    c. Leininger's cultural care theory: Mark would be treated as a caring being capable of being concerned about. The nurse would explore Mark's physical, psychocultural and social aspects and individualize care directed toward promoting and maintaining health behaviors or recovery from alcoholism.
    d. Levine's four conservation principles theory of nurs-ing: Mark would be treated as a living being who is constantly interacting with his environment and adapting to change. Treatment would focus on Mark's environment and his interaction with the peo-ple around him.
    e. Neuman's healthcare systems model: Mark would be treated as a total person with biologic, psychologic, sociocultural and developmental variables. Treatment would focus on Mark and all the variables affecting his response to his disease.
    f. Orem's self-care deficit theory of nursing: Mark would be treated as a human with physical, psycho-logic, interpersonal and social components. He would meet self-care needs through learned behavior.

Through education, he would learn to substitute wholesome activities (exercise, hobbies, diet) for negative actions (drinking).

   g. Peplau's psychodynamic nursing: Mark would be treated as a human being undergoing the four phases of the nurse–patient relationship—orientation, identification, exploitation, and resolution. The nurse would meet collaboratively with Mark to identify and clarify his problem. The nurse would then assist him to understand his illness by helping him to explore his feelings about himself and his behavior. A nursing goal would be Mark's feeling of belonging and capability of dealing with the problem.

   h. Roger's theory of unitary human beings: Mark would be treated as a unified being with individuality constantly exchanging energy with the environment. Treatment would be directed on unifying all aspects of Mark's persona with his environment to bring about change in behavior.

   i. Roy's adaptation model: Mark would be treated as a biopsychosocial person that is basically good. Mark must learn to adapt to the changing needs of his society and environment without resorting to alcohol to get him through the process.

   j. Watson's philosophy and science of caring: Mark would be treated as a person in need of the caring process to attain health. Treatment would focus on human care for Mark's spiritual dimension as well as physical dimension and knowledge, values, commitment, and actions would be explored.

6. Answers will vary with student's experience.

Chapter 6

MATCHING

1. g	2. d	3. a	4. f	5. i	6. b
7. e	8. c	9. d	10. a	11. c	12. e
13. d	14. b	15. a	16. c	17. b	18. e
19. d	20. c	21. d	22. e	23. a	24. c
25. b	26. e	27. d	28. a	29. c	

MULTIPLE CHOICE

1. c	2. b	3. a	4. b	5. c	6. a

COMPLETION

1. Sample Answers
   a. Values clarification: Have the mother state the three most important things in her life. Explore her answers with her and find out why she chose them and how her choices may affect her situation.
   b. Choosing: After exploring the mother's values have her choose her key values freely. She may choose her child or profession.
   c. Prizing: Reinforce the mother's choices and, if possible, involve the husband and child in decision-making.
   d. Acting: Assist the mother to plan new behaviors consistent with the values she has chosen and incorporate them into her life. For example, if she values her child, she may reduce the number of classes she takes at night and spend more time with her.

2. Sample Answers
   a. Cost containment issues
   b. End of life decisions
   c. Incompetent, unethical, or illegal practices of colleagues
   d. Pain management

3. a. Autonomy: Respect the decision-making capacity of autonomous persons—e.g., A patient has the right to refuse treatment he does not feel would be helpful to his condition.
   b. Nomaleficence: Avoid causing harm—e.g., Be sure you are fully knowledgeable of a procedure before performing it.
   c. Beneficence: Provide benefits and balance these benefits against risks and harms—e.g., Securing a patient with restraints who is at high risk for falls.
   d. Justice: Distribute benefits, risks and costs fairly—e.g., Give service to all patients regardless of their life circumstances.
   e. Fidelity: Be faithful to promises you made to the public to be competent and be willing to use your competence to benefit patients entrusted to your care.

4. a. Ethical sensibility: The nurse would recognize that a patient's right to confidentiality has been breached.
   b. Ethical responsiveness: The nurse can decide to ignore her superior's breach of confidence, or she can confront her superior or report her to a higher authority.
   c. Ethical reasoning: The nurse confides in her mentor and discusses the options available to her.
   d. Ethical accountability: The nurse is willing to accept the reprecussions of any actions she takes to rectify the situation.
   e. Ethical character: Since the nurse valued patient confidentiality, her course of action was obvious.
   f. Ethical valuing: The nurse could not ignore the situation because of good ethical character and personal integrity.
   g. Transformative ethical leadership: As a result of her confronting her superior, the nurse was able to impact positively on the hospital environment.

5. Answers will vary with student's experiences.

6. Answers will vary with student's experiences.

7. Sample Answers
   a. Gather as much data as possible to support your diagnosis.
   b. Identify the ethical problem and explore solutions to the problem.
   c. Plan a course of action you can justify, e.g., seeking assistance for the patient at a higher level.
   d. Implement your decision by speaking to your superiors and presenting your case in a competent manner.
   e. Evaluate your decision: What was the outcome; how does this make me feel; did I make the right decision?

8. a. Breach of confidentiality, incompetent practice
   b. Covering for another nurse who is not performing her job competently, short-staffing
   c. Physician incompetence, conflicts concerning the role of the nurse in certain situations
   d. Cost-containment vs. hospitalization, healthcare rationing

Chapter 7

MATCHING

1. g	2. e	3. a	4. c	5. h	6. f.
7. b	8. i	9. i	10. h	11. a	12. l
13. c	14. d	15. k	16. b	17. f	18. g
19. j	20. c	21. g	22. a	23. b	24. d
25. e					

MULTIPLE CHOICE

1. c	2. b	3. a	4. c	5. d	6. b
7. c	8. a	9. c	10. d		

COMPLETION

1. Sample Answers
   a. Failure to ensure patient safety: Update knowledge on patient safety and new interventions to prevent and reduce injury.
   b. Improper treatment or performance of treatment: Use proper techniques when performing procedures and follow agency procedures.
   c. Failure to monitor and report: Follow physician orders regarding monitoring of patient unless changes in the patient's condition necessitate a change in the frequency of monitoring; report need for change to the physician.
   d. Medication errors and reactions: Listen to patient's objections regarding medication and investigate patient concerns before administering the medication.
   e. Failure to follow agency procedure: Advise the appropriate person of procedures that need to be revised.
   f. Equipment use: Learn how to operate equipment in a safe and appropriate manner. Never operate equipment with which you are unfamiliar.
   g. Adverse incidents: Do not assume, voice, or record any blame for an incident.
   h. Patient with HIV: Know and follow agency policies and procedures for the care of patients with infectious disease.
2. a. Voluntary standards: Developed and implemented by the nursing profession itself; not mandatory; used for peer review. Example: professional nursing organizations.
   b. Legal standards: developed by legislative action; implemented by authority granted by the state (or province) to determine minimum standards for the education of nurses, set requirements for licensure or registration, and decide when to revoke or suspend nurse's licenses. Example: licensure.
3. a. For each specialized diagnostic procedure.
   b. For experimentation involving patients.
   c. On admission for routine treatment.
   d. For medical or surgical treatment.
4. Sample Answers
   a. Talking with patients in rooms that are not soundproof.
   b. Pressing the patient for information not necessary for care planning.
   c. Using tape recorders, dictating machines, computer banks, etc. without taking precautions to ensure patient's confidentiality.

5. a. Solid educational background
   b. Understanding of the legal aspects of nursing and malpractice liability
   c. Knowledge of the state (or province) nurse practice act and standard of nursing care where the incident occurred
6. A contract must contain real consent of the parties, a valid consideration, a lawful purpose, competent parties, and the form required by law.
7. Sample Answer
   Limit telephone orders to true emergency situations; repeat a telephone order back to the physician; document the order, its time and date, situation necessitating order, physician prescribing, reconfirming the order as it is read back, and signing name, and VO or TO. If possible, two nurses should listen to a questionable telephone order with both nurses countersigning the order.
8. a. Contraindicated by normal practice.
   b. Contraindicated by patient's present condition.
9. Sample Answer
   The nurse is liable for her actions and should file an incident report. The incident report should contain the name of the patient, all witnesses, a complete factual account of the incident, the date, time, and place of the incident; pertinent characteristics of the person involved and other relevant variables believed important to the incident.
   Answers will vary with student's experience.

Chapter 8

MATCHING

1. d	2. a	3. f	4. e	5. h	6. e
7. g	8. c	9. b	10. g	11. e	12. c
13. f	14. a	15. d	16. b		

CORRECT THE FALSE STATEMENT

1. True
2. False—regular and predictable
3. True
4. False—different
5. False—sexuality
6. False—id
7. True
8. True
9. False—assimilation
10. False—preconventional level, stage 1, punishment and obedience orientation

MULTIPLE CHOICE

1. a	2. c	3. d	4. a	5. a	6. b
7. c	8. c	9. d	10. d		

COMPLETION

1. Complete the following chart by filling in the missing information relevant to theorists, their theories and basic concepts (see next page).
2. a. Preconventional level: Follows intuitive thought and is based on external control as child learns to con-

Theorist and Theory	Basic Concepts of Theory	Stages of Development
EXAMPLE		
Sigmund Freud Psychoanalytic theory	Stressed the impact of instinctual drives on determining behavior: Unconscious mind, the id, the ego the superego, stages of development based on sexual motivation.	Oral stage Anal stage Phallic stage Latent stage Genital stage
Eric Erikson Psychosocial theory	Based on Freud, expanded to include cultural and social influences in addition to biologic processes; (1) stages of development, (2) developmental goals or tasks, (3) psychosocial crises, (4) process of coping	Trust vs. mistrust Autonomy vs. shame/doubt Initiative vs. guilt Industry vs. inferiority Identity vs. role confusion Intimacy vs. isolation Generativity vs. stagnation Ego integrity vs. despair
Robert J. Havighurst Developmental tasks	Living and growing are based on learning; person must continually learn to adjust to changing social conditions, developmental tasks	Infancy and early childhood Middle childhood Adolescence Young adulthood Middle adulthood Later maturity
Jean Piaget Cognitive development	Learning occurs as result of internal organization of an event, which forms a mental schemata and serves as a base for further schemata as one grows and develops.	Sensorimotor stage Preoperational stage Concrete operational stage Formal operational stage
Lawrence Kohlberg Moral development	Levels closely follow Piaget's; preconventional level, conventional level, postconventional level; moral development influenced by cultural effects on perceptions of justice or interpersonal relationships	Preconventional level Stage 1: punishment and obedience orientation Stage 2: instrumental relativist orientation conventioinal level Stage 3: "good boy–good girl" orientation Stage 4: "law and order" orientation Post-conventional level Stage 5: social contract, utilitarian orientation Stage 6: universal ethical principle orientation
Carol Gilligan Moral development	Conception of morality from female point of view (ethic of care); selfishness, goodness, nonviolence; female: morality of response and care; Male: morality of justice.	Level 1—selfishness Level 2—goodness Level 3—nonviolence
James Fowler Faith development	Theory of spiritual identity of humans; faith is reason one finds life worth living; six stages of faith.	Intuitive–projective faith Mythical–literal faith Synthetic–conventional faith Individuative–reflective faith Conjunctive faith Universalizing faith

form to rules imposed by authority figures. Sample example: Child learns that he will be sent to his room if he writes on the walls.

b. Conventional level: This level is obtained when person becomes concerned with identifying with significant others and shows conformity to their expectations. Sample example: A college student gets all "A's" in college, so his parents will think he is a good son.

c. Postconventional level: This level is associated with moral judgment that is rational and internalized into one's standards or values. Sample example: A bank teller resists the urge to steal money from a patient's account because it is against the law.

3. Sample Answers
   a. Freud: The 6-year-old is between the phallic and

latency stage and will be experiencing increased interest in gender differences and conflict and resolution of that conflict with parent of same sex.

b. Erikson: The 6-year-old is becoming achievement oriented and the acceptance of parents and peers is paramount.

c. Havighurst: The 6-year-old is ready to learn the developmental tasks of developing physical skills, wholesome attitudes towards self, getting along with peers, sexual roles, conscience, morality, personal independence, etc. An illness could stall these processes.

d. Piaget: The 6-year-old is in the preoperational stage; increased language skills, play activities allowing child to better understand life events and relationships.

Copyright © 2001 Lippincott Williams & Wilkins. **Study Guide to Accompany Fundamentals of Nursing: The Art and Science of Nursing Care**, fourth edition by Carol Taylor, Carol Lillis, Priscilla LeMone, and Marilee LeBon

e. Kohlberg: Moral development is influenced by cultural effects on perceptions of justice in interpersonal relationships. Moral development begins in early childhood and could be affected by traumatic illness.

f. Gilligan: Females develop a morality of response and care; level one being selfishness: a woman may tend to isolate herself to avoid getting hurt.

g. Fowler: The 6-year-old is in stage 1—intuitive–projective faith. Children imitate religious gestures and behaviors of others, primarily their parents, without a thorough understanding of them.

4. a. Superego
   b. Identity vs role confusion
   c. Formal operations stage
   d. Synthetic–conventional faith

5. Sample Answer
   The family plays a vital role in wellness promotion and illness prevention. Family values and cultural heritage influence interpretation of illness. A health problem of any family member can affect the remainder of the unit. Many health practices are shared by the family. Sometimes the family may be the cause of illness.

Chapter 9

MATCHING

1. f	2. d	3. d	4. f	5. a	6. c
7. b	8. e				

MULTIPLE CHOICE

1. c	2. a	3. b	4. b	5. c	6. b
7. b	8. b	9. a	10. c	11. c	12. b
13. d					

COMPLETION

1. Age group—Physiologic characteristics and behaviors.
   P—Motor abilities include skipping, throwing and catching, copying figures, and printing letters and numbers.
   A—Puberty begins.
   I—Brain grows to about half the adult size.
   N—Reflexes include sucking, swallowing, blinking, sneezing, yawning.
   N—Temperature control responds quickly to environmental temperatures.
   T—Walks forward and backward, runs, kicks, climbs, rides tricycle.
   T—Drinks from a cup and uses a spoon.
   A—Sebaceous and axillary sweat glands become active.
   S—Height increases 2–3 inches, weight increases 3–6 lb. a year.
   A—The feet, hands, and long bones grow rapidly, muscle mass increases.
   N—Alert to environment, sees color and form, hears and turns to sound.
   I—Birth weight usually triples.
   P—Full set of 20 deciduous teeth, baby teeth fall out and are replaced.

P—Body is less chubby and becomes leaner and more coordinated.
A—Primary and secondary development occurs with maturation of genitals.
T—Typically four times the birth weight and 23–37 inches in height.
I—Body temperature stablizes.
P—Average weight is 45 pounds.
S—Brain reaches 90%–95% of adult size, nervous system almost mature.
P—Head is close to adult size.
I—Motor abilities develop, allowing feeding self, crawling, and walking.
N—Can smell and taste, and is sensitive to touch and pain.
N—Eliminates stool and urine.
I—Deciduous teeth begin to erupt.
S—All permanent teeth present except for 2nd and 3rd molars.
T—Bladder control during the day and sometimes during the night.
S—Holds a pencil, and eventually writes in script and sentences.
A—Full adult size is reached.
N—Drinks breast milk, glucose water, and plain water.
I—Eyes begin to focus and fixate.
T—Turns pages in a book and by age 3, draws stick people.
I—Heart doubles in weight, heart rate slows, blood pressure rises.
T—Rapid brain growth; increase in length of long bones of the arms/legs.
T—Uses fingers to pick up small objects.
S—Sexual organs grow but are dormant until late in this period.

2. Age group—Psychosocial characteristics and behaviors.
   I—Is in oral stage (Freud); strives for immediate gratification of needs. Strong sucking need.
   S—Developmental task of learning appropriate sex's social role.
   A—In Freud's genital stage, libido reemerges in mature form.
   T—Is in anal stage (Freud); focus on pleasure of sphincter control.
   A—Self-concept is being stabilized, with peer group as greatest influence.
   I—Develops trust (Erikson) if caregiver is dependable to meet needs.
   S—Achieving personal independence, developing conscience, morality, and scale of values.
   A—Tries out different roles, personal choices, and beliefs (identity vs. role confusion).
   I—Meets developmental tasks (Havighurst) by learning to eat/walk/talk.
   S—Develops skill in reading, writing, and calculating, and concepts for everyday living.
   A—More mature relationships with both males and females of same age.
   T—Enters Erikson's stage of autonomy vs. shame and doubt.

P—Is in Erikson's stage of initiative vs. guilt.

A—Inner turmoil/examination of propriety of actions by rigid conscience.

P—Getting ready to read and learning to distinguish right from wrong.

A—One's personal appearance accepted; set of values internalized.

S—Freud's latency stage—strong identification with own sex.

T—Developmental tasks of learning to control elimination; begins to learn sex differences, concepts, learn language, learn right from wrong.

P—Focus on learning useful skills, emphasis on doing, succeeding, accomplishing.

P—Developmental tasks of describing social and physical reality through concept formation and language development.

P—Is in phallic stage (Freud) with biologic focus on genitals.

A—Superego and conscience begin to develop.

P—Developmental tasks of learning sex differences and modesty.

S—Developmental task of learning physical game skills.

S—Is in Erikson's Industry vs. inferiority stage.

3. a. Preembryonic stage: Lasts about 3 weeks; zygote implants in the uterine wall and has three distinct cell layers: ectoderm, endoderm, and mesoderm.

b. Embryonic stage: 4th through 8th week; rapid growth and differentiation of the germ cell layers, all basic organs established, bones ossify and human features are recognizable.

c. Fetal stage: 9 weeks to birth; continued growth and development of all body organs and systems take place.

4. a. Gross motor behavior and skills

b. Fine motor behavior and skills

c. Language acquisition

d. Personal and social interaction

5. Sample Answers

a. Infant sleeps, eats and eliminates easily; smiles spontaneously; and cries in response to significant needs.

b. Infant is more passive and distant than the "easy" infant.

c. Infant has volatile and labile responses, often is restless sleeper, is highly sensitive to noises and eats poorly.

6. a. Colic is acute abdominal pain caused by spasmodic contractions of the intestine during the first 3 months of life. The nurse should educate the parents about colic and teach them measures to help relieve the symptoms.

b. Failure to thrive is a condition thought to be related to a disturbed infant–primary caregiver interaction, which results in severely inadequate physiologic development. Underlying physical causes should be ruled out first; if the cause is psychosocial, specialized health interventions are warranted.

c. Sudden infant death syndrome is the sudden, unexpected death of an infant or young child in which a postmortem examination fails to reveal a cause of death. Parents should be aware that highest incidence occurs in families who are poor, or live in crowded housing in cold months of the year during sleep periods. Maternal health, smoking, and nutrition are being investigated; infants should sleep on their side or back.

d. Child abuse is the intentional, nonaccidental, physical or sexual abuse of a child by a parent or other caregiver. Healthcare professionals must recognize and report abuse of children and provide interventions for high-risk families.

7. Sample Answers

a. Toddler: A toddler begins to understand object permanence, following simple commands, and anticipating events. The perception of body image begins and the toddler uses short sentences. The nurse should be aware that the toddler may experience separation anxiety; parents should be included in the preparation; language should be clear and simple.

b. Pre-schooler: A pre-schooler may have fear of pain and body mutilation as well as separation anxiety that must be recognized by the nurse. The child needs much reassurance and parental support. A pre-procedure visit should be scheduled if possible; allowing the child to practice on a doll may be helpful.

c. School-age: Body image, self-concept and sexuality are interrelated. The school-age child has well-developed language skills and ability to store information in long-term memory. The procedure should be explained clearly and thoroughly to child and caregivers.

d. Adolescent: The adolescent tries out different roles, personal choices, and beliefs in the stage called identity versus role confusion. Self-concept is being stabilized, with peer group acting as the influential body. The nurse should be aware of the adolescent's need to understand the procedure and its benefits/risks.

8. Sample Answers

a. Infant: The most important role of the nurse is the prevention of illness and promotion of wellness through teaching family members. Teaching may range from scheduling immunizations to counseling parents who have a baby born with AIDS.

b. Toddler: The role of the nurse is in wellness promotion, helping caregivers find the means of helping toddlers through encouraging health independence while setting firm limits. Safety measures for parents of active toddlers should be taught.

c. Pre-schooler: Promoting wellness continues for the pre-schooler with emphasis on teaching accident prevention and safety, infection control, dental hygiene, play habits, and encouraging self-esteem.

d. School-age: Areas of concern for school-age children are traffic, bicycle and water safety. Substance abuse teaching should be included, and communicable conditions should be discussed. Nurses should work with parents and teachers to recognized mental health disorders, encourage physical fitness and positive self-identity.

e. Adolescent: Nurses should educate adolescents and family about substance abuse, motor vehicle accidents, nutrition, and sex education. Nurses and parents should be aware of the adolescent's need to belong to a peer group, be like everyone else, and try on different roles.

9. a. Prepubescence: Secondary sex characteristics begin to develop but the reproductive organs do not yet function.
   b. Pubescence: Secondary sex characteristics continue to develop and ova and sperm begin to be produced by the reproductive organs.
   c. Postpubescence: Reproductive functioning and the development of secondary sex characteristics reach adult maturity.

Chapter 10

MATCHING

1. b   2. e   3. g   4. i   5. a   6. c
7. f   8. d   9. j

MULTIPLE CHOICE

1. c   2. a   3. c   4. d   5. b   6. c
7. a   8. d   9. b   10. b

COMPLETION

1. a. Middle adulthood
   Physiologic development: The early years are marked by maximum physical development and functioning. As time passes, gradual internal and external changes occur.
   Psychosocial development: Usually a time of increased personal freedom, economic stability, and social relationships, increased responsibility, and awareness of one's own mortality.
   Cognitive, moral, and spiritual development: Intellectual abilities change from those of the young adult. There is increased motivation to learn. Problem-solving abilities remain, although response time may be slightly longer.
   b. Older adulthood:
   Physiologic development: The process of aging becomes more rapid. All organ systems undergo some degree of decline and body becomes less efficient.
   Psychosocial development: Most continue their activities from middle adulthood and adapt intuitively to gradual limitations of aging.
   Cognitive, moral, and spiritual development: Cognition does not change appreciably with aging; an older adult continues to learn and problem solve, and intelligence and personality remain consistent.
2. The children of the middle-aged adult are often independent and have children of their own. As involvement and responsibility for children decreases, there may be an increasing need to become involved in caring for aging parents.
3. Sample Answers
   a. Complete physical examination every 2 years.
   b. Annual dental examination.
   c. Eye examination every 1–2 years.
   d. Maintenance of current immunizations.
   e. Cancer screening for women.
4. a. Genetic theory: Explains that lifespan depends to a great extent on genetic factors.

   b. Immunity theory: Focuses on the functions of the immune system which declines steadily after young adulthood.
   c. Cross-linkage theory: As one ages, cross-links accumulate, leading to essential molecules in the cell binding together and interfering with normal cell function.
   d. Free radical theory: Free radicals formed during cellular metabolism are molecules with separated high-energy electrons that can have adverse effects on and attack adjacent molecules.
5. Alzheimer's disease affects brain cells, and is characterized by patchy areas of the brain that degenerate, or break down. At first, forgetfulness and impaired judgment may be evident; over a period of several years, the person becomes progressively more confused, forgetting family and becoming disoriented in familiar surroundings.
6. a. Disengagement theory: Maintains that an older adult withdraws from societal interactions because it is mutually desired and satisfying for both the individual and society.
   b. Activity theory: Successful aging involves the ability to maintain high levels of activity and functioning.
   c. Identity-continuity theory: Assumes that healthy aging is related to the ability of the older adult to continue similar patterns of behavior that existed in young to middle adulthood.
7. a. Integumentary: Wrinkling and sagging of skin occur with decreased skin elasticity; dryness and scaling are common.
   b. Musculoskeletal: Muscle mass and strength decrease.
   c. Neurologic: Temperature regulation and pain perception become less efficient.
   d. Cardiopulmonary: The body is less able to increase heart rate and cardiac output with activity.
   e. Gastrointestinal: Malnutrition and anemia become more common.
   f. Genitourinary: Blood flow to the kidneys decreases with diminished cardiac output.

Chapter 11

MATCHING

1. f   2. d   3. g   4. b   5. e   6. j
7. h   8. l   9. c   10. i   11. m   12. q
13. a   14. n   15. p   16. h   17. f   18. a
19. j   20. g   21. e   22. b   23. c   24. i
25. d

MULTIPLE CHOICE

1. a   2. b   3. a   4. d   5. c   6. c
7. d   8. b   9. a   10. a

COMPLETION

1. a. DRGs encourage early discharge from the hospital and have created a new acutely ill population who need skilled care at home.
   b. There are increasing numbers of older people living longer with multiple chronic illnesses who are not institutionalized.
   c. With more sophisticated technology, people can be kept alive and comfortable in their own homes.

d. Healthcare consumers demand that services be humane and provisions be made for a dignified death at home.

2. a. Primary care office: Make health assessments, assist physician and provide health education.

   b. Ambulatory care centers and clinics: A nurse practitioner may run these centers which usually provide walk-in services and are open at times other than traditional office hours.

   c. Mental health centers: Nurses who work in crisis intervention centers must have strong communication and counseling skills and must be thoroughly familiar with community resources specific to the need of patients being served.

   d. Rehabilitation centers: These centers use a healthcare team comprised of physicians, nurses, physical therapists, occupational therapists, and counselors.

   e. Long-term care centers: Help patients maintain patient function and independence with concern for the living environment as well as the healthcare provided. Provide direct care, supervise others, administrate, and teach.

3. With the trend toward discharging patients earlier in their hospital stay, hospitals more often focus on the acute care needs of the patient. Along with this focus has come a proliferation of services offered by the hospital aimed at the outpatient.

4. a. Surgical procedures
   b. Diagnostic tests
   c. Medications
   d. Physical therapy
   e. Counseling
   f. Health education

5. DRG: Diagnosis-related groups: this plan pays the hospital a predetermined, fixed amount that is determined by the medical diagnosis or specific procedure rather than by the actual cost of hospitalization and care. DRGs were implemented by the federal government in an effort to control rising healthcare costs. If the cost for hospitalization is greater than that assigned, the hospital must absorb the additional cost. However, if costs are less than that assigned, the hospital makes a profit.

6. See the following table.

7. When patients come in contact with many different healthcare providers (e.g., registered nurses, licensed practical nurses, nursing assistants, nurse specialists, physical therapists, dietitians, and students) and are frequently seen by other physician specialists called in on consultation or to do surgery, the patient may become confused about care and treatment. This *fragmentation of care* may result in the loss of continuity of care, resulting in conflicting plans of care, too much or too little medication, and higher healthcare costs.

Plan	Description	Advantages	Disadvantages
a. HMO	Prepaid group health care plans that allow enrollees to receive all medical services they require through a group of affiliated providers.	Often no additional out of pocket costs.	Patient does not have a choice about health care providers.
b. PPO	Third party payor contracts with a group of health care providers to provide services at a lower fee in return for prompt payment and guaranteed volume.	Patients have more choices than HMO; may seek care outside the panel.	May pay additional out-of-pocket expenses.
c. PPA	Type of PPO; contract is made with an individual health care provider rather than a group of providers.		
d. Private	Third-party payers; insurance company pays all or most of the cost of care.	Patient can choose own physician and services.	More expensive premiums
e. LTC	Long-term care. Most is paid for by Medicaid and out-of-pocket spending	Covers a variety of services such as nursing home care, home care, and adult day care centers.	
f. Medicare	Government program providing insurance for all citizens over 65 for hospital care, extended care and home health care.	Expanded to include catastrophic care costs	Based on DRGs. The full cost of some services is not covered; supplemental insurance is recommended.
g. Medicaid	Federally funded public assistance program for people of low income.	Free coverage for the disadvantaged	The rapid growth of aging population and increase of poor are draining the Medicaid budget, forcing reduced benefits.

Chapter 12

CORRECT THE FALSE STATEMENT
1. False—nurse
2. False—continuity of care
3. True
4. True
5. False—patient's name, I.D. number, and physician
6. False—decreasing
7. False—is indicated
8. True
9. False—remains at the hospital
10. False—physician's order

MULTIPLE CHOICE
1. c   2. a   3. d   4. a   5. b   6. c

COMPLETION
1. Sample Answers
   a. With patient's permission, check with relatives, neighbors, or fellow church or club members who could help; if necessary, check with social agencies available.
   b. Describe the procedure to the patient in detail so he/she will know what to expect.
   c. Check the patient's insurance status, Medicare, or Medicaid; see if procedures are covered and what amount the patient will be responsible for. Refer to the appropriate agencies if necessary.
   d. With patient's permission, check with family; if necessary, check into home healthcare possibilities, hospice, or extended care facilities.
2. a. Medications: Drug name, dosage, purpose, effect, times taken, stated verbally and in writing.
   b. Procedures and treatments: Demonstrate all steps, practice and put into writing. Caregivers should demonstrate procedures.
   c. Diet: Explain diet and purpose; give examples of meals and written plans.
   d. Referrals: Instruct patient and family how to make follow-up visits and who to call with problems.
   e. Health promotion: All aspects of the illness or effects of treatment should be described verbally and written materials supplied.
3. a. Discharge planning: Exchanges information among the patient, caregivers, and those responsible for home care while the patient is in the institution and after the patient returns home.
   b. Collaboration with other members of the healthcare team: Meets the patient's and family's physical, psychologic, sociocultural, and spiritual needs in all settings and at all levels of health.
   c. Involving patient and family in planning: Ensures that patient and family needs are consistently met as the patient moves from one level of care to another.
4. a. Assess the patient's need for nursing care related to admission.

b. Include consideration of biophysical, psychosocial, environmental, self-care, educational, and discharge planning factors in each patient's assessment.
   c. Involve the patient and family in care as appropriate.
   d. Nursing staff members should collaborate, as appropriate, with physicians and member of other clinical disciplines to make decisions regarding the patient's need for nursing care.
   e. Assess continuing care need in preparation for discharge and document referrals for such care in the patient's medical record.
5. a. Establish the health data base: Age; sex; height; weight; medical history, including any prior miscarriages; current medical treatment, follow-up treatment.
   b. Assess for personal data: Personal feelings about her miscarriage, effectiveness of personal coping methods.
   c. Explore husband's relationship with patient and ability to provide emotional support.
   d. Check if there are any support services, (e.g., support groups, fertility clinics) that would be available to this couple.
6. a. Transfer within the hospital setting: Patient's belongings and/or furniture are moved; patient's chart, Kardex, care plan, and medications must be correctly labeled for the new room, and other departments notified as appropriate. If transfer is to a new floor, the nurse at the original area gives a verbal report about the patient to the nurse at the new area.
   b. Transfer to a long-term facility: All of patient's belongings are carefully packed and sent to facility; prescriptions and appointment cards for return visits to the physician's office may be sent; patient is discharged from hospital setting but a copy of chart may be sent to long-term facility along with a detailed assessment and care plan.
   c. Discharge from a healthcare setting: Check patient discharge order; instructions; equipment and supplies and financial arrangements. Assist patient to dress and pack belongings; check for written order for future services; transport patient to car and assist as necessary; make necessary recordings on records and complete discharge summary.
7. A form must be signed that releases the physician and healthcare institution from any legal responsibility for the patient's health status; the patient is informed of any possible risk before signing the form; the signature of the patient must be witnessed, and the form becomes part of the patient's record.
8. Position the bed in its highest position; arrange the furniture in the room to allow easy access to the bed. Open the bed by folding back the top bed linens. Assemble necessary equipment and supplies. Assemble special equipment and supplies (e.g., oxygen therapy equipment) and make sure it is working properly. Adjust the physical environment of the room.

Chapter 13

MATCHING
1. a   2. c   3. c   4. b   5. b   6. a

CORRECT THE FALSE STATEMENT
1. False: hospital-based care to community-based care
2. True
3. False: chronic and acute
4. False: care must be adapted to patient's schedule
5. False: Mary Brewster
6. True
7. False: generalists
8. False: are responsible
9. True
10. True
11. False: short term
12. True
13. True

MULTIPLE CHOICE
1. d   2. c   3. a   4. b

COMPLETION
1. See the following table.
2. Sample Answers
   a. Home care nurses must have knowledge of legal regulations, physical assessment, body mechanics, nursing diagnoses, and infection control.
   b. Home care nurses enjoy practicing in an autonomous setting where they can use their expertise in an expanded role.
   c. Home care nurses are accountable to the patient, the family, and the primary healthcare provider.
3. a. Patient advocate: Protecting and supporting the patient's rights—The home care nurse helps a patient prepare a living will.
   b. Coordinator of services: The home care nurse is the coordinator of all other healthcare providers visiting the patient—The home care nurse helps arrange for rehabilitation services for a stroke patient.
   c. Educator: Home care nurses spend time teaching patients and families about the disease process, nutrition, medications, or treatment and care of wounds—Teaches a patient with diabetes about diet.
4. a. Wash hands before accessing supplies from the bag.
   b. Anything the nurse takes out of bag must be cleaned before returning it to the bag.
   c. Anytime the nurse needs to access the bag, handwashing must take place first.
   d. The bag should be placed on a liner before setting it down in the patient's home.
5. Teaching is geared to the patient's readiness to learn and adapted to the patient's physical and emotional status. Information that is essential to keep patients safe until the next visit is the major focus. Teaching is adapted to what works best in the home. Incentives to learn include knowledge of serious consequences as well as positive benefits of carrying through with certain behaviors.
6. As healthcare continues to shift from the hospital setting to community-based care, families will bear the burden associated with this change. Patients are discharged sooner with a higher acuity level; chronically ill patients will need continued long-term personal care at home not covered by Medicare.
7. Sample Answer:
The nurse would work with an interdisciplinary team of other health professionals such as social workers, pastoral counselors, home health aides, and volunteers to provide comprehensive palliative care. Emotional support would be provided for the husband and children as well as the patient, and pain and symptom management would be conducted. The focus is on improving the quality of life for the patient and preserving dignity for the patient in death. Bereavement care would continue for the family for 6 months after the death.

Date	Home Health Care Provider/Location	Type of Care
1893	Henry Street Settlement House, New York City	Visiting nurses cared for poor residents living in tenements.
Prior to WWII During and Post WWII	Physician Nurses	Often made home care visits to treat the sick. There was a shift in practice from the home to the hospital and office setting. Nurses provided most home care visits.
Mid 1960s	1965 Social Security Act	Home care services expanded to include the older population. The social security act provided program coverage for older adults participating in Medicare.
Post 1980	Home care specialists	Many home care nurses have specialized in advanced practice skills to meet the growing demands of acutely ill patients cared for at home.
2000s	Nurses and families	More complex services provided at home. Increasing numbers of surgical procedures performed on outpatient basis; families have more responsibility providing care.

Chapter 14

MATCHING

1. a	2. d	3. e	4. b	5. c	6. a
7. e	8. b	9. c	10. e	11. d	12. a
13. c	14. b	15. d	16. a	17. d	18. b
19. a	20. c	21. b	22. d		

MULTIPLE CHOICE

1. c	2. a	3. b	4. c	5. d	6. c
7. d	8. d				

COMPLETION

1. Patient:
   a. scientifically based, holistic, individualized care
   b. The opportunity to work collaboratively with nurses
   c. Continuity of care
   Nursing:
   a. Achievement of a clear and efficient plan of action by which the entire nursing team can achieve results for patients.
   b. Satisfaction that the nurse is making an important difference in the lives of their patients.
   c. Opportunity to grow professionally when evaluating the effectiveness of interventions and variables that contribute positively or negatively to the patient's goal achievement.

2. a. Determining the need for nursing care: The nursing process provides a framework that enables the nurse and patient to systematically collect patient data and clearly identify patient strengths and problems.
   b. Planning and implementing the care: The nursing process helps the nurse and patient develop a holistic plan of individualized care that specifies both the desired patient goals and nursing action most likely to assist the patient to meet those goals and execute the plan of care.
   c. Evaluating the results of the nursing care: The nursing process provides for evaluation of the plan of care in terms of patient goal achievement.

3. The nursing process is a systematic, patient-centered, goal-oriented method of caring that provides a framework for nursing practice.
   The goals of the nursing process are to help the nurse manage each patient's care scientifically, holistically, and creatively to promote wellness, prevent disease or illness, restore health, and facilitate coping with altered functioning.
   The skills necessary to use the nursing process successfully include intellectual, technical, interpersonal, and ethical/legal skills, as well as the willingness to use these skills creatively when working with patients.

4. Sample Answers
   a. Systematic: Each nursing task is a part of an ordered sequence of activities and each activity depends of the accuracy of the activity that precedes it and influences the actions that follow it.
   b. Dynamic: There is great interaction and interlapping among the five steps, no one step in the process is a one-time phenomenon; each step is fluid and flows into the next step.
   c. Interpersonal: The human being is always at the heart of nursing. The nursing process ensures that nurses are patient-centered, rather than task-centered.
   d. Goal-oriented: The nursing process offers a means for nurses and patients to work together to identify specific goals related to wellness promotion, disease and illness prevention, health restoration, and coping with altered functioning that are most important to the patient and match them with appropriate nursing actions.
   e. Universally applicable: Once nurses have a working knowledge of the nursing process, they can apply it to well or ill patients, young or old patients in any type of practice setting.

5. a. Purpose of thinking: This helps to discipline thinking by keeping all thoughts directed to the goal.
   b. Adequacy of knowledge: It is important to judge if the knowledge available to you is accurate, complete, and relevant. If you reason with false information or lack important data, it is impossible to draw a sound conclusion.
   c. Potential problems: As you become more skilled in critical thinking, you will learn to "flag" or remedy pitfalls to sound reasoning.
   d. Helpful resources: Wise professionals are quick to recognize their limits and seek help in remedying their deficiencies.
   e. Critique of judgment/decision: Ultimately you must identify alternative judgments or decisions, weigh their merits, and reach a conclusion.

6. Sample Answers
   a. Practice a necessary skill until you feel confident in its execution before performing it on a patient.
   b. Take time to familiarize yourself with new equipment before using it in a clinical procedure.
   c. Identify nurses who are technical experts and ask them to share their secrets.
   d. Never be ashamed to seek assistance when feeling unsure of how to perform a procedure or manage equipment.

7. Answers will vary with student's experience.

8. Answers will vary with student's experience.

9. Sample Answers
   a. I'm nurse Brown and I'll be your nurse this week. What would you like to accomplish with this time and how can I help you get through this period?
   b. What family members do you expect to see while you are here? Do you trust them to make decisions about your care if you were unable to do so yourself?
   c. What are your goals, hopes, and dreams in life? How do you hope to accomplish them? How will your hospitalization affect these goals?
   d. Tell me about your life at home/school/work. Is there anyone or anything in particular that you will miss during your recuperation?

10. a. Do I know the legal boundaries of my practice?
    b. Do I "own" my personal strengths and weaknesses and seek assistance as needed?
    c. Am I knowledgeable about, and respectful of, patient rights?
    d. Does my documentation provide a legally defensible account of my practice?

Chapter 15

MATCHING
1. f   2. j   3. e   4. c   5. g   6. i
7. k   8. a   9. b   10. d   11. a   12. b
13. a   14. a   15. b   16. b

MULTIPLE CHOICE
1. c   2. d   3. c   4. c   5. a   6. c
7. b   8. d   9. d

COMPLETION
1. a. Make a judgment about a patient's health status.
   b. Make a judgment about a patient's ability to manage his or her own healthcare.
   c. Make a judgment about a patient's need for nursing.
   d. Refer the patient to a physician or other healthcare professional.
   e. Plan and deliver individualized, holistic nursing care that draws on the patient's strengths.
2. a. Patient: Most patients are willing to share information when they know it is helpful in planning their care.
   b. Support people: Family members, friends, and caregivers are helpful sources of data when a patient is a child or has limited capacity to share information with the nurse.
   c. Patient record: A review of the records prepared by different members of the healthcare team provides information essential to comprehensive nursing care.
   d. Medical history, physical examination, and progress notes: Sources that record the findings of physicians as they assess and treat the patient.
   e. Reports of laboratory and other diagnostic studies: These sources (e.g., x-rays and diagnostic tests) can either confirm or conflict with data collected during the nursing history or examination.
   f. Reports of therapies by other healthcare professionals: Other healthcare professionals record their findings and note progress in specific areas (e.g., nutrition, physical therapy, or speech therapy).
   g. Other healthcare professionals: other nurses, physicians, social workers, etc., can provide information about a patient's normal health habits and patterns and response to illness.
   h. Nursing and other healthcare literature: If a nurse is unfamiliar with a disease, it is important for him or her to read about the clinical manifestations of the disease and its usual progression to know what to look for when assessing the patient.
3. a. Complete: All patient data need to be identified to understand a patient's health problem and develop a plan of care to maximize health promotion.
   b. Factual and accurate: Nurses concerned with accuracy and fact must continually verify what they hear with what they observe using other senses and validate all questionable data.
   c. Relevant: Because recording data can become an endless task, nurses must determine what type of data and how much data to collect for each patient.
4. Sample Answers
   a. What are the patient's current responses to his or her situation?
   b. What is the patient's current ability to manage his or her care?
   c. What is the immediate environment?
5. a. Patient should know the name of his/her primary nurse and what he/she can expect of nursing.
   b. Patient should sense that the nurse is competent and cares about him/her.
   c. Patient should know what is expected of him/her in terms of developing the plan of care and participating in its execution.
6. Sample Answers
   a. Closed questions:
      How long have you been experiencing these symptoms? How many children do you have at home?
   b. Open-ended questions:
      How will you modify your diet now that you have been diagnosed with diabetes? What do you know about insulin injections?
   c. Reflective questions:
      What effect will diabetes have upon your life? How do you feel about using insulin injections to control your diabetes?
7. a. Patient's health orientation: Patients must identify potential and actual health risks and explore habits, behaviors, beliefs, attitudes, and values that influence levels of health.
   b. Patient's developmental stage: Nursing assessments are modified according to the developmental stage of patients.
   c. Patient's need for nursing: Whether the nurse will interact with the patient for a short or long period and the nature of nursing care needs influence the type of data the nurse collects.
8. a. When there are discrepancies; e.g., when a patient claims he has no pain but grimaces when you touch his chest.
   b. When the data lack objectivity; e.g., when a patient claims to have 20/20 vision, but holds his reading material far away from his face.
9. Immediate communication of data is indicated whenever assessment findings reveal a critical change in the patient's health status that necessitates the involvement of other nurses or healthcare professionals.

Chapter 16

MATCHING
1. c   2. a   3. b   4. d   5. a   6. c
7. d

CORRECT THE FALSE STATEMENTS
1. False—nursing diagnosis
2. False—nursing diagnosis
3. False—standard or norm
4. True
5. False—cluster of significant data
6. True
7. False—etiology
8. True
9. False—potential
10. True
11. True
12. False—analyzes patient data
13. False—risk management diagnosis

MULTIPLE CHOICE
1. c   2. a   3. d   4. c   5. a   6. c

COMPLETION
1. a. Using legally inadvisable language.
   b. ✔
   c. Identifying responses not necessarily unhealthy.
   d. ✔
   e. Both clauses say the same thing.
   f. ✔
   g. Including value judgment.
   h. Identifying responses not necessarily unhealthy.
   i. ✔
   j. Including medical diagnosis.
   k. Identifying problems as signs and symptoms.
   l. Reversing clauses.
   m. ✔
   n. Both clauses say the same thing.
   o. Identifying problems/etiologies that cannot be altered.
   p. Both clauses say the same thing.
   q. ✔
   r. Writing diagnosis in terms of needs.
2. Sample Answers
   a. Were you able to pass urine this morning? Did you drink the fluids we brought you?
   b. Do you feel like talking to other patients who are undergoing the same treatment? Would you like to see your family today?
   c. Do you feel helpless to put your life back in order? Are you overwhelmed by the changes in your life?
   d. Were you able to get some sleep last night? Did the noise on the unit keep you awake?
3. a. No problem: Reinforce patient's health habits and patterns; initiate health promotion activities to prevent disease or illness or promote higher level of wellness.
   b. Possible problem: Collect more data to confirm or disconfirm suspected problem.
   c. Actual or potential nursing diagnosis: Unable to treat because patient denies problem or refuses treatment;

begin planning, implementing, and evaluating care designed to prevent, reduce, or resolve problem.
   d. Clinical problem other than nursing diagnosis: Consult with appropriate healthcare professional and work collaboratively on problem; refer to medicine.
4. Sample Answers
   a. An infant who is below the normal growth standards for his age group may be experiencing "failure to thrive."
   b. A mother who has a history of mental illness shows little or no interest in her baby.
   c. A patient placed in a nursing home by her son becomes incontinent without physical cause.
5. Mr. Klinetob, aged 86, has been seriously depresssed since the death of his wife of 52 years, 6 months ago. While he suffers from *degenerative joint disease* and has talked for years about having "just a touch of arthritis," this never kept him from being up and about. Recently, however, he spends all day sitting in a chair and seems to have no desire to engage in self-care activities. He tells the visiting nurse that *he doesn't get washed up anymore because he's "too stiff" in the morning to bathe and "just doesn't seem to have the energy."* The visiting nurse notices that *his hair is matted and uncombed, his face has traces of previous meals, and he has a strong body odor.* His adult children have complained that their normally fastidious father seems not to care about personal hygiene any longer.

   Nursing Diagnosis: Bathing/Hygiene Self-Care Deficit, related to decreased strength and endurance, discomfort, and depression, as evidence by matted and uncombed hair, new beard, food particles on face, and strong body odor.
6. Miss Ebenezer sustained a right-sided cerebral infarct that resulted in *left hemiparesis* (paralysis on left side of body) and *left "neglect."* She ignores the left side of her body and actually denies its existence. *When asked about her left leg, she stated that it belonged to the woman in the next bed*—this while she was in a private room. *This patient was previously quite active; she walked for 45–60 minutes four or five times a week and was an avid swimmer.* At present *she cannot move either her left arm or leg.*

   Nursing Diagnosis: Body Image Disturbance, related to left hemiparesis (paralysis), as evidenced by her ignoring the left side of her body following her inability to move it.
7. Ted and Rosemary Hines tried to conceive a child, unsuccessfully, for 11 years. At this time, they sought the assistance of a fertility specialist who was highly recommended by a friend. It was determined that Ted's sperm was inadequate, and Rosemary was inseminated with sperm from an anonymous donor. The Hines were told that the donor was healthy and that he was selected because he resembled Ted. Rosemary became pregnant after the second in vitro fertilization attempt and delivered a healthy baby girl named Sarah.

   At the time they present for counseling, their child is 7 years old, and Ted and Rosemary have learned from blood tests that their fertility specialist is the biologic father of their child. It seems that he lied to some couples about using sperm from anonymous donors, and deceived others into thinking the wives had become pregnant when he had simply injected them with hormones. Ted and Rosemary have joined other couples in pressing charges against this physician.

Rosemary informs the nurse in her pediatrician's office that she is concerned about how all this is affecting her family. *"Ted and I both love Sarah and would do nothing to hurt her*, but I am so angry about this whole situation that I am afraid I may be taking it out on her."* Questioning reveals that Rosemary *has found herself yelling at Sarah for minor disobediences and spanking her—something she rarely did before.* Both Ted and Rosemary had commented before about Sarah's striking physical resemblance to the fertility specialist but attributed this to coincidence. *"Whenever I see her now I can't help but see Dr. Clowser and everything inside me clenches up and I want to scream."* Both Ted and Rosemary express great remorse that Sarah, who is innocent, is bearing the brunt of something that is in no way her fault.

Nursing Diagnosis: Parental Role Conflict, related to unexpected discovery about their daughter's biologic father, as evidenced by parental concern about increased incidence of parental yelling and spanking and the anger the child evokes in her parents because of her physical resemblance to the fertility specialist who deceived them.

Chapter 17

MATCHING
1. a	2. e	3. f	4. b	5. d	6. c
7. g	8. b	9. b	10. a	11. b	12. c
13. a	14. c	15. b	16. a	17. b	18. c
19. c	20. a				

MULTIPLE CHOICE
1. d	2. a	3. c	4. b	5. c	6. b
7. c					

COMPLETION
1. a. Teach patient the proper technique and application for inhaler.
    b. Walk with patient the length of the hallway every 5 hours, encouraging her to rely on the walker for support.
    c. Teach patient the importance of a well-balanced diet and daily exercise; have patient monitor daily caloric intake.
    d. Help patient sit up and dangle legs over side of bed; gradually help patient to stand and take several steps around the room.
2. a. Establishing priorities: Before developing or modifying the plan of care, the prioritized list of nursing diagnoses should be reviewed to determine if they are correctly ranked as high priority, medium priority, and low priority.
    b. Writing goals/outcomes that determine the evaluative strategy: For each nursing diagnosis in the plan of care, at least one goal must be written that, if

achieved, demonstrates a direct resolution of the problem statement.
    c. Selecting appropriate nursing interventions: Nursing interventions should be consistent with standards of care, realistic, compatible with patient's values, beliefs, and psychosocial background, valued by patient and family, and compatible with other planned therapies.
    d. Communicating the plan of care: Nursing orders describe in writing, and thus communicate to the entire nursing staff and healthcare team, the specific nursing care to be implemented for the patient.
3. Sample Answers
    a. Informal planning: A postpartum nurse learns that a patient is complaining of soreness related to unsuccessful attempts to breastfeed her infant and plans to spend more time with her. A home healthcare nurse quickly assesses safety in the home of a patient prone to accidents.
4. A formal plan of care allows the nurse to individualize care; set priorities; facilitate communication among nursing personnel; promote continuity of high quality, cost-effective care; coordinate care; evaluate patient's response to nursing care; and promote the nurse's professional development.
5. a. Assess effectiveness of pain medication for patient every 4 hours.
    b. Speak to parents of patient to assess their ability to support patient.
    c. Assess patient's room for variety of colors, textures, visual stimulation.
    d. Teach patient to perform daily exercises and learn to ambulate with a walker.
6. a. Basic human needs: The nursing care plan should concisely communicate to caregivers data about the patient's usual health habits and patterns obtained during the nursing history that are needed to direct daily care (e.g., requires assistance setting up food tray).
    b. Nursing diagnoses: The plan should contain goals/outcomes and nursing interventions for every nursing diagnosis, as well as a place to note patient responses to the plan of care; e.g., if the nursing diagnosis is Impaired Skin Integrity related to mobility deficit, a goal should be written to turn patient frequently and assess for skin breakdown.
    c. Medical plan of care: The plan of care should record current medical orders for diagnostic studies and specified related nursing care; e.g., if a diagnostic test is scheduled for the morning, appropriate fasting measures should be included in the plan of care.
7. a. Have changes in the patient's health status influenced the priority of nursing diagnoses?
    b. Have changes in the way the patient is responding to health and illness or the plan of care affected those nursing diagnoses that can be realistically addressed?
    c. Are there relationships among diagnoses that require that one be worked on before another can be resolved?
    d. Can several patient problems be dealt with together?
8. a. Mrs. Myers learns one lesson on nutrition per day, beginning 2/16/02.

b. After viewing film on smoking, Mrs. Gray identifies three dangers of smoking.

c. ✔

d. ✔

e. By next visit, patient will list three benefits of psychotherapy.

f. ✔

9. Sample Answers

a. By 11/12/02, patient will reestablish fluid balance as evidenced by (1) an approximate balance between fluid intake and fluid output, to average approximately 2500 mL; and (2) urine specific gravity within the normal range—1.010–1.025.

b. By next visit, patient will report a resumption of usual level of sexual activity following her acceptance of her new body image.

c. By 6/4/02, patient will report a decrease in the number of stress incontinent episodes (less than one per day), following her use of Kegel exercises.

d. By 8/10/02, patient reports that he has sufficient energy to carry out the priority activities identified 8/2/02.

e. By end of shift, patient reports better pain management (pain decreased to less than 3 on a scale of 10), related to new administration schedule.

Chapter 18

MATCHING

1. a   2. b   3. a   4. c   5. b   6. c

CORRECT THE FALSE STATEMENTS

1. False—nurse
2. True
3. True
4. False—protocols
5. False—nurse
6. True
7. False—nothing about the plan of care is fixed
8. True
9. False—is not sufficient
10. False—reassess the strategy
11. True
12. True
13. False—nursing

MULTIPLE CHOICE

1. b   2. c   3. d   4. c   5. b

COMPLETION

1. a. Interpret the specialists' findings for patients and family members.

b. Prepare patients to participate maximally in the plan of care before and after discharge.

c. Serve as a liaison among the members of the healthcare team.

2. Sample Answers

a. Nurse variable: a nurse with overwhelming outside concerns.

b. Patient variable: a patient who gives up.

c. Understaffing causes overworked nurses.

3. a. If patients and their families want to participate actively in seeking wellness, preventing disease and illness, recovering health, and learning to cope with altered functioning, they must possess effective self-care behavior.

b. The nursing actions planned to promote patient goal/outcome achievement and the resolution of health problems should be carefully executed. It is important that the nurse use time wisely to maximize each patient encounter to help the patient achieve his or her goals/outcomes.

4. Sample Answer

Mr. Franks may be in need of a psychologic evaluation to assess his adjustment to his new environment. Efforts should be made to get Mr. Franks involved in his new life so he shows interest in himself and others.

5. Sample Answer

As well as treatment for pregnancy, this patient should receive counseling on planning economical, nutritious meals and should be alerted to any social services in her community that could provide some relief in this area.

6. a. the patient's condition

b. the complexity of the activity

c. the potential for harm

d. the degree of problem-solving and innovation necessary

e. the level of interaction required with the patient

f. the capabilities of the UAP

g. the availability of professional staff to accomplish the unit workload

7. a. The *right* task: The task should be one that can be delegated.

b. The *right* person: The person should be qualified to do the job.

c. The *right* communication: The communication should be a clear, concise description of the objective and expectations.

d. The *right* feedback: Evaluation should be done in a timely manner during and after the task is completed.

e. The *right* time: This intervention should be evaluated to be sure it does not require professions nurses and can be safely delegated.

Chapter 19

MATCHING

1. e   2. c   3. a.   4. d   5. b   6. a
7. b   8. b   9. a.   10. a

MULTIPLE CHOICE

1. a   2. c   3. b   4. d   5. b   6. d
7. d   8. d

COMPLETION

1. Sample Answers

a. Cognitive goals: Ask the patient to repeat the information or ask the patient to apply the new knowledge to their everyday situations.

b. Psychomotor goals: Ask the patient to demonstrate the new skill.

c. Affective goals: Observe the patient's behavior and conversation for signs that the goals are achieved.

2. a. Identifying evaluative criteria: Evaluative criteria are the patient goals/outcomes developed during the planning step and must be identified to determine if they can be met by the patient.

b. Determining if goals and criteria are met: Because evaluative criteria reflect desired changes or outcomes in patient behavior, and because nursing actions are directed toward these outcomes, they become the core of evaluation to determine if the plan has been effective.

c. Terminating, continuing, or modifying the plan: Reviewing each step of the nursing process helps to determine whether goals have been met and the plan should be terminated, continued, or modified.

3. a. Patient: Is the patient motivated to learn new health behaviors?

b. Nurse: Do the nurses come to work well rested and ready to help their patients?

c. Healthcare system: Is a healthy nurse/patient ratio important to the institution?

4. The nurse should reevaluate each preceding step of the nursing process for accuracy. After this is done, it may become necessary to collect new assessment data, add or revise diagnoses, modify or rewrite patient goals/outcomes, and change nursing orders. In addition, patient evaluations may have to be targeted more frequently.

5. a. Structure: An audit focused on the environment in which care is provided. Evaluation is based on physical facilities and equipment, organizational characteristics, policies and procedures, fiscal resources, and personnel resources.

b. Process: An audit that focuses on the nature and sequence of activities carried out by the nurse implementing the nursing process. Evaluation is based on acceptable levels of performance of nursing actions related to patient assessment, diagnosis, planning, implementation, and evaluation.

c. Outcome: Outcome evaluations focus on measurable and demonstrable changes in the health status of the patient or the results of nursing care.

7. a. Delete or modify the nursing diagnosis: After evaluating the data, the nurse may decide the nursing diagnosis is inadequate and delete or change the diagnosis.

b. Make the goal statement more realistic: The nurse should determine the effectiveness of the goal and adjust the goal to meet the patient's needs.

c. Adjust time criteria in goal statement: If the time period was too short to accomplish the goal, it may need to be extended.

d. Change nursing interventions: Reevaluate the nursing interventions and change the ones that were ineffective; tailor the interventions to the patient's needs.

8. Answers will vary according to the student's experience.

Chapter 20

MATCHING
1. c	2. f	3. i	4. e	5. h	6. a
7. g	8. b	9. j	10. k		

MULTIPLE CHOICE
1. d	2. d	3. c	4. a	5. b	6. b
7. c	8. a	9. c			

COMPLETION

1. a. Nursing care data related to patient assessments
   b. Nursing diagnoses or patient needs
   c. Nursing interventions
   d. Patient outcomes

2. a. Change-of-shift reports: Given by a primary nurse to the nurse replacing him/her or by the charge nurse to the nurse who assumes responsibility for continuing care of the patient. Can be written, oral, or audiotaped.

b. Telephone reports: Telephones can link healthcare professionals immediately and enable nurses to receive and give critical information about patients in a timely fashion.

c. Telephone orders: Policy must be followed regarding telephone orders; they must be transcribed on an order sheet and co-signed by the physician within a set time.

d. Transfer and discharge reports: Nurses report a summary of a patient's condition and care when transferring or discharging patients.

e. Reports to family members and significant others: Nurses must keep the patient's family and significant others updated about the patient's condition and progress toward goal achievement.

f. Incident reports: A tool used by healthcare agencies to document the occurrence of anything out of the ordinary that results in or has potential to result in harm to a patient, employee, or visitor.

g. Conferring about care: To consult with someone to exchange ideas or to seek information, advice, or instructions.

h. Consultations and referrals: When nurses detect problems they cannot resolve because they lie outside the scope of independent nursing practice they make referrals to other professionals.

i. Nursing care conference: Nurses and other healthcare professionals frequently confer in groups to plan and coordinate patient care.

j. Nursing care rounds: Procedures in which a group of nurses visit selected patients individually at each patient's bedside to gather information, evaluate nursing care, and provide the patient with an opportunity to discuss his care.

3. a. Communication: The patient record helps healthcare professionals from different disciplines who interact with the same patient at different times to communicate with one another.

b. Care planning: Each professional working with the patient has access to the patient's baseline and updated data and can see how he/she is responding to the treatment plan from day to day. Modifications of the plan are based on these data.

c. Quality review: Charts may be reviewed to evaluate the quality of nursing care and the competence of the nurses providing that care.

d. Research: The record may be studied by researchers to determine the most effective way to recognize or treat specific health problems.

e. Decision analysis: Information from records review often provides data needed by strategic planners to identify needs and the means and strategies most likely to address these needs.

f. Education: Healthcare professionals and students reading a patient's chart can learn a great deal about the clinical manifestations of health problems, effective treatment modalities, and factors that affect patient goal achievement.

g. Legal documentation: Patient records are legal documents that may be entered into court proceedings as evidence and play an important role in implicating or absolving health practitioners charged with improper care.

h. Reimbursement: Patient records are used to demonstrate to payers that patients received the care for which reimbursement is being sought.

i. Historical document: Because the notations in patient records are dated, they provide a chronologic account of services provided.

4. a. Nurses should identify themselves and the patient, and state their relationship to the patient.

b. Nurses should report concisely and accurately the change in the patient's condition and what has already been done in response to this change.

c. Nurses should report the patient's current vital signs and clinical manifestations.

d. Nurses should have the patient record at hand so that knowledgeable responses can be made to the physician's inquiries.

e. Nurses should record concisely the time and date of the call, what was said to the physician, and the physician's response.

5. See the chart on page 323.

Chapter 21

MATCHING

1. b	2. d	3. g	4. a	5. c	6. e
7. b	8. c	9. a	10. a	11. c	12. b
13. c	14. a	15. b	16. b	17. c	18. a
19. e	20. d	21. c			

MULTIPLE CHOICE

1. d	2. a	3. b	4. a	5. c	6. b
7. c	8. d	9. d	10. c	11. c	12. c

COMPLETION

1. a. Touch: the nurse gently squeezes a patient's hand prior to surgery: The patient's response to this touch may express fear, gratitude, acceptance, etc.

b. Eye contact: A patient avoids eye contact: The patient may be expressing defenselessness or avoidance of communication.

c. Facial expressions: A patient grimaces when looking at his surgical incision: The patient may be experiencing anxiety over the alteration in his/her physical appearance.

d. Posture: A patient stands erect with good body alignment: The patient may be experiencing good health.

e. Gait: A patient walks slightly bent over: The patient may be accommodating an illness.

f. Gestures: A patient gives you a thumbs-up sign after receiving test results: The patient is most likely happy with the results.

g. General physical appearance: A patient is sweating and having difficulty breathing: The patient may be experiencing a life-threatening condition.

h. Mode of dress and grooming: A patient who has been bedridden for a week asks to take a shower and get dressed: The patient is probably feeling better.

i. Sounds: A patient sighs whenever you mention her significant other: The patient may be experiencing difficulty with this relationship.

j. Silence: A patient who has undergone a mastectomy remains silent when asked how she is feeling: The patient may be overwhelmed with emotion and unable to express her feelings.

2. a. An 8-year-old boy: An 8-year-old has limited understanding of surgical procedures. Therefore, the nurse must explain the procedure in simple terms so that the child will cooperate without being frightened.

b. A 16-year-old girl: Adolescents are developing their ability to think abstractly, and can understand fairly detailed descriptions of clinical procedures.

c. A 65-year-old man with a hearing impairment: The nurse should talk directly to the patient while facing him. When necessary, nonverbal communication should be used, e.g., sign language or finger spelling, or by writing any ideas that cannot be conveyed in another manner.

3. Occupation may reveal a person's abilities, talents, interests, and economic status.

4. a. Assessing: Verbal and nonverbal communication are essential nursing tools because the major focus of patient assessment is information gathering. Written words, patient records, spoken words, and observational skills are employed.

b. Diagnosing: Once a nurse formulates a diagnosis, it must be communicated through the spoken and written word to other nurses as well as to the patient.

c. Planning: The patient, nurse, and other healthcare team members must communicate with each other as patient goals and outcomes are developed and interventions selected.

d. Implementing: Verbal and nonverbal communication allows nurses to enhance basic care giving measures and to teach, counsel, and support patients and their families.

e. Evaluating: Nurses often rely on the verbal and nonverbal clues they receive from their patients to determine whether patient objectives or goals have been achieved.

Documentation Method	Description/Advantages/Disadvantages
Source-oriented Record	Each health care group keeps data on its own separate form. Notations are entered chronologically, with most recent entry being nearest the front of the record. **Advantages:** Each discipline can easily find and chart pertinent data. **Disadvantages:** Data are fragmented, making it difficult to track problems chronologically with input from different groups of professionals.
Problem-oriented Medical Records	Organized around a patient's problems; contributes collaboratively to plan of care. SOAP is used to organize data entries in the progress notes. **Advantages:** Entire health care team works together in identifying a master list of patient problems and contributes collaboratively to plan of care. **Disadvantages:** Some nurses believe that SOAP method focuses too narrowly on problems and advocates a return to the traditional narrative format.
PIE—Problem, Intervention, Evaluation	Unique in that it does not develop a plan of care; the plan of care is incorporated into the progress notes in which problems are identified by a number. A complete assessment is performed and documented at the beginning of each shift. **Advantages:** It promotes continuity of care and saves time since there is no separate plan of care. **Disadvantages:** Nurses need to read all the nursing notes to determine problems and planned interventions before initiating care.
Focus Charting	Its purpose is to bring the focus of care back to the patient and the patient's concerns. A focus column is used that incorporates many aspects of a patient and patient care. The focus may be a patient strength, problem, or need. **Advantages:** Holistic emphasis on the patient and patient's priorities; ease of charting. **Disadvantages:** Some nurses report that DAR categories (Data, Action, Response), are artificial and not helpful when documenting care.
Charting by Exception	Shorthand documentation method that makes use of well-defined standards of practice; only significant findings or "exceptions" to these standards are documented in the narrative notes. **Advantages:** Decreased charting time, greater emphasis on significant data, easy retrieval of significant data, timely bedside charting, standardized assessment, greater communication, better tracking of important responses and lower costs. **Disadvantages:** None noted.
Case Management Model	Interdisciplinary documentation tools clearly identify those outcomes that select groups of patients are expected to achieve on each day of care. Collaborative pathway is part of a computerized system that integrates the collaborative pathway and documentation flowsheets designed to match each day's expected outcomes. **Advantages:** Reduced charting time by 40% and increased staff satisfaction with the amount of paperwork from 0–85%. **Disadvantages:** Works best for "typical" patients with few individualized needs.
Variance Charting	Variances from the plan are documented; e.g., when a patient fails to meet an expected outcome or a planned intervention is not implemented in the case management model. **Advantages:** Decreased charting time; only variances are charted. **Disadvantages:** Loss of individualized care.
Computerized Records	Comprehensive computer systems have revolutionized nursing documentation in the patient record. **Advantages:** The nurse can call up the admission assessment tool and key in the patient data, develop the plan of care using computerized care plans, add to the patient data base new data, receive a work list showing treatments, procedures and medications, and document care immediately. **Disadvantages:** Policies should specify what type of patient information can be retrieved, by whom, and for what purpose (privacy).

f. Documenting: The documentation of data promotes the continuity of care given by nurses and other healthcare providers.

5. a. Having specific objectives: Having a purpose for an interaction guides the nurse toward achieving a meaningful encounter with the patient.

b. Providing a comfortable environment: A comfortable environment in which the patient and nurse are at ease helps to promote meaningful interactions. Effective relationships are enhanced when the atmosphere is relaxed and unhurried.

c. Providing privacy: Every effort should be made to provide privacy during nurse–patient conversations.

d. Maintaining confidentiality: The patient should know his/her right to specify who may have access to clinical or personal information.

e. Maintaining patient focus: Communication in the nurse–patient relationship should focus on the patient and the patient's need, not on the nurse or an activity in which the nurse is engaged.

f. Using nursing observations: Observation is especially valuable in validating information and helping the nurse become aware of patient's nonverbal communication. It also demonstrates the nurse's caring and interest in the patient.

g. Using optimal pacing: The nurse must consider the pace of any conversation or encounter with a patient and let the patient set the pace.

h. Providing personal space: Nurses must try to determine each patient's perception of personal space because their invasion of this zone can evoke uncomfortable feelings.

i. Developing therapeutic communication skills: Nurses must train and practice using therapeutic skills by controlling the tone of their voices, being knowledgeable about the topic, being flexible, being clear and concise, avoiding words that may be interpreted differently, being truthful and open-minded and taking advantage of available opportunities for communicating.

j. Developing listening skills: Nurses should sit when communicating with a patient, be alert and relaxed, keep the conversation natural, maintain eye contact if culturally correct, indicate they are paying attention, think before responding to the patient and listen for themes in the patient's comments.

k. Using silence as a tool: The nurse can use silence appropriately by taking the time to wait for the patient to initiate or continue speaking. Nurses should be aware of the different possible meanings of silence (the patient is comfortable with the nurse, the patient is demonstrating stoicism or exploring inner thoughts, the patient may be fearful, etc.).

6. Sample Answers
   a. Tell me about the night you had.
   b. Let's try walking on that foot now.
   c. What things prompted you to stop taking your insulin?
   d. Tell me what makes you afraid of taking the test.
   e. Your procedure has been performed successfully every time here.
   f. Should not be said at all.

7. Mrs. Clarke is a 42-year-old woman postmastectomy. She has a husband and two children, ages 10 and 5. When the nurse enters Mrs. Clarke's room, she finds her patient's *eyes are teary* and a *worried expression on her face*. When asked how she is feeling, Mrs. Clarke replies "fine," although *her face is rigid and mouth drawn in a firm line*. She is *moving her foot back and forth under the covers*. On further investigation, the nurse finds out Mrs. Clarke is worried about her children and her own ability to be a healthy, functioning wife and mother again. With prompting, Mrs. Clarke states: "I don't know if my husband will still love me like this." She *sighs and falls silent*, reflecting upon her recovery. The nurse tries to make Mrs. Clarke comfortable and *puts her hand over Mrs. Clarke's hand*. She *establishes eye contact* with Mrs. Clarke and reassures her that things have a way of working out and to give her situation some time.

8. Sample Answers
   a. Orientation phase:
      1. By 8/6/02, Mr. Uhl will call Nurse Parish by her name.
      2. By 8/6/02, Mr. Uhl will describe his freedoms/responsibilities within the institute.
   b. Working phase:
      1. By 8/10/02, Mr. Uhl will list various classes/activities available to patients.

2. By 8/10/02, Mr. Uhl will express any anxieties he may have in his new environment to the nurse.
   c. Termination phase:
      1. By 8/25/02, Mr. Uhl will be introduced to the new nurse in charge of his case by Nurse Parish, who will continue to oversee the new relationship until her departure.
      2. By 8/27/02, Mr. Uhl will report feeling good about his past care and look forward to his new relationship.

9. Sample Answers
   a. Warmth and friendliness: A nurse who greets a patient with a pleasant smile.
   b. Openness: A nurse who provides an honest explanation of a procedure.
   c. Empathy: A nurse who listens to a woman's lament over her miscarriage while helping her bathe.
   d. Competence: A nurse who competently and smoothly inserts a heplock into a patient's vein.
   e. Consideration of patient variables: A nurse who finds another nurse who speaks Spanish for her Hispanic patient.

10. Sample Answers
    a. Emphatic component: "Mr. Johnson, you've always been so independent, it must be difficult for you to accept the fact that you need medical care."
    b. Description: "Mr. Johnson, you have been diagnosed as having prostate cancer. There are several options for treatment."
    c. Expectation: "Mr. Johnson, your prognosis for leading a normal life is good, but we need your cooperation to make this treatment work."
    d. Consequence: "When you are discharged on Tuesday, we'll set you up with a schedule for your radiation treatments and let you know what you can expect. I'd like to work with you to help you understand your illness and its treatments better."

11. Sample Answers
    a. Failure to perceive the patient as a human being: The nurse should focus on the whole person, not simply the illness or dysfunction.
    b. Failure to listen: The nurse should be open to valuable opportunities for important communication by keeping an open mind and focusing on the patient's needs instead of their own needs.
    c. Use of inappropriate comments or questions: The nurse should avoid certain types of comments and questions (cliches, questions that probe for information, leading questions, comments that give advice, judgmental comments) that tend to impede effective communication.
    d. Changing the subject: The nurse should avoid changing the subject as the patient may be at a point of readiness to discuss something and may be frustrated if put off by a change in topic.
    e. Giving false assurance: The nurse should not try to convince the patient that things are going to turn out well when knowing the chances are not good. False assurance may give the patient the impression the nurse is not interested in their problems.

Chapter 22

MATCHING
1. b	2. a	3. d	4. h	5. f	6. g
7. e	8. g	9. d	10. c	11. c	12. b
13. a	14. d	15. b	16. a,b	17. d	18. c
19. b	20. d	21. b	22. a	23. b	24. c
25. c	26. a				

MULTIPLE CHOICE
1. a	2. c	3. b	4. d	5. a	6. c
7. b	8. d	9. c	10. c		

COMPLETION
1. a. Promoting wellness: Nurses can teach/counsel patients concerning health practices that lead to a higher level of wellness.
   b. Preventing illness: Nurses can teach patients health practices that help prevent specific illnesses or dangerous situations.
   c. Restoring health: Nurses can teach patients self-care practices that will facilitate recovery.
   d. Facilitating coping: Nurses can teach patients and their families to come to terms with the patient's illness and necessary lifestyle modifications.
2. a. The sensitivity and concern of the nurse in the helping relationship are the foundation for a nonthreatening learning environment for the adult patient.
   b. Honest and open communication can provide the adult learner with a realistic preview of what will be involved and allow them to retain some control over what is taught.
   c. New information must be presented clearly and in amounts that the patient can comprehend to prevent him from becoming discouraged or overwhelmed.
3. Sample Answers
   a. Demonstration: Take Mr. Lang through the exercises and have him demonstrate them in return.
   b. Print material: Give Mr. Lang a brochure that explicitly describes and diagrams the exercises you wish him to learn.
   c. Discussion: Have a conversation with Mr. Lang about the exercises and his desire and ability to perform them.
4. a. Content must be prioritized such that essential information is taught thoroughly and promptly and less important content is saved for last or for another time.
   b. Teamwork and cooperation allow nurses to meet deadlines for teaching. If teaching continues beyond hospitalization, the nurse can schedule additional learning opportunities through outpatient programs or referrals to community-based programs.
5. a. Formal: Planned teaching that is provided to fulfill learner objectives; e.g., viewing a film on diabetes.
   b. Informal: Unplanned teaching that comprises the majority of nurse-patient interactions; e.g., a nurse showing a mother the proper way to hold an infant.
6. a. Cognitive domain: oral questioning
   b. Affective domain: patient's response
   c. Psychomotor domain: return demonstration

7. A summary of the learning need, plan, implementation of the plan, and evaluated results should be documented in the patient chart. The evaluative statement should indicate whether the patient has displayed concrete evidence of learning how to bathe her infant.
8. a. Short-term counseling: Situational crisis; e.g., a nurse counsels a house-bound patient after a fire destroys her bedroom.
   b. Long-term counseling: Developmental crisis; e.g., a nurse counsels an adolescent about the dangers of drugs and alcohol.
   c. Motivational counseling: Discussion of feelings and incentives with the patient; e.g., a nurse counsels a woman in a shelter to leave her abusive spouse.
9. a. Identifying the new knowledge, attitudes or skills that are necessary for patient and family to manage their healthcare.
   b. Assessing learning readiness
   c. Assessing the ability of the patient to learn
   d. Identifying patient strengths and personal resources the nurse can tap
10. Answers will vary with student's experience.

Chapter 23

MATCHING
1. d	2. b	3. a	4. d	5. e	6. c
7. b	8. c	9. a	10. a		

CORRECT THE FALSE STATEMENTS
1. True
2. False—mentorship
3. False—a profession
4. False—traditional knowledge
5. True
6. True
7. False—advocacy
8. False—for nearly all patients
9. True
10. False—facilitate patient's decision-making
11. False—intertwined
12. False—explicit
13. True

MULTIPLE CHOICE
1. c	2. b	3. c	4. a	5. c	6. b
7. d	8. c				

COMPLETION
1. Answers will vary with student's experience.
2. Sample Answers
   a. Communication skills: The nurse explains to Mr. Eng that she realizes he is in a lot of pain, and she will be available to administer medication if he feels he needs more pain relief.
   b. Problem-solving skills: When the nurse learns that Mr. Eng's pain is not being relieved by the medication prescribed by his doctor, she calls the doctor to have it adjusted. She also teaches Mr. Eng some visualization exercises to help take his mind off the pain.

c. Management skills: The nurse meets with Mr. Eng's family to involve them in his care. She also instructs the staff to monitor Mr. Eng for signs of stress due to pain.

d. Self-evaluation skills: The nurse realizes she is being effective in relieving Mr. Eng's suffering and vows to research more techniques for pain management.

3. Sample Answer

Step 1. Identify problems with the old system and specific processes that need to be changed.

Step 2. Analyze several potential solutions to the problems, including a computerized system, and discuss the advantages and disadvantages of each.

Step 3. Select a course of action to initiate change.

Step 4. Plan for changes by developing specific objectives and a timetable to meet them, and identifying the people who will be involved in the change process.

Step 5. Implement the change, evaluate its effects, and revise accordingly to stabilize the new system.

Resistance to change: Determine why resistance exists and what technique will be most effective in helping employees overcome it.

4. a. Threat to self: Loss of self-esteem: belief that more work will be required and that social relationships will be disrupted. Explain the proposed change to everyone affected in simple, concise language so they know how they will be affected by it.

b. Lack of understanding: The people who will be affected by the change should be involved in the change process. When they understand the reason for, and benefits of the change, they are more likely to accept it.

c. Limited tolerance for change: Some people do not like to function in a state of flux or disequilibrium: Expedite the change so there is only a short period of confusion and explain this tactic to the employees involved.

d. Disagreements about the benefits of the change: Resistance may occur when the information available to the change agent is different than that received by individuals resisting the change. If the information available to the resisters is more accurate and relevant than information available to the change agent, then resistance may be beneficial.

e. Fear of increased responsibility: People often worry about having more complex responsibilities placed on them, particularly if they are unprepared for them. Since communication is the key to understanding, opportunities should be provided for open communication and feedback. Incentives may be helpful in obtaining a commitment to change.

5. a. Observing all nursing care activities to look for any area that needs improvement.

b. Questioning practices to see if the rationale behind caregiving activities is sound.

c. Participating in patient-care research done by colleagues or nurse researchers.

d. Making suggestions for specific topics to be researched.

6. Sample Answer

Nurses can change negative portrayals of nursing in the media by organizing, monitoring the media, reacting to the media, and fostering an improved image.

7. Informed consent protects the patient's right to knowledgeably agree to participate in the study without coercion, or to refuse to participate without jeopardizing the care that he or she will receive, the right to confidentiality, and the right to be protected from harm.

8. Sample Answers

a. Obtain a translator and make sure the patient understands her diagnosis, prognosis, and treatment options.

b. Make sure the patient understands the consequences of refusing treatment, and make her wishes known to the doctor. If the patient wants to formulate an advance directive, offer to secure legal assistance.

9. Sample Answers

a. Planning: Identify the problem and establish goals and a timeline for effecting change.

b. Organizing: Mobilize all available people and resources to educate the students about the dangers of binge drinking.

c. Directing: Lead organized groups dedicated to stop binge drinking on campus.

d. Controlling: Evaluate the plan of action and degree of effectiveness.

10. Answers will vary with student experience.

11. a. Observing all nursing care activities to look for any areas that need improvement.

b. Questioning practices to see if the rationale behind care giving activities is sound.

c. Participating in patient-care research done by colleagues or nurse researchers.

d. Making suggestions for specific topics to be researched.

Chapter 24

MATCHING

1. b	2. i	3. d	4. g	5. a	6. h
7. e	8. j	9. c	10. f	11. l	12. i
13. g	14. d	15. a	16. f	17. j	18. h
19. e	20. c	21. k	22. e	23. g	24. f
25. a	26. c	27. d			

a. temporal
b. carotid
c. brachial
d. femoral
e. posterior tibial
f. popliteal
g. radial
h. dorsalis pedis

MULTIPLE CHOICE

1. a	2. c	3. c	4. d	5. b	6. a
7. b	8. d	9. b	10. b		

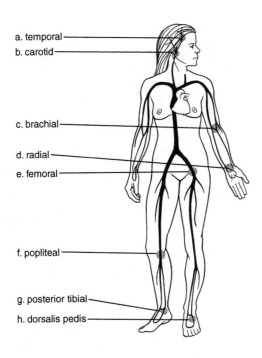

a. temporal
b. carotid
c. brachial
d. radial
e. femoral
f. popliteal
g. posterior tibial
h. dorsalis pedis

e. Environmental temperature: Exposure to extreme cold without adequate protective clothing can result in heat loss severe enough to cause hypothermia. Exposure to extreme heat may result in hyperthermia.
2. See table below.
3. a. The middle three fingers may be used to palpate all peripheral pulse sites.
   b. A stethoscope may be used to auscultate the apical pulse.
   c. Doppler ultrasound may be used to assess pulses that are difficult to palpate or auscultate.
4. a. Pumping action of the heart: When the amount of blood pumped into the arteries increases, the pressure of blood against arterial walls also increases.
   b. Blood volume: When blood volume is low, blood pressure is also low because there is less fluid within the arteries
   c. Viscosity of blood: The more viscous the blood, the higher the blood pressure.
   d. Elasticity of vessel walls: The elasticity of the walls, in addition to the resistance of the arterioles, helps to maintain normal blood pressure.
5. a. Make sure that there are no air leaks in the rubber bladder or sphygmomanometer connectors, tubing, or valve.
   b. Check the mercury meniscus and the needle on the aneroid manometer to make sure they are exactly on zero when the cuff is deflated.
   c. The mercury manometer should be cleaned and checked at least annually to make sure that the mercury is free of foreign matter and air.
   d. The calibration of the aneroid manometer must be checked frequently for accuracy against an accurate mercury manometer.
6. a. Impaired gas exchange: Excess or deficit in oxygenation and/or carbon dioxide elimination at the alveolar–capillary membrane.
   b. Ineffective airway clearance: Inability to clear secretions or obstructions from the respiratory tract to maintain a clear airway.
   c. Ineffective breathing pattern: Inspiration and/or expiration that does not provide adequate ventilation.
   d. Inability to sustain spontaneous ventilation: A state in which the response pattern of decreased energy reserves results in an individual's inability to maintain breathing adequate to support life.

COMPLETION

1. a. Circadian rhythms: Predictable fluctuations in measurements of body temperature and blood pressure exhibit a circadian rhythm; e.g., body temperature is usually approximately 0.6°C lower in the early morning than in later afternoon and early evening.
   b. Age: Body temperatures of infants and children respond more rapidly to heat and cold air temperatures than in adults. The older adult loses some thermoregulatory control and is at risk for harm from extremes in temperature.
   c. Gender: Body temperature tends to fluctuate more in women than in men, probably as a result of normal, cyclic fluctuations in the release of their sex hormones.
   d. Stress: The body responds to both physical and emotional stress by increasing the production of epinephrine. As a result, the metabolic rate increases, raising the body temperature.

Type of Thermometer	Brief Description	Contraindication	Normal Reading
a. Glass oral	Calibrated in degrees Centigrade or Fahrenheit	Unconscious, irrational, seizure-prone, infants, oral disease	98.6°F 37.0°C
rectal	Calibrated in degrees Centigrade or Fahrenheit	Newborns, diseases of Rectum, certain heart diseases	99.5°F 37.5°C
b. Electronic	Two nonbreakable probes, disposable probe covers		
c. Tympanic Membrane	Infrared sensors off membrane	Infants to 3 months Tympanic membrane damage	99.5°F 37.5°C
d. Temperature sensitive patch	Forehead or abdomen; changes color at different temperatures	Newborns	94.0°F 34.4°C
e. Automated monitoring device	Measure body temperature, pulse and blood pressure automatically		

7. a. Altered tissue perfusion: A decrease in oxygen resulting in the failure to nourish the tissues at the capillary level.
b. Risk for fluid volume imbalance: A risk of a decrease, increase, or rapid shift from one to the other of intravascular, interstitial, or intracellular fluid.
c. Fluid volume excess: The state in which an individual experiences increased isotonic fluid retention.
d. Fluid volume deficit: The state in which an individual experiences decreased intravascular, interstitial, or intracellular fluid.
e. Decreased cardiac output: A state in which the blood pumped by the heart is inadequate to meet the metabolic demands of the body.
8. a. Stethoscope: Used to auscultate and assess body sounds, including the apical pulse and blood pressure. The acoustical stethoscope has an amplifying mechanism connected to ear pieces by tubing.
b. Sphygmomanometer: Consists of a cuff and the manometer. The cuff contains an airtight, flat, rubber bladder covered with cloth, which is closed around the limb with contact closures. Two tubes are attached to the bladder within the cuff; one is connected to a manometer, the other is attached to a bulb used to inflate the bladder.

Chapter 25

MATCHING

1. a	2. b	3. a	4. d	5. c	6. b
7. e	8. d	9. c	10. a	11. b	12. d
13. c	14. a	15. b	16. e	17. g	18. d
19. h	20. f	21. f	22. b	23. d	24. j
25. a	26. c	27. e	28. h	29. i	30. g
31. d	32. f	33. a	34. c	35. b	36. e
37. g	38. a	39. b	40. s	41. n	42. f
43. s	44. l	45. m	46. k	47. i	48. o
49. c	50. h	51. p	52. q	53. e	54. d
55. r	56. t	57. u			

MULTIPLE CHOICE

1. b	2. c	3. a	4. c	5. d	6. b
7. a	8. d	9. c	10. a	11. c	12. b
13. d	14. a	15. c	16. a	17. d	18. b

COMPLETION

1. a. Establish a nurse–patient relationship
b. Gather data about the patient's general health status, integrating physiologic, psychologic, cognitive, sociocultural, developmental, and spiritual dimensions.
c. Identify patient strengths.
d. Identify existing and potential health problems.
e. Establish a base for the nursing process.
2. a. Ophthalmoscope: Lighted instrument used for visualization of interior structures of the eye.
b. Otoscope: Lighted instrument used for examining external ear canal and tympanic membrane.
c. Snellen chart: Screening test for vision
d. Nasal speculum: Instrument that allows visualization of lower and middle turbinates of the nose.
e. Vaginal speculum: Two-bladed instrument used to examine vaginal canal and cervix.
f. Tuning fork: Two-pronged metal instrument used for testing auditory function and vibratory perception.
g. Percussion hammer: Instrument with a rubber head, used to test reflexes and determine tissue density.
3. It is important to consider the patient's age, physical condition, energy level, and need for privacy.
4. a. Patient: Consider physiologic and psychologic needs of the patient. Explain that a physical assessment will be done by the nurse, that body structures will be examined, and that such assessments are painless. Have patient put on a gown and empty bladder.
b. Environment: The time of the assessment should be mutually agreed on and should not interfere with meals or daily routines. The patient should be as free of pain as possible; and the room should be quiet and private.
5. See table below.
6. a. Pitch—ranging from high to low
b. Loudness—ranging from soft to loud
c. Quality—e.g., swishing or gurgling
d. Duration—short, medium, or long
7. a. Edema: Palpate edematous area with the fingers; an indentation may remain after the pressure is released.
b. Dehydration: Pick up the skin in a fold; when dehydration exists, normal elasticity and fullness are decreased and skin fold returns to normal slowly.
8. a. Reaction to light: Ask patient to look straight ahead, bring the penlight from side of patient's face, and shine the light on one of the pupils. Observe pupil's reaction; normally it will constrict. Repeat procedure in the same eye, and observe the other eye—normally it too will constrict. Repeat the entire procedure with the other eye.
b. Accommodation: Hold the forefinger about 10–15 cm in front of the bridge of the patient's nose. Ask the patient to first look at the forefinger, then at a

Technique	Definition	Assessment/Observation
a. Inspection:	Process of deliberate, purposeful observations performed in a systematic manner.	Body size, color, shape, position, symmetry, norms, and deviations from norm.
b. Palpation:	Technique that uses sense of touch.	Temperature, turgor, texture, moisture, vibrations, shape.
c. Percussion:	The act of striking an object against another object to produce a sound.	Location, shape, size, and density of tissues.
d. Ascultation:	The act of listening to sound produced in the body, using stethoscope.	Lung and bowel sounds; heart and vascular sounds

distant object, then the forefinger again. Normally, the pupil constricts when the patient looks at the finger and dilates when he/she looks at a distant object.

   c. Convergence: Move a finger toward the patient's nose. Normally, the patient's eyes converge.

9. a. Weber: Hold the tuning fork at its base and strike it against the palm of the opposite hand so that the fork vibrates. Place the base of the fork on the center of the top of the patient's head; ask patient where the sound is heard. Normal findings: sound is heard in both ears or in midline.

   b. Rinne: Activate tuning fork. Hold the base of fork against patient's mastoid process and ask him/her to tell you when the sound can no longer be heard. Immediately place the still-vibrating fork close to the external ear canal and ask the patient if he/she can hear the sound. A normal ear will hear the sound. Repeat procedure with the other ear.

10. Equipment: Vials of aromatic substances, visual acuity chart, penlight, sharp object, cotton balls, vials of solution to test taste, tuning fork, tongue depressor, reflex hammer, and familiar objects. Position: sitting.

11. a. Orientation: What is today's date?

   b. Immediate memory: What did you eat for lunch today?

   c. Past memory: When is your wedding anniversary?

   d. Abstract reasoning: Explain the proverb: A stitch in time, saves nine.

   e. Language: Would you read this passage from this book?

12. a. Biceps reflex: Patient's arms should be partially flexed at the elbow, with palms down. Place a thumb or finger firmly on the patient's biceps muscle and strike with hammer, aimed directly toward finger. Observe for flexion at elbow and feel for contraction of biceps muscle.

   b. Brachioradialis or supinator reflex: Rest patient's forearm on abdomen with palm facing downward. Strike tendon on patient's radius 1–2 inches above wrist. Observe for flexion and supination of forearm.

   c. Patellar or knee reflex: Place patient in a sitting or supine position with the knees in a flexed position. Briskly tap patellar tendon just below patella and observe for contraction of quadriceps with knee extension.

   d. Achilles tendon reflex: Patient's leg should be slightly flexed at the knee, with the foot in dorsiflexion at the ankle joint. Strike achilles tendon and observe for plantar flexion at the ankle.

13. a. lub; b. mitral; c. tricuspid; d. ventricular; e. S1; f. apical; g. S2; h. systole; i. aortic, j. pulmonic; k. dub; l. one

Chapter 26

MATCHING
1. d. Give syrup of ipecac to induce vomiting, perform gastric lavage, give chelating agent.
2. b. Never induce vomiting; dilute poison with milk or water. Take to ER immediately.
3. a. Give syrup of ipecac to induce vomiting, fluids, IV fluids, sodium bicarbonate.
4. e. Chelating therapy.
5. c. Never induce vomiting; perform gastric lavage.
6. d 7. g 8. e 9. a 10. f 11. c 12. b

CORRECT THE FALSE STATEMENTS
1. True
2. False—motor vehicle accidents
3. True
4. False—increased
5. True
6. True
7. False—home
8. False—children
9. True
10. True
11. False—preschooler
12. False—falls
13. False—unjustified; a variety of alternative options can be used
14. False—children under five
15. True
16. False—15 mL orally

MULTIPLE CHOICE
1. a 2. c 3. d 4. b 5. a 6. b 7. a

COMPLETION
1. a. Neonates and infants: mother who smokes; mother who drinks alcohol
   b. Toddler and preschooler: child abuse; expanded environment
   c. School-age child: accidents, fire
   d. Adolescent: drug and alcohol consumption; motor vehicle accidents
   e. Adults: spousal abuse; using alcohol to relieve stress
   f. Older adult: motor impairment; elder abuse
2. Sample Answers
   a. Developmental considerations: A teenager who drinks and drives is at risk for accidents; an adult who is under stress at work is at risk for drug or alcohol abuse.
   b. Lifestyle: A person who lives in a high-crime neighborhood is at risk for violence; a person who has a dangerous job is at risk for accidents.
   c. Limitation in mobility: An older patient with an unsteady gait is at risk for falls; recent surgery or prolonged illness can temporarily affect mobility.
   d. Limitation in sensory perception: Visual changes may cause a person to stumble, lose balance and fall; a hearing deficit interferes with normal communication and may result in patient who is insensitive to alarms, horns, sirens, etc.

e. Limitation in knowledge: A mother who does not know how to childproof her home puts her toddler at risk for accidents; an elderly person who does not know how to use her walker is at risk for falls.

f. Limitation in ability to communicate: Fatigue or stress, certain medications, aphasia, and language barriers are factors that can affect personal interchange and compromise the patient's ability to express urgent safety concerns.

g. Limitation in health status: A patient recovering from a stroke may have muscle impairment; many patients who fall also have a primary or secondary diagnosis of cardiovascular disease.

h. Limitation in psychosocial state: Depression may result in confusion and disorientation, accompanied by reduced awareness of environmental hazards; social isolation may be responsible for a reduced level of concentration.

3. a. Nursing history: The nurse must be alert for any history of falls because a person with a history of falling is likely to fall again. Assistive devises should be noted. A history of drug or alcohol abuse should also be noted.

b. Physical assessment: Nurses need to assess patient's mobility status, ability to communicate, level of awareness or orientation, and sensory perception.

c. Accident-prone behavior: Some people seem to be more likely than others to have accidents.

d. The environment: The nurse must assess every setting in which the patient is at risk for injury, including the home, community, and healthcare agency.

4. Sample Answers
a. Age older than 65 years.
b. Documented history of falls.
c. Slowed reaction time.
d. Disorientation or confusion.

5. Sample Answer
The mother should be informed about safety for toddlers, and a plan should be devised to help her childproof her home. The plan should include the installation of cabinet locks; electrical outlet covers; moving medications, cleaners, poisonous plants, etc. to higher levels; and keeping small or sharp objects out of reach.

6. Sample Answer
a. Do your children's toys have small or loose parts?
b. Have you ever left your infant in the bathtub to answer the phone?
c. Do you have soft pillows or thick blankets in your infant's crib?

7. a. Risk for injury related to refusal to use child safety seat.
b. Risk for poisoning related to reduced vision.
c. Risk for aspiration or trauma (burns) related to child left unattended in bathtub.
d. Risk for trauma related to history of previous falls.
e. Impaired home maintenance related to insufficient finances.

8. a. Screening programs for vision and hearing
b. Fire prevention programs
c. Drug and alcohol prevention programs

9. Sample Answer
a. Impaired circulation

b. Pressure ulcers and diminished bone mass
c. Fractures
d. Altered nutrition and hydration
e. Incontinence

10. Documentation should include alternative strategies that were ineffective, the reason for restraining the patient, the type of restraint and time it was applied, pertinent nursing assessments, and regular intervals when restraints were removed.

11. The nurse completes the incident report immediately after an accident and is responsible for recording the occurrence of the accident and its effect on the patient in the medical record. The report should objectively describe the circumstances of the accident and provide details concerning the patient's response and the examination and treatment of the patient after the incident.

12. a. Respond to the present, not the past.
b. Evaluate the potential for injury.
c. Speak with family members or caregivers.
d. Try alternative measures first.
e. Reassess the patient to determine if alternatives are successful.
f. Alert the physician and the patient's family if restraints are indicated
g. Individualize restraint use.
h. Note important information on the patient's chart.
i. Put a time limit on the use of restraints.

Chapter 27

MATCHING

1. k	2. f	3. a	4. b	5. j	6. i
7. m	8. c	9. e	10. g	11. d	12. n

13. c. blood, semen, vaginal secretions
14. e. ticks
15. d. sputum
16. a. skin surface
17. b. blood, feces, body fluids
18. a. mouth
19. a. throat

20. d	21. a	22. c	23. b

CORRECT THE FALSE STATEMENTS

1. True
2. False—medical asepsis
3. False—5%
4. True
5. False—washing hands
6. False—transient bacteria
7. True
8. True
9. False—does not eliminate
10. True
11. True
12. False—surgical asepsis
13. True

MULTIPLE CHOICE

1. b	2. d	3. c	4. b	5. a	6. d
7. c	8. b	9. c	10. a	11. a	12. c

COMPLETION

1. a. Number of organisms
   b. Virulence of the organism
   c. Competence of a person's immune system
   d. Length and intimacy of the contact between a person and the microorganism
2. Sample Answers
   a. Other humans: tuberculosis
   b. Animals: rabies
   c. Soil: gas gangrene
3. a. Gastrointestinal
   b. Genitourinary tracts
   c. Blood and tissue
4. Sample Answers
   a. Direct contact: transmission of disease through touching, kissing, sexual contact.
   b. Indirect contact: personal contact with contaminated blood, food, water, etc.
   c. Vectors: mosquitoes, ticks, and lice transmit organisms from one host to another.
   d. Airborne: spread of droplet nuclei through coughing, sneezing, talking.
5. a. Inflammatory response: A protective mechanism that eliminates the invading pathogen and allows for tissue repair to occur.
   b. Immune response: Involves specific reactions in the body as it responds to an invading foreign protein such as bacteria or, in some cases, the body's own proteins. The body responds to an antigen by producing an antibody.
6. a. Intact skin and mucous membranes protect the body against microbial invasion.
   b. The normal pH levels of gastric secretions and of the genitourinary tract help to ward off microbial invasion.
   c. The body's white blood cells influence resistance to certain pathogens.
   d. Age, sex, race, and hereditary factors influence susceptibility.
7. a. Assessing: Early detection and surveillance techniques are critical. The nurse should inquire about immunization status and previous or recurring infections, observe nonverbal cues, and the history of the current disease.
   b. Diagnosing: The direction or focus of nursing care depends on a nursing diagnosis that accurately reflects the patient's condition.
   c. Planning: Effective nursing interventions can control or prevent infection. Nurses should review assessment data and consider the cycle of events that results in infection control as patient goals are formulated.
   d. Implementing: The nurse uses principles of aseptic technique to halt the spread of microorganisms and minimize the threat of infection.
   e. Evaluating: The nurse can intervene in and positively affect a patient's outcome by assessing the person at risk, selecting appropriate nursing diagnoses, planning and intervening to maintain a safe environment and evaluating the plan of care to determine if it is working.
8. Sample Answers
   a. Patient's home: Wash hands before preparing food and before eating; use individual personal care items, such as washcloths, towels, toothbrushes, etc.
   b. Public facilities: Wash hands after using any public bathroom; use individually wrapped drinking straws.
   c. Community: Use sterilized combs and brushes in beauty and barber shops; examine food handlers for evidence of disease.
   d. Healthcare facility: Use standard aseptic techniques to prevent further spread of a present organism and prevent nosocomial infections
9. a. Instituting constant surveillance by infection-control committees and nurse epidemiologists.
   b. Having written infection prevention practices for all agency personnel.
   c. Using practices that help promote the best possible physical condition in patients.
10. a. Nature of organisms present: Some organisms are easily destroyed, whereas others are able to withstand certain commonly used sterilization and disinfection methods.
    b. Number of organisms present: The more organisms present on an item, the longer it takes to destroy them.
    c. Type of equipment: Equipment with narrow lumens, crevices, or joints requires special care. Certain items may be damaged by sterilization methods.
    d. Intended use of equipment: The need for medical or surgical asepsis influences methods used in the preparation and cleaning of equipment.
    e. Available means for sterilization and disinfection: The choice of chemical or physical means of sterilization and disinfection takes into consideration the availability and practicality of the means.
    f. Time: Time is a key factor. Failure to observe recommended time periods for disinfection and sterilization significantly increases the risk for infection and is grossly negligent.
11. a. Put VRE-infected patients in single rooms or in the same room as other VRE patients.
    b. Wear clean gloves and a gown when entering room; remove protective items before leaving the room.
    c. Wash hands immediately with an antiseptic or antimicrobial soap.
    d. Keep equipment that will be used with patient in the patient's room.
    e. Keep patient in VRE isolation until at least three cultures—taken 3 weeks apart—are negative.
12. a. Hospital: The infection-control nurse is responsible for educating patients and staff about effective infection-control techniques and for collecting statistics about infections.
    b. Home: The infection-control nurse's duties include surveillance for agency-associated infections, as well as education, consultation, performance of epidemiological investigations and quality improvement activities, and policy and procedure development.
13. Infectious agent; reservoir; portal of exit; means of transmission; portal of entry; susceptible host
14. a. Risk of Infection related to altered skin integrity/burns.
    b. Effective nursing interventions can control or prevent

infection. The nurse should review patient data, consider the cycle of events that result in the development of an infection, and incorporate infection control as a patient goal.

15. Use standard precautions for the care of all patients in the ER. The additional concern with TB necessitates using airborne precautions in addition to standard precautions.

Chapter 28

MATCHING

1. b	2. e	3. a	4. c	5. d	6. f
7. a	8. c	9. k	10. b	11. j	12. d
13. g	14. i	15. h	16. l	17. c	18. i
19. b	20. e	21. f	22. d	23. g	24. a
25. e	26. d	27. a	28. g	29. f	30. b
31. c					

MULTIPLE CHOICE

1. d	2. a	3. c	4. d	5. b	6. a
7. b	8. d	9. b	10. a	11. c	12. d
13. b	14. c	15. b	16. d	17. a	18. d

COMPLETION

1. Drugs may be classified by body systems, by the symptom relieved by the drug, or by the clinical indication for the drug.
2. a. Drug–receptor interactions: The drug interacts with one or more cellular structures to alter cell function.
   b. Drug–enzyme interactions: The drug combines with enzymes to achieve the desired effect.
3. Sample Answers
   a. Route of administration: Injected medications are usually absorbed more rapidly than oral medications.
   b. Drug solubility: Liquid medications are absorbed more rapidly than solid preparations. When in solution, the nonionized form is more readily absorbed.
   c. pH: The efficiency with which a drug is absorbed varies with the pH in that part of the body. Acidic drugs are well absorbed in the stomach. Basic drugs remain insoluble in a highly acid environment.
   d. Local conditions at the site of administration: The more extensive the absorbing surface, the greater the amount of the drug absorbed and the more rapid its effect.
   e. Drug dosage: A loading dose is higher than body capacity; a maintenance dose is a lower dosage that becomes the usual or daily dosage.
4. Sample Answers
   a. Developmental considerations: A child's dose of medication is smaller than an adult's dose.
   b. Weight: Drug doses for children should be calculated on weight or body surface area. Doses for adults are based on a reference adult, i.e., a healthy adult of 18–65 years weighing 150 lbs.
   c. Sex: Hormonal fluctuations can affect drug action.
   d. Genetic factors: Asian patients may require smaller doses of a drug because they metabolize it at a slower

rate. Cultural: herbal remedies may interfere with or counteract the action of prescribed medication.
   e. Psychologic factors: Patients may have the same effect with a placebo as with an active drug.
   f. Pathology: Liver disease may affect drug action by slowing down metabolism of drugs.
   g. Environment: The lower oxygen concentration of air at high altitudes may increase sensitivity to some drugs.
   h. Time of administration: The presence of food in the stomach delays the absorption of oral medications.
5. a. Patient's name
   b. Date and time the order is written
   c. Name of drug to be administered
   d. Dosage of the drug
   e. Route by which the drug is to be administered
   f. Frequency of administration of the drug
   g. Signature of person writing the order
6. Sample Answers
   a. The nurse knows that the patient is allergic to the drug.
   b. The nurse has difficulty reading the order.
   c. The nurse knows the drug will be harmful to the patient.
7. a. Stock supply system: Large quantities of medications are kept on the nursing unit.
   b. Individual supply system: Each patient is supplied with the medication needed for a period of time.
   c. Unit dose system: The pharmacist simplifies medication preparation by packaging and labeling each dosage for a 24-hour period.
8. a. Three checks: The medication label should be checked (1) when the nurse reaches for the container, (2) immediately before pouring or opening the medication, and (3) when replacing the container to the drawer or shelf or before administering the dose to the patient.
   b. Five rights: (1) Give the right medication (2) to the right patient (3) in the right dosage (4) through the right route (5) at the right time.
9. Sample Answers
   a. Crush the medication or add it to food.
   b. Allow the patient to suck on a piece of ice to numb the taste buds.
   c. Give the medication with generous amounts of water.
10. Sample Answers
    a. Route of administration: A longer needle is needed for an intramuscular injection than for an intradermal or subcutaneous injection.
    b. Viscosity of the solution: Some medications are more viscous than others and require a large-lumen needle to be injected.
    c. Quantity to be administered: The larger the amount of medication to be injected, the greater the capacity of the syringe.
    d. Body size: An obese person requires a longer needle to reach muscle tissue than a thin person.
    e. Type of medication: There are special syringes for certain uses.
11. a. Check the patient's condition immediately when the error is noted. Observe for adverse effects.
    b. Notify the nurse manager and the physician to discuss possible courses of action based on the patient's condition.

c. Write a description of the error on patient's medical record, including remedial steps that were taken.

d. Complete a special form for reporting errors, as dictated by agency policy.

12. a. Ampules: An ampule is a glass flask that contains a single dose of medication for parenteral administration. Medication is removed from an ampule after its thin neck is broken.

b. Vials: A vial is a glass bottle with a self-sealing stopper through which medication is removed. The nurse can remove several doses from the same container.

c. Prefilled cartridges: These provide a single dose of medication. The nurse inserts the cartridge into a reusable holder and clears the cartridge of excess air.

13. a. 1.5 cc
b. tab i
c. 0.5 tab
d. 3 tabs
e. 0.5 tab
f. 3 tabs
g. 0.5 tab (1/2 tab)
h. 0.5 tab (1/2 tab)
i. 2 tabs
j. 4 cc

14. See table below.
15. See table below.

Method	Xanax	Zantac	Cipro
Dosage	0.25–0.5 mg	150–300 mg	250–750 mg
Route of administration	PO	PO	PO
Frequency/schedule	tid	bid	bid
Desired effects	Relief of anxiety	Cure/relief peptic ulcer	Cure/treat infection
Possible adverse effects	Drowsiness, lightheadedness, dry mouth, constipation	Malaise, rash, GI upset	GI upset, nausea, diarrhea
Signs and symptoms of toxic drug effects	Diminished reflexes, somnolence, confusion	Tachycardia, GI upset	CNS stimulation
Special instructions	No alcohol	None	No antacids
Recommended course of action with problems	Gastric lavage	None	None

Medical Administration Record

Ord date	PRN MEDS.		
2/24/02	Dalmane 30 mg	**Date**	
	PO hs prn	**Time**	
		Init / **Site**	
2/24/02	Tylenol with codeine #2	**Date**	2/24/02
	PO q4h prn	**Time**	10 AM
		Init / **Site**	CL/PO

SINGLE ORDERS–PREOPERATIVES

Ord date	Medication–Dosage–Route of Admin	Date/Time	Site/Initials
2/24/02	Regular Insulin U-100	2/24/02	® thigh/CL
	10U SQ STAT		

INJECTION SITES MUST BE CHARTED

	ROUTINE MEDICATIONS		Date/Time						
Ord date	Medication–Dosage–Route of Admin	Hr	2/25	2/26	2/27	2/28	3/1	3/2	3/3
2/24/02	Tenormin 50 mg PO od	10AM	CL						
2/24/02	Hydrodiuril 50 mg PO od	10AM	CL						
			130/90						
2/24/02	NPH Insulin U-100 45U	7:30AM	CL						
	SQ daily in AM		Ⓛ arm						
2/24/02	Cipro 500 mg PO q12h	10AM	CL						
		10PM							
2/24/02	Timoptic 0.25% † gtt	10AM	CL						
	OD bid	6PM							
2/24/02	Nitropaste 1/2" q8h	8AM	CL $\frac{130}{90}$						
	to chest wall	4PM							
		12PM							
2/24/02	Colace 100 mg PO od	10AM	CL						

CL: Claire Long, RN

Chapter 29

MATCHING

1. c	2. a	3. b	4. c	5. b	6. a
7. c	8. d	9. a	10. e	11. b	12. a
13. c	14. d	15. b	16. d	17. b	

MULTIPLE CHOICE

1. a	2. c	3. b	4. d	5. b	6. a
7. c	8. c	9. a	10. c	11. b	12. d
13. b	14. a	15. c	16. a		

COMPLETION

1. a. Preoperative phase: Begins with the decision that surgical intervention is necessary and lasts until the patient is transferred to the operating room table.
   b. Intraoperative phase: Extends from admission to the surgical department to transfer to the recovery area.
   c. Postoperative phase: Lasts from admission to the recovery area to the complete recovery from surgery.
2. a. Based on urgency: May be classified as elective surgery (preplanned; patient choice), urgent surgery (necessary for patient's health; not emergency), and emergency surgery (preserves patient's life, body part, or body function).
   b. Based on degree of risk: May be classified as minor (performed in physician's office, same-day surgery setting, or outpatient clinic), or major (requires hospitalization, is prolonged and has higher degree of risk, involves major body organs)
   c. Based on purpose: Descriptors include diagnostic, ablative, palliative, reconstructive, transplant, and constructive.
3. a. Induction: Begins with administration of the anesthetic agent and continues until the patient is ready for the incision.
   b. Maintenance: Continues from point of incision until near the completion of the procedure.
   c. Emergence: Starts as the patient begins to "emerge" from the anesthesia and usually ends when the patient is ready to leave the operating room.
4. a. Description of the procedure or treatment
   b. Name and qualifications of the person performing the procedure or treatment
   c. Explanation of the risks involved, including potential for damage, disfigurement or death
   d. Patient's right to refuse treatment and withdraw consent.
5. a. Cardiovascular disease: Increased potential for hemorrhage and hypovolemic shock, hypotension, venous stasis, thrombophlebitis, and overhydration with IV fluids.
   b. Pulmonary disorders: Increased possibility of respiratory depression from anesthesia, postoperative pneumonia, atelectasis, and alterations in acid-base balance.
   c. Kidney and liver function disorders: Influence the patient's response to anesthesia, affect fluid and electrolyte as well as acid-base balance, and alter metabolism and excretion of drugs, and impair wound healing.

d. Metabolic disorders: Increased potential for hypoglycemia or acidosis and slow wound healing.
6. a. Fear of the unknown: Encourage the patient to identify and verbalize fears; identify and correct incorrect knowledge; identify patient strengths.
   b. Fear of pain and death: Support the patient's spiritual needs through acceptance, participation in prayer, or referral to clergy or chaplain.
   c. Fear of changes in body image and self-concept: Identify the need for support systems during initial interview; arrange a preoperative visit from a person who has had the same operation and adapted successfully.
7. The nurse is responsible for ensuring that the tests are ordered and done, that the results are recorded in the patient's record before surgery, and that abnormal findings are reported.
8. a. Surgical events and sensations: Tell the patient and family when surgery is scheduled; how long it will last; what will be done before, during, and after surgery; and what sensations the patient will be experiencing during the perioperative period.
   b. Pain management: The patient should be informed that pain reported by the patient is the determining factor of pain control; pain will be assessed as often as every 2 hours after major surgery; there is little danger of addiction to pain medications; and non-pharmacologic methods of pain control (relaxation techniques, TENS and PCA) are available.
9. a. Hygiene and skin preparation: Clean the skin with antibacterial soap to remove bacteria. The patient can do this in a bath or shower, shampoo the hair, and clean the fingernails. Remove hair from incisional area with depilatory cream or hair clipper if indicated.
   b. Elimination: Emptying the bowel of feces is no longer a routine procedure, but the nurse should use preoperative assessments to determine the need for an order for bowel elimination. If indwelling catheter is not in place, the patient should void immediately before receiving preoperative medications.
   c. Nutrition and fluids: Diet depends on the type of surgery; patients need to be well nourished and hydrated before surgery to counterbalance fluid, blood, and electrolyte loss during surgery.
   d. Rest and sleep: The nurse can facilitate rest and sleep in the immediate preoperative period by meeting psychologic needs, carrying out teaching, providing a quiet environment, and administering prescribed bedtime sedative medication.
10. a. Maintain intact skin surfaces
    b. Remain free of neuromuscular damage
    c. Have symmetric breathing patterns
11. a. Unconsciousness
    b. Response to touch and sounds
    c. Drowsiness
    d. Awake but not oriented
    e. Awake and oriented
12. Sample Answer
    The person(s) who will be changing the patient's dressing at home should demonstrate proper techniques in wound care and dressing change. Teaching should include the fol-

lowing information: (1) where to buy dressing materials and medical supplies, (2) signs and symptoms of infection, (3) need to eat well-balanced meals and drink fluids, (4) how to modify activities of daily living (as needed), (5) need to wear disposable gloves when changing the dressing and wash hands before and after donning gloves, (6) how to dispose of old dressings.

13. Sample Answers
    a. Developmental considerations: Infants and older adults are at a greater risk from surgery than are children and young or middle-aged adults.
    b. Medical history: Pathologic changes associated with past and current illnesses increase surgical risk.
    c. Medications: Use of anticoagulants before surgery may precipitate hemorrhage.
    d. Previous surgery: Previous heart or lung surgery may necessitate adaptations in the anesthesia and in positioning during surgery.
    e. Perceptions and knowledge of surgery: The patient's questions or statements are important for meeting psychologic and family needs when preparing the patient for surgery.
    f. Lifestyle: Cultural and ethnic background of the patient may affect surgical risk.
    g. Nutrition: malnutrition and obesity increase surgical risk.
    h. Use of alcohol, illicit drugs, nicotine: Patients with a large habitual intake of alcohol require larger doses of anesthetic agents and postoperative analgesics, increasing risk of drug-related complications.
    i. Activities of daily living: Exercise, rest, and sleep habits are important for preventing postoperative complications and facilitating recovery.
    j. Occupation: Surgical procedures may require a delay in returning to work.
    k. Coping patterns: Information and emotional support for the patient are necessary to successfully recover from surgery.
    l. Support systems: Family members should be encouraged to provide support before and after surgery.
    m. Sociocultural needs: The patient's cultural background may require that nursing interventions be individualized to meet needs in such areas as language, food preferences, family interaction and participation, personal space, and health beliefs and practices.

14. a. Vital signs: Assess temperature, blood pressure, pulse and respiratory rates, note deviations from preoperative and PACU data as well as symptoms of complications.
    b. Color and temperature of skin: Assess for warmth, pallor, cyanosis, and diaphoresis.
    c. Level of consciousness: Assess for orientation to time, place, and person as well as reaction to stimuli and ability to move extremities.
    d. Intravenous fluids: Assess type and amount of solution, flow rate, securement and patency of tubing, and infusion site.
    e. Surgical site: Assess dressing and dependent areas for drainage. Assess drains and tubes and be sure they are intact, patent and properly connected to drainage systems.
    f. Other tubes: Assess indwelling urinary catheter, gas-

trointestinal suction, and so forth, for drainage, patency, and amount of output.
    g. Comfort level: Assess for pain and determine if analgesics were given in the PACU. Assess for nausea and vomiting.
    h. Position and safety: Place patient in an ordered position, or if the patient is not fully conscious, place him or her in the side-lying position. Elevate the side rails and place the bed in low position.
    i. Comfort: Cover the patient with a blanket, reorient him or her to the room as necessary, and allow family members to remain with the patient after the initial assessment is completed.

15. Sample Answers
    a. Nausea and vomiting: Provide oral hygiene as needed, avoid strong-smelling food.
    b. Thirst: Offer ice chips, maintain oral hygiene.
    c. Hiccups: Rebreathe into paper bag, eat a teaspoon of granulated sugar.
    d. Surgical pain: Assess pain frequently, offer nonpharmacologic measures to supplement medications.

Chapter 30

MATCHING

1. a	2. d	3. h	4. e	5. f	6. c
7. g	8. d	9. b	10. c	11. a	12. d
13. b	14. c	15. d	16. a		

MULTIPLE CHOICE

1. b	2. a	3. b	4. c	5. d	6. c
7. c	8. a	9. a			

COMPLETION

1. Sample Answers
   Nurses interacting with older adults need to understand that simple measures such as addressing older patients respectfully, communicating that you take their concerns seriously, noticing and affirming their personal strengths, and interacting with them as individuals.
2. Answers will vary with student's experiences.
3. Sample Answers
   a. Significance: Do you feel loved and appreciated by the key people in your life?
   b. Competence: Does anything interfere with your ability to do your life work?
   c. Virtue: How would you describe your ability to follow your moral code?
   d. Power: Do you feel you are in control of your life?
4. Sample Answers
   a. Developmental considerations: A teenager needs to be trusted and guided to make good choices that affect his/her life.
   b. Culture: As a child internalizes the values of parents and peers, culture begins to influence his/her sense of self.
   c. Internal and external resources: The amount of money a person earns may influence his/her self-concept.
   d. History of success or failure: A child who repeatedly fails in school may have difficulty succeeding in life.

e. Stressors: Self-concept determines the way a person perceives stressors in his/her life and reacts to them.

f. Aging, illness, or trauma: A paralyzing injury will most likely affect self-concept.

5. Sample Answers

a. Nurses must accept the fact that they must constantly learn new theories and procedures to keep up with medicine.

b. A periodic review of a nurse's skills, strengths, and weaknesses should be built into the practice.

c. Nurses should not dwell upon the one mistake they may have made, but should recall what they did right and learn from their mistakes.

d. If a nurse has weak technical skills in one area, she should focus on this area and strengthen her knowledge and competency through research, study, and practice.

e. Congratulate colleagues and celebrate when the nursing team is successful.

f. Nurses should be aware of their impact on society, and the image they project should be positive.

6. Answers will vary with student's experience

7. Sample Answers

a. Personal identity: How would you describe yourself to others?

b. Patient strengths: What special talents and abilities do you have?

c. Body image: What are your positive physical attributes?

d. Self-esteem: What do you like most about yourself?

e. Role performance: What major roles describe you?

8. Sample Answers

a. Diagnosis: Anxiety related to unwelcome change in body image (mastectomy)

Patient goal: Patient will express satisfaction with ability to live with altered body image.

b. Diagnosis: Anxiety related to inability to accept or manage new role.

Patient goal: Patient reports feeling less anxious about being pregnant.

c. Diagnosis: Altered Health Maintenance related to low self-esteem and inability to cope with grief.

Patient goal: Patient will acknowledge his own self-worth and express a desire to take care of himself despite his grief.

d. Diagnosis: Knowledge Deficit: How to Help Child Develop Self-Esteem, related to lack of experience with parenting.

Patient goal: Patient will describe methods of developing self-esteem in children.

e. Diagnosis: High Risk for Violence, Domestic Abuse, related to low self-esteem and sense of hopelessness.

Patient goal: Patient will verbalize that self is liked and deserves to live without fear of abuse.

f. Diagnosis: Altered Sexuality Patterns related to changed body image, disturbance in self concept.

Patient goal: Patient will describe self realistically, identifying strengths that make her desirable to husband.

9. a. Encourage patients to identify their strengths.

b. Notice and reinforce patient strengths.

c. Encourage patients to will for themselves the strengths they desire and to try them on.

10. a. Using looks, touch, and speech to communicate worth.

b. Speaking respectfully to the patient and addressing the patient by preferred name.

c. Moving the patient's body respectfully if the patient is unable to move on his/her own.

11. Sample Answers

a. Help her find meaning in the experience, regain mastery to the extent that this is possible, and realistically evaluate the adequacy of her coping strategy. Teach her to develop a game plan for confronting anxiety-producing situations. Identify and secure interventions for treatable depression. Remedy treatable causes of self-identity disturbances, such as pain or substance abuse.

b. Notice and affirm positive physiologic characteristics of the patient. Teach preventive self-care measures that reduce discomforting signs of aging. Explore new activities (which may include old hobbies) that are within the changing physical abilities of the patient.

c. Help patient identify and utilize personal strengths. Let him know that you value him, simply for who his is. Use the name he prefers. Ask him questions about his life, interests, and values. Engage him in activities in which he can be successful. Empower him to meet his needs. Provide necessary knowledge, teach new behaviors, and instill in him the belief that he can change.

d. Explore with patient the many roles she has fulfilled throughout her lifetime. Encourage her to reminisce. Facilitate grieving over valued roles that she can no longer perform.

CHAPTER 30: PATIENT CARE STUDY

1. Objective data are underlined; subjective data are in boldface.

An English teacher asks you, the school nurse, to see one of her students whose grades have recently dropped and who no longer seems to be interested in school—or anything else. "She was one of my best students, and I can't figure out what's going on. She seems reluctant to talk about this change." When Julie, a 16-year-old junior, walks into your office, you are immediately struck by her stooped posture, unstyled hair and sloppy appearance. Julie is attractive, but at 5'3" and 150 lbs, she is overweight. Although Julie is initially reluctant to talk, she breaks down at one point and confides that for the first time in her life she feels **"absolutely awful"** about herself. **"I've always concentrated on getting good grades and achieved this easily. But right now, this doesn't seem so important. I don't have any friends. All I hear the girls talking about is boys, and** I was never even asked out by a boy**—which I guess isn't surprising. Look at me."** After a few questions, it becomes clear that Julie has new expectations for herself based on what she observes in her peers, and she finds herself falling far short of her new, ideal self. Julie admits that in the past, **once she set a goal for herself, she was always able to achieve it because she is strongly self-motivated.**

Although she has withdrawn from her parents and teachers, she admits that she does know adults she can trust who have been a big support to her in the past. "If only I could become the kind of teenager other kids like and have lots of friends!"

2. Nursing Process Worksheet

Health Problem:

Situational low self-esteem.

Expected Outcome:

In one month, 10/10/02, patient will report that she feels "better" about herself, based on new socialization experiences with peers and improved body image.

Etiology:

Perceived inability to meet newly accepted peer standards regarding socialization/dating.

Nursing Interventions:

1. Help patient develop workable self-care strategies to decrease weight and enhance physical appearance.
2. Explore patient's interest in activities that will serve two goals: (1) enable patient to develop friendships, and (2) improve her body image, e.g., sports, dancing, hiking clubs.
3. Counsel patient about peer relationships/sexuality/dating.

Signs & Symptoms (Defining Characteristics):

Feels "absolutely awful" about herself; 5'3", 150 lbs; "I don't have any friends"; never dated; grades have dropped recently; new lack of interest/vitality; stooped posture; unstyled hair; sloppy appearance.

Evaluative Statement:

10/10/02: Goal partially met—patient states that she feels great about losing weight (150 lbs, down to 145) and likes her "new look," but still feels shy with peers and is not dating. Revision: Celebrate new self-care behaviors and reevaluate efforts to enhance peer relationships.

M. Stenulis, RN

3. Patient strengths: Physically attractive; past history of achieving personal goals; strongly self-motivated; has trusting relationships with adults (parents and teachers).

   Personal strengths: Ability to establish trusting nurse-patient relationships with high school students; knowledge of teen social "norms"; successful history of motivating teens to develop and take pride in health self-care behaviors.

4. 10/10/02: Met with patient one month after initial meeting. In that time, she lost 5 lbs, which she attributes to decreased snacking and increased activity (joined field hockey team). She walked into the office with erect posture and exhibited more interest/vitality than at last meeting. She reports still feeling very shy with her peers and is uncomfortable with boys. She is very interested, however, in participating in group activities in which she can overcome her shyness, and will hopefully make new friends.

M. Stenulis, RN

Chapter 31

MATCHING

1. c	2. i	3. l	4. f	5. b	6. e
7. a	8. d	9. g	10. h	11. j	12. c
13. i	14. b	15. h	16. a	17. e	18. f
19. g					

MULTIPLE CHOICE

1. a	2. c	3. b	4. b	5. a	6. d
7. c	8. c	9. a	10. a	11. d	12. a
13. b					

COMPLETION

1. a. Mind–body interaction: Humans react to threats of danger as if they were real. The person perceives the threat on an emotional level, and the body prepares itself to either resist it or turn away and avoid the danger. For example: An executive has an important presentation to make in the morning and is restless the night before, unable to eat breakfast, and has feelings of apprehension and rapid heartbeat prior to the presentation.
   b. Local adaptation syndrome: A localized response of the body to stress. It does not involve the entire body, only a body part. LAS is an adaptive response, primarily homeostatic, and short-term. For example: Reflex pain response and inflammatory response.
   c. General adaptation syndrome: A biochemical model of stress developed by Hans Selye which describes the body's general response to stress and serves as part of the knowledge base essential to all areas of nursing care. For example: Alarm reaction—various defense mechanisms are activated; resistance—body attempts to adapt to the stressor; exhaustion—the body either rests and mobilizes its defenses to return to normal or reaches total exhaustion and dies.
2. a. Bleeding is controlled initially by vasoconstriction of blood vessels at injury site. Histamines are released and capillary permeability increases, allowing increased blood flow and increased white blood cells to area; blood flow returns to normal.
   b. Exudate is released from the wound; amount depends on size, location, and severity of wound.
   c. Damaged cells are repaired by either regeneration or formation of scar tissue.
3. a. Severity and duration of the stressor
   b. Previous health of the person
   c. Immediacy and effectiveness of healthcare interventions
4. a. Mild anxiety: Present in day-to-day living; increases alertness and perceptual fields, and motivates learning and growth.
   b. Moderate anxiety: Narrows person's perceptual fields so that the focus is on immediate concerns, with inattention to other details.
   c. Severe anxiety: Creates a very narrow focus on specific detail; causes all behavior to be geared toward relief.
   d. Panic: Causes the person to lose control and experience dread and terror; characterized by increased

physical activity, distorted perceptions and relations, and loss of rational thought.

5. Answers will vary with student's experience
6. Sample Answers
   a. Stressors in health facilitate normal growth and development.
   b. Fear of developing cardiovascular disease can motivate a person to exercise regularly.
   c. Fear of failure in business can motivate a person to attend classes.
7. Sample Answers
   a. Developmental stress: An infant learns that his hunger will be taken care of in a timely manner; a school-age child learn the rewards of studying; an elderly male accepts the limitations of age on his social life.
   b. Situational stress: A child contracts a life-threatening illness; a spouse loses her job; a spouse asks for a divorce.
8. Sample Answers
   a. It must have been frightening being in an automobile accident.
   b. I notice that you seen distracted; would you care to talk about it?
9. Sample Answers
   Confront the mother in an understanding manner and question her about her daily schedule and ability to do all the things necessary to take care of her family. Refer the mother to outside agencies, e.g., day care programs, supportive friends and family members, or resources for hired help to give her a break from her responsibilities. Help the mother arrange her daily care to schedule in some time for herself, if possible.
10. a. Exercise: The benefits of exercise include an improved musculoskeletal system, more effective cardiovascular function, weight control, and relaxation. It improves one's sense of well-being, relieves tension, and enables one to cope with life better.
    b. Rest and sleep: Allows the body to maintain homeostasis and restore energy levels; provides insulation against stress.
    c. Nutrition: Plays an active role in maintaining the body's homeostatic mechanisms and in increasing resistance to stress.
11. a. Identify the problem.
    b. List alternatives.
    c. Choose from among the alternatives.
    d. Implement a plan.
    e. Evaluate the outcome.
12. a. Age affects the ability to adapt; nutrition and sleep affect stress levels; social factors and life events affect stress level.
13. a. Provide social support.
    b. Provide emotional and physical support.
    c. Help with problem solving and teaching–learning activities.

CHAPTER 31: PATIENT CARE STUDY ANSWERS

a. (a) On a scale of 1–10, with 10 being most able to control this situation, how would you rate yourself at this time? What does that number mean to you?
   (b) Who do you talk to when you feel sad or nervous?
   (c) What has helped you handle stressful situations in the past? (Also see samples of questions in text.)
b. Heart palpitations, dry mouth, difficulty breathing, increased perspiration, nausea, tremors, increased pulse rate, increased blood pressure, crying, sleep disturbances, eating disturbances
c. (a) Anxiety related to multiple stressors occurring in relatively short period of time.
   (b) Altered Thought Processes related to severe anxiety
   (c) Risk for Altered Nutrition: Less than Body Requirements related to decreased food intake
   (d) Risk for Social Isolation related to perceived need to be family caregiver.
d. (a) Verbalize a decrease in anxiety with increased feelings of comfort.
   (b) Develop effective coping skills through problem-solving and anxiety-reducing techniques.
   (c) Maintain or slightly increase body weight.
   (d) Actively participate in at least one social activity outside the home each week.
e. A crisis occurs when previous coping and defense mechanisms are no longer effective. This failure causes high levels of anxiety, disorganized behavior, and an inability to function adequately.
f. Identify the problem, list alternatives, choose from among alternatives, implement a plan, evaluate the outcome.
g. Exercise: Exercise helps maintain physical and emotional health; it also improves ability to cope with stressors. Recommend an exercise program of 30–45 minutes of enjoyable exercise 3–4 times a week.
   Rest and sleep: Rest and sleep restore energy levels and provide insulation against stress. Relaxation techniques are often helpful in inducing sleep.
   Nutrition: Nutrition plays an active role in increasing resistance to stress. Follow recommended guidelines for amounts and types of foods to eat. (See Chapter 41 for more information about nutrition.)
h. Mrs. Brent will meet expected outcomes if she verbalizes the causes of stress and anxiety, identifies and uses sources of support, uses problem-solving techniques to reduce the number of stressors, practices healthy lifestyle habits, and verbalizes a decrease in anxiety and an increase in comfort.

Chapter 32

MATCHING

1. h	2. e	3. a	4. g	5. b	6. d
7. c	8. d	9. a	10. e	11. b	12. c
13. f					

CORRECT THE FALSE STATEMENTS

1. False—unresolved grief
2. False—anger
3. True
4. False—durable power of attorney for healthcare
5. True
6. False—no-code or do-not-resuscitate order
7. True
8. False—mortician
9. False—nurse
10. False—mortician/family member (custom dictates this ritual)
11. True

MULTIPLE CHOICE

1. c	2. d	3. b	4. c	5. a	6. d
7. b	8. a				

COMPLETION

1. a. Care of the body: Place body in normal anatomic position; remove soiled dressings/tubes (unless an autopsy is being performed); place ID tags on shroud, ankle, and prostheses.
   b. Care of the family: Be an attentive listener; attend funeral (if family permits); make follow-up call to assess family's well-being.
   c. Discharging legal responsibilities: Ensure death certificate has been signed by physician; review organ donation arrangements.
2. a. Heart–lung death: The irreversible cessation of spontaneous respiration and circulation; the acceped criterion for death until the 1960s, this definition emerged from the historical idea that the flow of body fluids was essential for life.
   b. Whole brain death: The irreversible cessation of all functions of the entire brain, including the brain stem, this definition emerged in the 1960s from the belief that neocortical functioning is the key to the definition of a human being.
   c. Higher brain death: The irreversible loss of all higher brain functions, or cognitive function; this definition was suggested in the 1970s and emerged from the belief that the brain is more important than the spinal cord and that the critical functions are the individual's personality, conscious life, uniqueness, capacity for remembering, judging, reasoning, acting, enjoying, worrying.
3. a. Denial and isolation: The patient denies that he or she will die, may repress what is discussed, and may isolate self from reality.
   b. Anger: The patient expresses rage and hostility and adopts a "why me?" attitude.
   c. Bargaining: The patient tries to barter for more time.

   d. Depression: The patient goes through a period of grief before death.
   e. Acceptance: The patient feels tranquil; she/he has accepted death and is prepared to die.
4. The patient should be told her diagnosis and prognosis as soon as possible, how the disease is likely to progress and what this will mean for her.
5. Inability to swallow; pitting edema; decreased gastrointestinal and urinary tract activity; bowel and bladder incontinence; loss of motion, sensation, and reflexes; elevated temperature; cyanosis; lowered blood pressure; noisy or irregular respiration; and Cheyne–Stokes respirations.
6. Answers will vary with student's experiences.
7. Nursing's role is to participate in the decision-making process by offering helpful information about the benefits and burdens of continued ventilation and description of what to expect if it is initiated. Supporting the patient's family and managing sedation and analgesia are critical nursing responsibilities.
8. Sample Answers
   a. Communicate openly with patients about their losses and invite discussion of the adequacy of their coping mechanisms.
   b. Respond genuinely to the concerns and feelings of dying patients and their families; do not be afraid to cry with patient and to allow feelings to show.
   c. Value time spent with patients and family members in which supportive presence is the primary intervention.
9. Sample Answers
   a. The patient shall make healthcare decisions reflecting his values and goals.
   b. The patient shall experience a comfortable and dignified death.
   c. The patient and family shall accept need for help as appropriate and use available resources.
10. Sample Answers
   a. In favor of: It is a beneficent and compassionate act. It takes the matter outside the reach of "medical power" and scrupulosity. It respects autonomy by preserving the patient's control of the manner, method, and timing of death.
   b. Against: It undermines the value of, and respect for, all human life. A focus on euthanasia will deviate attention from other valuable palliative techniques. If legalized, it is predicted patients will feel a subtle pressure to conform in order to relieve the economic and emotional burdens they impose on family and friends.
11. a. No-code: If a physician has written DNR on the chart of a patient, the patient or surrogate has expressed a wish that there be no attempts to resuscitate the patient in the event of cardiopulmonary emergency. The nurse must clarify the patient's code status.
   b. Comfort measures only: Nurses should be familiar with the forms used to indicate patient preferences about end-of-life care. The goal of a comfort measures only order is to indicate that the goal of treatment is a comfortable dignified death and that further life-sustaining measures are no longer indicated.

c. Do not hospitalize orders: These orders are used by patients in nursing homes and other residential settings who have elected not to be hospitalized for further aggressive treatment. The nursing responsibilities would be the same as for comfort measures only.

d. Terminal weaning: The nurse's role is to participate in the decision-making process by offering helpful information about the benefits and burdens of continued ventilation and a description of what to expect if terminal weaning is initiated.

12. a. Durable power of attorney: Nurses must facilitate dialogue about this advance directive that appoints an agent the person trusts to make decisions in the event of the appointing person's subsequent incapacity.

b. Living will: Nurses must also facilitate dialogue about this advance directive that provides specific instructions about the kinds of healthcare that should be provided or foregone in particular situations.

CHAPTER 32: PATIENT CARE STUDY

1. Objective data are underlined; subjective data are in boldface.

LeRoy is a 40-year-old architect whose life partner, Michael, is dying of AIDs. Although both LeRoy and Michael did the bathhouse scene in the early 1980s and had multiple unprotected sexual encounters, they have been in a monogamous relationship for the last 14 years. Michael has been in and out of the hospital during the last 3 years, and is now dying of end-stage AIDs at home. He is enrolled in a hospice program. LeRoy has been very supportive of Michael throughout the different phases of his illness, but at present seems to be "losing it." Michael noticed that LeRoy is sleeping at odd times and seems to be losing weight. He suspects that **LeRoy may be drinking more than usual and using recreational drugs.** He also says that he is "acting strangely," that **he seems emotionally withdrawn and unusually uncommunicative.** "I don't think he's able to deal with the fact that I am dying. He won't let me talk about it at all." The hospice nurse noted that LeRoy is now rarely home when he comes to visit. When the hospice nurse called to arrange a meeting with LeRoy, LeRoy informed him that he was **"managing quite well,** thank you," and that **he had no concerns or problems to discuss.**

2. Nursing Process Worksheet

Health Problem:

Anticipatory grieving

Expected Outcome:

LeRoy will openly express his grief over Michael's impending death and participate in decision making for the future.

Etiology:

Inability to even allow himself to think about what his life will be like without his life partner; history of using denial as a coping mechanism.

Nursing Interventions:

1. Determine what is making this anticipated loss so "unthinkable."

2. Encourage patient to share concerns. Normalize the experience of grieving by sharing experiences of other gay partners who have successfully grieved over the death of their friends and loved ones. Respect patient's use of denial to make time to work things through. Let him know you are available to help at a later date, if necessary.

3. Help the patient explore his usual strategies for adjusting to loss (i.e., denial) and determine how they are serving him now. If he feels they are inadequate, help him develop new strategies.

4. Promote grief work through each phase of the grieving process: denial, isolation, depression, anger, guilt, fear, rejection. Help Michael understand LeRoy's grief and need to move in and out of each stage at his own pace.

5. Refer patient to community-based support groups.

Signs and Symptoms:

Partner reports that LeRoy is sleeping at odd times and seems to be losing weight. He suspects that LeRoy is drinking more than usual and using recreational drugs. He also says that he is "acting strangely," that he seems emotionally withdrawn and unusually uncommunicative. LeRoy is now rarely home when the hospice nurse visits. When the nurse called to arrange a meeting with him, LeRoy informed him that he was "managing quite well, thank you," and that he had no concerns or problems to discuss.

Evaluative Statement:

5/1/02: Goal not met. LeRoy is still denying that he is experiencing any difficulty dealing with Michael's impending death; appears fearful of even discussing this subject. Revision: Reiterated stages of grieving and importance of grief work; offered a listening "ear," should he decide he wishes to talk about this later.

C. Taylor, RN

3. Patient strengths: LeRoy's longstanding relationship with Michael and desire to be present and supportive is a powerful motivator for getting him to address his inability to consciously work through his grief. LeRoy is intelligent and trusts healthcare professionals, with whom he has had good experiences in the past.

Personal strengths: Knowledge about stages of grief and grief work; strong interpersonal skills; teaching and counselling skills.

4. 5/13/02: LeRoy, the patient's life partner and significant other, called today to arrange a time to meet. He noted that he finally had a long talk with Michael and is able to see that he hasn't been able to deal with his dying in a conscious manner at all. "I guess I just kept hoping that if I didn't think about it, it wouldn't happen." He now states that he realizes that if he continues in this manner, he won't be able to provide Michael the support he needs. He also admits feeling "totally overwhelmed." Brief discussion of stages of grieving and grief work, and appointment made for 5/20/02.

C. Taylor, RN

Chapter 33

MATCHING

1. h	2. d	3. a	4. c	5. b	6. f
7. e	8. a	9. c	10. d	11. b	12. c
13. d	14. b	15. a			

MULTIPLE CHOICE

1. c	2. d	3. b	4. a	5. b	6. d	7. b

COMPLETION

1. a. A stimulus, an agent, act, or other influence capable of initiating a response by the nervous system.
   b. A receptor or sense organ must receive the stimulus and convert it into a nerve impulse.
   c. The nerve impulse must be conducted along a nervous pathway from the receptor or sense organ to the brain.
   d. A particular area in the brain must receive and translate the impulse into a sensation.
2. a. Environment: A patient with AIDS in isolation is at high risk for sensory deprivation.
   b. Impaired ability to receive environmental stimuli: A patient who is visually impaired is at high risk for sensory deprivation.
   c. Inability to process environmental stimuli: A patient who is confused cannot process environmental stimuli.
3. a. Perceptual responses: Inaccurate perception of sights, sounds, tastes, smells, and body position; poor coordination and equilibrium; mild to gross distortions in perception, ranging from daydreams to hallucinations.
   b. Cognitive responses: Inability to control the direction of thought content; decreased attention span and ability to concentrate; difficulty with memory, problem-solving, and task performance.
   c. Emotional responses: Inappropriate emotional responses-apathy, anxiety, fear, anger, belligerence, panic, depression; rapid mood changes.
4. Sample Answers
   a. A patient is disoriented by the strange sights, odors, and sounds in a CCU.
   b. A burn victim is in constant pain and cannot concentrate on his environment.
   c. A confused patient panics at the sight of doctors and nurses probing his body.
5. Cultural care deprivation is a lack of culturally assistive, supportive or facilitative acts, e.g., touching is viewed as a natural and welcome custom in certain cultures, while in other cultures it may be taboo.
6. Sample Answers
   a. Infant: Soothing sounds, rocking, holding and changing position, changing patterns of light and shade, developing appropriate play.
   b. Adult: The use of music, poetry, drama to alleviate boredom.
   c. Elderly: The use of art classes or organizing a book club in a nursing home.
7. a. Patient will report feeling safe and in control of his/her environment.
   b. Patient will verbalize acceptance of the sensory deficit.
8. Sample Answer
   This patient is suffering from sensory deprivation.

Measures should be taken to stimulate as many senses as possible. The curtains could be drawn to allow light into the room; soft music could be played to stimulate auditory functioning; flavorful meals could be prepared to stimulate taste; flowers, cards, and pictures could be displayed to stimulate visual functioning.

9. a. Avoid damage from UV rays.
   b. Use caution with aerosol sprays.
   c. Have regular eye examinations and tests for glaucoma.
   d. Know the danger signals that indicate serious eye problems.
10. Sample Answers
    a. Visual: Read different types of books to the child; limit television; plan various outings.
    b. Auditory: Teach the child songs; play records; join a storytelling group.
    c. Olfactory: Have child identify different odors; prepare enticing meals and savor the aromas.
    d. Gustatory: Encourage the child to experiment with different foods with varying colors, tastes, shapes and textures; introduce finger foods into diet.
    e. Tactile: Use games and sports to increase body contact with child; demonstrate affection by hugging, holding child in lap, etc.
11. Sample Answers
    a. Developmental considerations: The adult may experience the need to compensate for the loss of one type of stimulation by increasing other sources of sensory stimuli.
    b. Culture: An individual's culture may dictate how much sensory stimulation is considered normal.
    c. Personality and lifestyle: Different personality types demand different levels of stimulation.
    d. Stress: Increased sensory stimulation may be sought during periods of high stress.
    e. Illness and medication: Illness can affect the reception of sensory stimuli; medications that alert or depress the central nervous system may interfere with the perception of sensory stimuli.
12. a. Stimulation: Assess for recent changes in sensory stimulation, if the type of stimulation present is developmentally appropriate.
    b. Reception: Assess for anything that may interfere with sensory reception and prescribe any corrective devices the patient uses for sensory impairment.
    c. Transmission–perception–reaction: High-risk patients include confused patients and patients with nervous system impairments. Assess patient's abilities to transmit, perceive, and react to stimuli during everyday interactions.
13. Sample Answers
    a. Visually impaired patients: Acknowledge your presence in the patient's room, identify yourself by name, speak in a normal tone of voice.
    b. Hearing impaired patients: Avoid excessive noise, avoid excessive cleaning of ears, know the symptoms of hearing loss.
    c. Unconscious patients: Be careful of what is said in the patient's presence, assume the person can hear you, speak to the person before touching him.

CHAPTER 33: PATIENT CARE STUDY

1. Objective data are underlined; subjective data are in bold-face.

   Mr. Gibson, an <u>81-year-old married African-American</u>, with much prodding from his wife, reluctantly reports that **he seems not to be hearing as well as he used to be. "I don't know what the trouble is. I'm in perfect health; always have been. More and more people just seem to be mumbling instead of talking."** You notice that <u>he is seated on the edge of his chair and bends toward you when you speak to him. His wife reports that he has stopped going out and pretty much stays in his room whenever people come to the house to visit</u> because **he is embarrassed** by his inability to hear. **"This is really a shame because** <u>George was always the life of the party."</u> You ask Mr. Gibson if he has ever had his hearing evaluated and he tells you, <u>**"no,"**</u> that until now **he's been trying to convince himself that nothing's wrong with his hearing.**

2. Nursing Process Worksheet

Health Problem:

Sensory/perceptual alteration: auditory.

Etiology:

Reluctance to accept that he has an auditory problem and to seek help.

Signs & Symptoms (Defining Characteristics):

Leans forward to hear speaker; attempts to deny hearing loss and attributes problem to others who are "mumbling"; has greatly reduced opportunities for conversation; has not sought help until now.

Expected Outcome:

After medical evaluation of hearing loss and treatment, patient demonstrates better coping skills by increasing amount of time he spends socializing with others.

Nursing Interventions:

1. Explain that hearing loss often accompanies aging and that a medical evaluation is important to provide proper treatment.
2. Help patient make an appointment for evaluation.
3. Explore strategies for improving his communication skills and prevent social isolation.

Evaluative Statement:

12/5/02: Goal partially met—hearing aid has enabled patient to comprehend most one-to-one conversations, but ability to hear well in groups is still impaired. Is willing to investigate possibility of learning how to lip-read. No longer avoids company, especially if it is only one or two people.

D. Mason, RN

3. Patient strengths: Healthy until now; wife is supportive; previous history of strong interactional skills.
   Personal strengths: Recognize significance of sensory/perceptual alterations; able to distinguish changes in perceptual abilities normally related to aging from those indicating treatable medical problems; able to establish trusting relationship with older patients.

4. 12/5/02: Patient presents after auditory examination revealed a partial sensorineural loss, which was distorting his perception of certain frequencies and which was partially correctable with amplification. Patient still leans close to speaker, but in a one-to-one conversation his responses demonstrate his ability to correctly interpret most of what the speaker is saying. He reports that he still has great difficulty listening in groups. His wife noted with delight that he seems more like "his old self" when one or two friends come to visit. He expresses an interest in learning how to lip-read.

D. Mason, RN

Chapter 34

MATCHING

1. f	2. m	3. e	4. n	5. g	6. o
7. d	8. l	9. k	10. a	11. j	12. h
13. b	14. c	15. i	16. d	17. a	18. h
19. b	20. g	21. e	22. c	23. f	

MULTIPLE CHOICE

1. a	2. c	3. c	4. b	5. d	6. c
7. b	8. b	9. c			

COMPLETION

1. Sample Answers
   a. Chronic pain: Teach altered or modified positions for coitus.
   b. Diabetes: Some men may be candidates for penile prosthesis; pharmacologic management of erectile dysfunction may be indicated.
   c. Cardiovascular disease: Teach gradual resuming of sexual activity, comfortable position for affected partner.
   d. Loss of body part: Teach acceptance of body image.
   e. Spinal cord injuries: Promote stimulation of other erogenous zones.
   f. Mental illness: Counseling for depression.
   g. Sexually transmitted diseases: Educate the public about the prevention and treatment of STDs.
2. a. Follicular phase: Days 4–14; a number of follicles mature but only one produces a mature ovum; at the same time, in the uterus the endometrium is becoming thick and velvety in preparation of the fertilized egg.
   b. Proliferation phase: Ovulation occurs on day 14; the mature ovum ruptures from the follicle and the surface of the ovary is swept into the fallopian tube. If sperm are present, the ovum is fertilized at this time.
   c. Luteal phase: Days 15–28; the leftover empty follicle fills up with a yellow pigment and is then called the corpus luteum, which produces hormones that encourage a fertilized egg to grow. If fertilization does not occur, the corpus luteum disintegrates.
   d. Secretory phase: The endometrial lining becomes thick; in the absence of fertilized egg, corpus luteum

dies and endometrial lining disintegrates; menses begins at day 28 as result of the uterus shedding the endometrial lining.

3. a. Excitement phase:

Female: The breasts of the woman swell and nipples become erect; vaginal lubricant seeps out of body; upper two thirds of vagina expand; clitoris enlarges and emerges slightly from clitoral hood; labia enlarge and turn deep rosy red.

Male: Erection of the penis caused by increased congestion with blood; scrotum noticeably elevates, thickens, and enlarges. The skin of the penis and scrotum turns deep reddish-purple; male nipples may harden and become erect.

b. Plateau:

Female: The clitoris retracts and disappears under clitoral hood; intensity is greater than that of excitement phase, but not enough to begin orgasm.

Male: Secretions from Cowper's glands may appear at the glans of the penis during this phase.

c. Orgasm:

Female: The orgasm phase begins with a heightened feeling of physical pleasure followed by overwhelming release and involuntary contractions of the genitals. Loss of muscular control can cause spastic contractions.

Male: Involuntary spasmodic contractions of the genitals occur in the penis, epididymis, vas deferens, and rectum; most often accompanied by ejaculation.

d. Resolution:

Female: Return to normal body functioning; feelings of relaxation, fatigue, and fulfillment; the woman is physiologically capable of immediate response to sexual stimulation and may achieve multiple orgasms.

Male: Return to normal body functioning accompanied by same feelings as above; men experience a refractory period, during which they are incapable of sexual response.

4. a. Confrontation: Look the harasser in the eye and tell him or her you do not like this behavior and want it to stop.

b. Documentation: Document specific instances of harassment; put details in a letter and send it to the harasser indicating you do not like this behavior and want it to stop. Send the letter by way of registered mail.

c. Written complaint: If behavior does not stop, submit a written complaint to administration (use appropriate channels).

d. Government complaint: If all else fails, file a complaint with the Equal Employment Opportunity Commission.

5. a. Any inpatient or outpatient who is receiving care for pregnancy, an STD, infertility, or conception.

b. Any patient who is currently experiencing a sexual dysfunction or problem.

c. Any patient whose illness will affect sexual functioning and behavior in any way.

6. a. "How would you describe this problem?"

b. "What do you think caused the problem, or what was happening when you first noticed it?"

c. "What have you tried in the past to correct the problem?"

7. a. A change in knowledge

b. A change in patient attitude

c. A change in behavior

8. See table below.

Method	Advantages	Disadvantages
a. Natural family planning	Methods can be effective in avoiding pregnancy if mutual understanding, support, and motivation exist between the woman and her partner. There are no side effects (as in hormonal methods) and no messy devices to insert.	Requires abstinence during ovulation and complete understanding of the signs and symptoms of ovulation.
b. Barrier Methods	Condoms help to prevent STDs; appropriate for women with sensitivity to the pill; effective when used correctly; relatively inexpensive methods.	Devices must be applied before intercourse; not all women can wear them; threat of toxic shock syndrome with vaginal sponge.
c. Intrauterine Devices	High rate of effectiveness; little care or motivation on part of patient is necessary; excellent method for women who have completed their families but are not ready for sterilization.	Serious side effects and complications.
d. Hormonal Methods	Many beneficial noncontraceptive effects, e.g., protecting women against development of breast, ovarian, and endometrial cancer; almost 100% effective when taken as directed.	Cost may be prohibitive to some; compliance is necessary; some women should not take the pill due to physiologic disorders or diseases.
e. Sterilization	After initial surgery and recheck, no further compliance is necessary; almost 100% effective.	Should be considered permanent irreversible.

CHAPTER 34: PATIENT CARE STUDY

1. Objective data are underlined; subjective data are in bold-face.

Anthony Piscatelli, a <u>6-foot-tall, muscular, healthy 19-year-old college freshman in the School of Nursing</u> confides to his nursing advisor that "everything is great" about college life, with one exception. **"All of a sudden I find myself questioning the values I learned at home about sex and marriage.** My mom was really insistent that each of her sons should respect women and that intercourse was something you saved until you were ready to get married. If she told us once she told us a hundred times that we'd save ourselves, the girls in our lives, and her and dad a lot of heartache if we could just learn to control ourselves sexually. Problem is that no one here seems to subscribe to this philosophy. **I feel like I'm abnormal in some way to even think like this.** There's a lot of sexual activity in the dorms, and no one even thinks you're serious if you talk about virginity positively. What do you think? Did my mom sell me a bill of goods? Is it true that if you take the proper precautions, no one gets hurt and everyone has a good time?" Tony reports that **he is a virgin and that he really misses his close family back home. "I do get lonely at times, and would love to just cuddle with someone or even give and get a big hug, but no one seems to understand this."**

2. Nursing Process Worksheet:

Health Problem:

High risk for altered sexuality patterns.

Etiology:

Discrepancy between his family's values about sex and marriage and those he is discovering in peer group.

Signs & Symptoms (Defining Characteristics):

"All of a sudden I find myself questioning the values I learned at home about sex and marriage"; feels like he is "abnormal" in some way to value virginity; lonely—wants intimacy; "Is it true that if you take the proper precautions, no one gets hurt and everyone has a good time?"

Expected Outcome:

By next meeting, 11/17/02, patient will report personal satisfaction with the results of his reevaluation of his beliefs/values concerning sex and marriage.

Nursing Interventions:

1. Assess patient's knowledge of sexual development and need for intimacy and belonging, and correct any misinformation.
2. Explore with the patient the source of the beliefs/values he learned at home and assist in determining the role he wants these beliefs/values to play in his life.
3. Compare the options of abstinence and becoming sexually active, and perform related sexual teaching.
4. Refer to appropriate on-campus sexuality classes, counseling center or seminars, as indicated.

Evaluative Statement:

11/17/02: Goal not met. Patient reports that his confusion has only deepened and he now feels like "my head is warring with my body." Reports sleeping with his girlfriend but feeling very guilty afterwards—now ignores this girl. Revision: See if he's willing to talk with a peer or professional counselor regarding sexual concerns.

R. LeBon, RN

3. Patient strengths: Healthy; caring family; ability to voice his concerns; very "likeable" person.
   Personal strengths: Sound knowledge of sexuality; respect for and appreciation of sexuality; understanding of developmental challenges of young adults and self-identity and intimacy needs; ability to create trusting relationships with young adults.

4. 11/17/02: Patient states he is "more confused now" than when we last met. He yielded to peer pressure and slept with girlfriend; used condom. While he "enjoyed this experience," he has been "wracked with guilt" ever since. He cannot reconcile this behavior with what he learned at home and continues to feel "unsure" of who he wants to be. He definitely wants some resolution of this conflict and is interested in speaking with a professional sexuality counselor. Referral made.

R. LeBon, RN

Chapter 35

MATCHING

1. b	2. c, d	3. a	4. f	5. g	6. e
7. d	8. a	9. e	10. b	11. g	12. c
13. a	14. d	15. c	16. b	17. a	18. d
19. c					

MULTIPLE CHOICE

1. b	2. d	3. c	4. a	5. b	6. d
7. b	8. a				

COMPLETION

1. a. Need for meaning and purpose
   b. Need for love and relatedness
   c. Need for forgiveness
2. Sample Answers
   a. Offering a compassionate presence.
   b. Assisting in the struggle to find meaning and purpose in the face of suffering, illness and death.
   c. Fostering relationships with God/humans that nurture the spirit.
   d. Facilitating the patient's expression of religious or spiritual beliefs and practices.
3. a. Life-affirming influences enhance life, give meaning and purpose to existence, strengthen feeling of self-worth, encourage self-actualization, and are health-giving and life-sustaining.
   b. Life-denying influences restrict or enclose life patterns, limit experiences and associations, place bur-

dens of guilt on individuals, encourage feelings of unworthiness, and are generally health-denying and life-inhibiting.

4. a. Many religions prescribe dietary requirements and restrictions.
   b. Some religious faiths restrict birth control practices.
5. a. A guide to daily living: Religions may specify dietary requirements or birth control measures.
   b. A source of support: It is common for people to seek support from religious faith in times of stress; this support is often vital to the acceptance of an illness. Prayer, devotional reading, and other religious practices often do for the person spiritually what protective exercises do for the body physically.
   c. A source of strength and healing: People have been known to endure extreme physical distress because of strong faith; patients' families have taken on almost unbelievable rehabilitative tasks because they had faith in the eventual positive results of their effort.
   d. A source of conflict: There are times when religious beliefs conflict with prevalent healthcare practices; for example, the doctrine of Jehovah's Witnesses prohibits blood transfusions. For some, illness is viewed as punishment for sin, and inevitable.
6. a. Developmental considerations: As a child matures, life experiences usually influence and mature spiritual beliefs. With advancing years, the tendency to think about life after death prompts some individuals to reexamine and reaffirm their spiritual beliefs.
   b. Family: A child's parents play a key role in the development of the child's spirituality.
   c. Ethnic background: Religious traditions differ among ethnic groups. There are clear distinctions between Eastern and Western spiritual traditions as well as among those of individual ethnic groups; such as Native Americans.
   d. Formal religion: Each of the major religions have several characteristics in common.
   e. Life events: Both positive and negative life experiences can influence spirituality and in turn are influenced by the meaning a person's spiritual beliefs attribute to them.
7. Answers will vary with student's experiences.
8. a. Basis of authority or source of power
   b. Scripture or sacred word
   c. An ethical code that defines right and wrong
   d. A psychology and identity that allows its adherents to fit into a group and the world to be defined by the religion
   e. Aspirations or expectations
   f. Some ideas about what follows death
9. Sample Answers
   a. Spiritual pain: This seems to be a source of deep pain for you....
   b. Spiritual alienation: Does it seem like God is far away from your life?
   c. Spiritual anxiety: Are you afraid that God might not be there for you when you need him?
   d. Spiritual anger: I sense a great deal of anger in your statements about God taking away your daughter. Can you share more about this?
   e. Spiritual loss: Tell me more about how your inability to get to the synagogue is affecting you.
   f. Spiritual despair: So you are saying that no matter how hard you try, you'll never be able to be close to God?
10. Diagnosis: Hopelessness related to belief that God doesn't care.
    Nursing care plan: The nurse should offer a supportive presence, facilitate patient's practice of religion, counsel the patient spiritually, or contact a spiritual counselor.
11. Answers will vary with student's experiences.
12. a. The room should be orderly and free of clutter.
    b. There should be a seat for the counselor at the bedside or near the patient.
    c. The top of the bedside table should be free of items and covered with a clean, white cover if a sacrament is to be administered.
    d. The bed curtains should be drawn to provide privacy, or the patient should be moved to a private setting.
13. Sample Answers
    a. Deficit: Meaning and Purpose: Explore with the patient what has given his life meaning and purpose to the present, sources of meaning for other people and possible meaning of illness. Refer the patient to a spiritual advisor and appropriate support groups.
    b. Deficit: Love and relatedness: Treat the patient at all times with respect, empathy, and genuine caring.
    c. Deficit: Forgiveness: Offer a supportive presence to the patient that demonstrates your acceptance of him/her. Explore the patient's self-expectations and assist the patient in determining how realistic they are. Explore the importance of learning to accept oneself and others.

CHAPTER 35: PATIENT CARE STUDY

1. Objective data are underlined; subjective data are in boldface.

Jeffrey Stein is a 31-year-old attorney who is presently in a step-down unit following his transfer from the cardiac care unit, where he was treated for a massive heart attack. "Bad hearts run in my family, but I never thought it would happen to me. I jog several times a week and work out at the gym, eat a low fat diet, and I don't smoke." Jeffrey is 5'7", weighs about 150 lbs, and is well-built. During his second night in the step-down unit, he is unable to sleep and tells the nurse, "I've really got a lot on my mind tonight. I can't stop thinking about how close I was to death. If I wasn't with someone who knew how to do CPR when I keeled over, I probably wouldn't be here today." Gentle questioning reveals that Mr. Stein is worried about what would have happened had he died. "I don't think I've ever thought seriously about my mortality, and I sure don't think much about God. My parents were semi-observant Jews, but I don't go to synagogue myself. I celebrate the holidays, but that's about all. If there is a God, I wonder what he thinks about me." He asks if there is a rabbi or anyone he can talk with in the morning who could answer some questions for him and perhaps help him get himself back on track. "For the last couple of years, all I've been concerned about is paying off my school debts and making money. I guess there's a whole lot more to life, and maybe this was my invitation to sort out my priorities."

2. Nursing Process Worksheet

Health Problem:

Spiritual distress: spiritual anxiety.

Expected Outcome:

After meeting with Rabbi White 2/12/02, patient reports feeling "less anxious" about his religious belief system and reevaluated sense of priorities.

Etiology:

Challenged belief and value system.

Nursing Interventions:

1. Encourage patient to continue to share concerns about his religious beliefs and value system.
2. Arrange for patient to talk with the hospital's Jewish chaplain in the morning.
3. Normalize this experience by sharing with the patient that serious illness often prompts a life review.
4. Recommend that the patient begin to list the things in life that are most important to him.

Signs & Symptoms (Defining Characteristics):

Recent massive heart attack; unable to sleep; raised in semi-observant Jewish family but "for the last couple of years only concerned about paying off school debts and making money"; questions about afterlife.

Evaluative Statement:

Patient slept last two nights after meeting with Rabbi White and reports being "less anxious" about "religion." He says there are some things he wants to change about his life, and that this is a good time to start.

T. Michael Gray, RN

3. Patient strengths: Healthy; practices healthy self-care behaviors; strongly motivated to attain life goals. Knows himself well enough to "name his problems" and cares enough about himself to seek the assistance he needs.

   Personal strengths: Belief that meeting spiritual needs is an important component of good nursing; excellent rapport with the hospital's pastoral care department; history of establishing therapeutic relationships with patients.
4. 2 AM, 2/14/02: Before patient fell asleep, he thanked me for arranging for him to meet with Rabbi White. "I guess I did what a lot of people do—forget all about God while they try to make a living." He appears less anxious about his religious beliefs and feels that his "recent bout with death" was a timely reminder to evaluate his priorities in life and make some needed changes. Sleeping peacefully at present.

T. Michael Gray, RN

Chapter 36

MATCHING
1. d   2. c   3. h   4. j   5. a   6. i
7. f   8. b   9. e   10. g   11. k

CORRECT THE FALSE STATEMENTS
1. True
2. False—dermis
3. False—ceruminal glands
4. True
5. False—yellowish
6. True
7. False—phlebitis, thrombi formation
8. False—lowest position
9. True
10. False—oily skin
11. False—lack of blood circulation
12. True
13. True
14. False—pediculus humanus corpus
15. False—podiatrist
16. True
17. false—dermis
18. false—morning care

MULTIPLE CHOICE
1. d   2. c   3. a   4. c   5. b   6. b
7. d

COMPLETION
1. a. Protect the body
   b. Regulate body temperature
   c. Sense stimuli from the environment and transmit these sensations
   d. Excrete waste products
   e. Help maintain water and electrolyte balance
   f. Produce and absorb vitamin D
2. a. Children: A child's skin becomes increasingly resistant to injury and infection; however, the skin requires special care because of toilet and play habits.
   b. Adolescents: Ordinarily have enlarged sebaceous glands and increased glandular secretions caused by hormonal changes; predisposed to acne.
   c. Adults: Secretions from the skin glands are at their maximum during adolescence and up to around 50 years.
   d. Older adult: The skin becomes thinner and less elastic and less supple; dryness, wrinkles, and liver spots are common.
3. a. Culture: Many people in North America place a high value on personal cleanliness, shower frequently, and use many products to mask odors. Culture may also dictate whether bathing is private or communal.
   b. Socioeconomic class: Financial resources often define the hygiene options available to individuals. The availability of running water and finances for soap, shampoo, etc. affects hygiene.
   c. Spiritual practice: Religion may dictate ceremonial washings and purifications, which may be a prelude to prayer or eating.

d. Developmental level: Children learn different hygiene practices while growing up. Family practices may dictate morning or evening baths, frequency of shampooing, feelings about nudity, frequency of clothing changes, etc.

e. Health state: Disease or injury may adversely affect an individual's ability to perform hygiene measures or motivation to follow usual hygiene habits.

f. Personal preference: Different people have different personal preferences with regard to shower vs. tub baths, bar soap vs. liquid soap, etc.

4. a. Feeding
   b. Bathing and hygiene
   c. Dressing and grooming
   d. Toileting

5. Bathing/Hygiene Deficit related to mother's lack of knowledge on bathing infants.
   The mother must be educated on the proper method of bathing her infant. She should be made aware of the need for good hygiene for her baby, and a bath should be demonstrated with a return demonstration.
   Investigate whether the mother has the financial means to buy the materials necessary for baby's hygiene (baby shampoo, baby oil, powder, diaper rash ointment, etc.).

6. a. Early morning care: The patient should be assisted with toileting and provided comfort measures designed to refresh the patient and prepare him/her for breakfast. The face and hands should be washed and mouth care provided.

   b. Morning care: After breakfast, the nurse offers assistance with toileting, oral care, bathing, back massage, special skin care measures, hair care, cosmetics, dressing, and positioning. Bed linens are refreshed or changed.

   c. Afternoon care: The nurse should ensure the patient's comfort after lunch and offer assistance with toileting, handwashing, and oral care to nonambulatory patients.

   d. Hour of sleep care: The nurse again offers assistance with toileting, washing of face and hands, and oral care. A back massage helps the patient relax and fall asleep. Soiled bed linens or clothing should be changed and patient positioned comfortably.

   e. As needed care: The nurse offers individual hygiene measures as needed. Some patients require oral care every 2 hours. Patients who are diaphoretic may need their clothing or linens changed several times a shift.

7. Bathing cleanses the skin, acts as a conditioner, relaxes a restless person, promotes circulation, serves as musculoskeletal exercise, stimulates the rate and depth of respirations, promotes comfort, provides sensory input, improves self-esteem and strengthens nurse–patient relationship.

8. Provide the patient with articles for bathing and a basin of water that is at a comfortable temperature; place these items conveniently for the patient. Provide privacy for the patient, remove top linens on patient's bed and replace with a bath blanket. Place cosmetics in a convenient place with a mirror and light, and supply hot water and a razor for a patient who wishes to shave. Assist patients who cannot bathe themselves completely.

9. a. A towel bath can be accomplished with little fatigue to the patient.
   b. The towel remains warm during the short procedure.
   c. Patients state that they feel clean and refreshed.
   d. The oil in the bathing solution eliminates dry, itchy skin.

10. a. A back rub acts as a body conditioner.
    b. Giving a back rub provides an opportunity for the nurse to observe the skin for signs of breakdown.
    c. A back rub improves circulation and provides a means of communication with the patient through the use of touch.

11. a. Ventilation: It is wise to air the room when the patient is away for a diagnostic or therapeutic procedure in order to remove pathogens and unpleasant odors associated with body secretions and excretions.

    b. Odors: Odors can be controlled by promptly emptying bedpans, urinals, and emesis basins, and by being careful not to dispose of soiled dressings or anything with a strong odor in the waste receptacle in the patient's room. Deodorizers may need to be used.

    c. Room temperature: Whenever possible, patient preference should be followed regarding room temperature. In general, the temperature should fall between 20°C and 23°C.

    d. Lighting and noise: The nurse should reduce harsh lighting and noises whenever possible. Conversations should not be carried on immediately outside patient's room.

12. Sample Answer
    a. Rinse off soaps or detergents well when they are used for cleaning the skin.
    b. Add moisture to the air through a humidifier.
    c. Increase fluid intake.
    d. Use an emollient after cleansing the skin.

13. a. Lips: color, moisture, lumps, ulcers, lesions, and edema
    b. Buccal mucosa: color, moisture, lesions, nodules, and bleeding
    c. Gums: lesions, bleeding, edema, and exudate; loose or missing teeth
    d. Tongue: color, symmetry, movement, texture, and lesions
    e. Hard and soft palates: intactness, color, patches, lesions, and petechiae
    f. Eye: position, alignment, and general appearance; presence of lesions, nodules, redness, swelling, crusting, flaking, excessive tearing, or discharge; color of conjunctivae; blink reflex; visual acuity
    g. Ear: position, alignment, and general appearance; build-up of wax; dryness, crusting, discharge, or foreign body; hearing acuity
    h. Nose: position and general appearance; patency of nostrils; presence of tenderness, dryness, edema, bleeding, and discharge or secretions.

14. a. Eye: Clean the eye from the inner canthus to the outer canthus using a wet, warm washcloth, cotton ball, or compress to soften crusted secretions. Avoid cross contamination.
    b. Ear: Clean the ear with a washcloth-covered finger, instructing patient never to insert objects into the ear for cleaning purposes.

c. Nose: Clean the nose by instructing patient to blow nose while both nares are patent (nasal suctioning may be indicated), remove crusted secretions around the nose, and apply petroleum to tissue.

15. a. Contact lenses: Wash hands before touching eye surfaces or lenses; remove the lenses by gently grasping the lens near the lower edge and lifting it from eye. Soft lenses are cleaned, rinsed, and placed in a container of solution for storage. Identify as right or left lens.

b. Artificial eye: Assemble a small basin, soap, and water, and solution for rinsing the prosthesis. Ask the patient how he/she cleans the eye area (usually flushed with normal saline before replacing the eye).

c. Hearing aids: Batteries should be checked routinely and earpieces cleaned daily with mild soap and water.

d. Dentures: Dentures should not be wrapped in tissue or disposable wipes. Dentures should be stored in water to prevent drying and warping of plastic materials. A deodorant solution of water and a few drops of essence of peppermint may be added. Don gloves and hold dentures over a basin of water or soft towel. Cleanse with cool or lukewarm water with a brush and nonabrasive powder or paste. Dentures can be soaked with special preparations to remove stain and hardened particles. Rinse well after cleaning; rinse mouth before replacing dentures.

16. Deficient self-care abilities, vascular disease, arthritis, diabetes mellitus, history of biting nails or trimming them improperly, frequent or prolonged exposure to chemicals or water, trauma, ill-fitting shoes, or obesity.

CHAPTER 36: PATIENT CARE STUDY

1. Objective data are underlined; subjective data are in boldface.

Dominic Gianmarco is a 78-year-old retired man with a history of Parkinson's disease, who lives alone in a small twin home. He was recently hospitalized for problems with cardiac rhythm, and a pacemaker was installed. The home healthcare nurse made a scheduled visit 1 week after the hospitalization to monitor his recovery and compliance with his medication regimen. The nurse observed that his appearance was disheveled and multiple stains were apparent on his clothing. A variety of food items were in various stages of preparation on the kitchen counter, and some appeared to have spoiled. Mr. Gianmoarco had several days' growth of beard and a body odor was apparent. He was pleasant and oriented to place and person, but unable to identify the time or day of the week. "I lose track of what day it is. Time's not important when you're my age. The most important thing to me right now is to be able to take care of myself and stay in this house near my friends." A walker was visible in a corner of the living room, but Mr. Gianmarco ambulated slowly around the house with a minimum of difficulty and did not use the walker. He commented that he keeps busy "reading, watching old movies, and going to Senior Citizen activities with friends who stop by for me."

His daughter, who lives several hours away, visits him every weekend and prepares his medications for the week in a plastic container that is easy for him to open. The nurse observed that all medications appeared to have been taken to date. "I don't mess around with my medicines. One helps my ticker and the others keep me from shaking so much."

2. Nursing Process Worksheet

Health Problem:

Self Care Deficit: Bathing/Hygiene, Dressing/Grooming

Etiology:

Neuromuscular impairment secondary to Parkinson's disease, effects of aging.

Signs & Symptoms (Defining Characteristics):

Inability to bathe and groom self independently (disheveled appearance, stains on clothing, unshaven, presence of body odor).

Expected Outcome:

Within 2 weeks, patient will be able to perform self-care grooming activities with assistance of home healthcare aide.

Nursing Interventions:

1. Assess patient's ability to care for self in home setting.
2. Explore availability of home healthcare aide to visit patient and assist with personal hygiene activities on a regular basis.
3. Maintain safe environment.
4. Encourage patient's independent activities.
5. Investigate need for any adaptive equipment.

Evaluative Statement:

3/28/02: Expected outcome partially met. Home healthcare aide assisting patient for several hours, three mornings/week. Continue to evaluate patient's ability to manage treatment regimen and need for any adaptive equipment.

M. Gomez, RN

3. Patient strengths: Has previously been able to care for self, motivated to maintain independence, caring family member able to visit on a regular basis.

Personal strengths: Commitment to caring, experienced home healthcare nurse, strong interpersonal skills, good knowledge of gerontologic nursing.

4. 3/28/02: Revisited patient 2 weeks after initial visit. Patient alert and oriented. Neat personal appearance—clean-shaven, absence of body odor, hair shampooed and combed, wearing clean clothes. Stated "my girlfriends love me now." Conforming to medication schedule and participating in social activities. Continue periodic observations.

M. Gomez, RN

Chapter 37

MATCHING

1. a	2. f	3. q	4. j	5. e	6. n
7. k	8. p	9. i	10. m	11. o	12. c
13. d	14. h	15. l	16. f	17. a	18. g
19. a	20. b	21. d	22. c	23. e	24. g
25. e					

26. f. Generally used for leg ulcers, burns, abrasions, skin tears, and chronic wounds.
27. a. Used for wounds with minimal drainage and can remain in place 24–72 hours.
28. c. Used for wounds with moderate to heavy exudate, and require a second dressing to hold them in place.
29. g. This procedure is used on chronic open wounds, dehisced surgical incisions, and stage III and IV pressure ulcers.
30. b. Most often used for deep wounds with heavy drainage.
31. d. Used for shallow wounds with minimal drainage and may remain in place for 3—7 days.
32. e. Used for wounds with minimum exudate.

MULTIPLE CHOICE

1. b	2. d	3. a	4. c	5. d	6. c
7. b	8. d	9. a	10. c	11. d	12. a
13. b	14. c				

COMPLETION

1. a. External pressure: Compresses blood vessels and causes friction.
   b. Friction and shearing forces: Tear and injure blood vessels.
2. a. Nutrition: Poorly nourished cells are easily damaged, e.g., vitamin C deficiency causes capillaries to become fragile, and poor circulation to the area results when they break.
   b. Hydration: Dehydration can interfere with circulation and subsequent cell nourishment.
   c. Moisture on the skin: Moisture associated with urinary incontinence increases the risk of skin damage more than chemical irritation from the ammonia in urine.
   d. Mental status: The more alert a patient is, the more likely he/she will relieve pressure periodically and manage adequate skin hygiene.
   e. Age: Older people are good candidates for developing pressure ulcers because the skin is susceptible to injury.
3. Sample Answer
   Provide the caregivers with a simple, easy-to-understand list of instructions about caring for the pressure ulcer; address the causative factor for the pressure ulcer before proceeding with the plan of care; consult frequently with the physician about the progress of wound healing and products being used; use clean dressings; teach caregivers good handwashing technique; review signs of infection with caregivers and encourage them to contact a physician or home health nurse about any problems.

4. a. Inflammatory phase: Begins with the incision for surgery and lasts through the third or fourth postoperative day. The two major physiologic activities are hemostasis and phagocytosis. The inflammatory response is immediate and prepares the tissues for healing. Fibroplasia phase: Begins about day 3 or 4 and can last up to day 21. Fibroblasts rapidly synthesize collagens and ground substance, forming the scaffold for the final repair of the wound. Capillaries grow across the wound; fibroblasts migrate from bloodstream into the wound depositing fibrin; granulation tissue forms. Maturation phase: Begins about three weeks after injury for as long as 1—2 years. Collagen is remodeled, making the healed wound stronger and more like adjacent tissue. New collagen is deposited so that scar eventually becomes a flat, thin white line.
5. Sample Answer
   a. The patient will participate in the prescribed treatment regimen to promote wound healing.
   b. The patient will remain free of infection at the site of the pressure ulcer.
   c. The patient will demonstrate self-care measures necessary to prevent the development of pressure ulcer.
6. Sample Answers
   a. Overall appearance of skin: Are there any areas on your body where your skin feels paper-thin?
      How does your skin feel in relation to moisture—dry, clammy, oily?
   b. Recent changes in skin: Have you noticed any sores anywhere on your body?
      Do you ever notice any redness over a bony area when you stay in one position for a while?
   c. Activity/mobility: Do you need assistance to walk to the bathroom?
      Can you change your position freely and painlessly?
   d. Nutrition: Have you lost weight lately?
      Do you eat well-balanced meals?
   e. Pain: Do you have any painful sores on your body?
      Do you take any medications for pain?
   f. Elimination: Do you have any problems with incontinence?
      Have you ever used any briefs or pads for incontinence problems?
7. a. Appearance: Assess for the approximation of wound edges, color of the wound and surrounding areas, drains or tubes, sutures, and signs of dehiscence or evisceration.
   b. Wound drainage: Assess the amount, color, odor, and consistency of wound drainage.
      Drainage can be assessed on the wound, the dressings, in drainage bottles or reservoirs, or under the patient.
   c. Pain: Assess if the pain has increased or is constant; pain may indicate delayed healing or the presence of an infection.
   d. Sutures and staples: Assess the type of suture and whether enough tensile strength has developed to hold the wound edges together during healing.
   e. Drains and tubes: Assess the type of drain or tube that was inserted during surgery and the patency and placement of the tubes or drains.

8. Provide physical, psychologic, and aesthetic comfort, remove necrotic tissue, prevent eliminate or control infection, absorb drainage, maintain a moist wound environment, protect the wound from further injury, and protect the skin surrounding the wound.

9. a. R = red = protect: Red wounds are in the proliferative stage of healing, and are the color of normal granulation and need protection by gentle cleansing, using moist dressings, applying a transparent or hydrocolloid dressing, and only changing the dressing when necessary.

   b. Y = yellow = cleanse: Yellow wounds are characterized by oozing from the tissue covering the wound, often accompanied by purulent drainage. They need to be cleansed using irrigation, wet-to-moist dressings, using nonadherent, hydrogel, or other absorptive dressings; and topical antimicrobial medication.

   c. B = black = debride: Black wounds are covered with thick eschar which is usually black but may also be brown, gray or tan in color. The eschar must be debrided before the wound can heal by using sharp, mechanical, chemical, or autolytic debridement.

10. a. Hot water bags or bottles: Relatively inexpensive and easy to use, may leak, burn, or make the patient uncomfortable from their weight.

    b. Electric heating pad: Can be used to apply dry heat locally, it is easy to apply relatively safe and provides constant and even heat. Improper use can result in injury.

    c. Aquathermia pad: Commonly used in healthcare agencies for various problems including back pain, muscle spasms, thrombophlebitis, and mild inflammation. Safer than a heating pad, but still must be checked carefully.

    d. Heat lamps: Provide dry heat to increase circulation to a small area, such as a pressure ulcer. Assess skin exposed to the heat every five minutes.

    e. Heat cradles: A heat cradle is a metal half-circle frame that encloses the body part to be treated with heat. Precautions should be taken to prevent burning.

    f. Hot packs: Commercial hot packs provide a specified amount of dry heat for a specific period.

    g. Warm moist compresses: Used on wounds to promote circulation and wound healing and to reduce edema. Must be changed frequently and covered with a heating agent.

    h. Sitz baths: Patient is placed in a tub filled with sufficient water to reach the umbilicus; the legs and feet remain out of water.

    i. Warm soaks: The immersion of a body area into warm water or a medicated solution to increase blood supply to a locally infected area, to aid in cleaning large sloughing wounds, such as burns, to improve circulation and to apply medication to a locally infected area. Makes manipulation of a painful area much easier because of the buoyancy.

CHAPTER 37: PATIENT CARE STUDY

1. Objective data are underlined; subjective data are in boldface.

   Mrs. Chijioke, an 88-year-old woman who lived alone for years, was brought to the hospital after neighbors found her lying at the bottom of her cellar steps. She had broken her hip and is now 3 days after hip repair surgery. The nurse assigned to care for Mrs. Chijioke noticed during the patient's bath that the skin of her coccyx, heels, and elbows was reddened. The skin did return to a normal color when pressure was relieved in these areas. There was no edema, nor was there induration or blistering. While Mrs. Chijioke was able to be lifted out of bed into a chair, she spent most of the day in bed, lying on her back with an abductor pillow between her legs. At 5'0" and 89 lbs, Mrs. Chijioke looked lost in the big hospital bed. Her eyes were bright and she usually attempted a warm smile, but she had little physical strength and would lie seemingly motionless for hours. Her skin was wrinkled and paper thin, and her arms were already bruised from unsuccessful attempts at intravenous therapy. Dehydrated on admission, since **she had spent almost 48 hours crumpled at the bottom of her steps before being found by her neighbors,** Mrs. Chijioke was clearly in need of nutritional, fluid, and electrolyte support. A long-time diabetic, Mrs. Chijioke is now spiking a temperature (39.0°C/102.2°F), which concerns her nurse.

2. Nursing Process Worksheet

Health Problem:

Risk for impaired skin integrity.

Etiology:

Immobility; effects of aging, dehydration, and illness.

Signs & Symptoms (Defining Characteristics):

Skin of her coccyx, heels, and elbows is reddened—returns to normal color when pressure is relieved; lies motionless on her back when unattended; skin is wrinkled and thin; elevated temperature: 39°C.

Expected Outcome:

Whenever observed, the patient's skin will appear clean and intact (no redness, blistering, indurations).

Nursing Interventions:

1. Reposition patient in correct alignment at least every 1–2 hours and ensure protection of pressure points where possible; examine skin for signs of breakdown with each position change.
2. Massage pressure points and keep skin clean and dry.
3. Keep bed linens dry and free of wrinkles.
4. Monitor high-risk factors: dehydration, effects of illness.

Evaluative Statement:

10/6/02: Goal met—patient's skin is clean and intact and shows no signs of breakdown. Continue prevention program.

M. Wong, RN

3. Patient strengths: Concerned neighbors; until now has been able to care for herself and keep herself in good health.

   Personal strengths: Ability to recognize patients at high risk for problems such as impaired skin integrity. Strong commitment to meeting the needs of geriatric patients. Experienced clinician.

4. 10/6/02: Patient remains on a 2-hour positioning regimen. The protective heel and elbow pads have resulted in intact skin in these areas—no redness. The skin on her coccyx appears reddened after she lies on her back, but the redness disappears when the pressure is relieved. No constant redness, edema, or induration. Skin remains dry; lotion applied with each position change.

M. Wong, RN

Chapter 38

MATCHING

1. e	2. c	3. f	4. b	5. a	6. a
7. f	8. d	9. b	10. c	11. e	12. a
13. c	14. d	15. e	16. l	17. a	18. g
19. o	20. d	21. k	22. b	23. n	24. c
25. m	26. j	27. h	28. e	29. i	30. b
31. e	32. f	33. a	34. i	35. c	36. d
37. g					

CORRECT THE FALSE STATEMENT

1. False—irregular bones
2. True
3. True
4. True
5. False—body mechanics
6. True
7. False—wider
8. False—propriocepter or kinesthetic
9. False—basal ganglia
10. True
11. True
12. True
13. False—facing
14. True
15. False—slide, roll, push or pull

MULTIPLE CHOICE

1. b	2. a	3. c	4. d	5. a	6. c
7. b	8. c	9. d	10. c	11. a	12. a
13. b	14. d	15. d	16. a		

COMPLETION

1. See table on effects of exercise and immobility on body systems.
2. a. Motion
   b. Maintenance of posture
   c. Heat production

Body System	Effects of Exercise	Effects of Immobility
Cardiovascular System	↑Efficiency of heart ↓Resting heart rate and blood pressure ↑Blood flow and oxygenation of all body parts	↑Cardiac workload ↑Risk for orthostatic hypotension ↑Risk for venous thrombosis
Respiratory System	↑Depth of respiration ↑Respiratory rate ↑Gas exchange at alveolar level ↑Rate of carbon dioxide excretion	↓Depth of respiration ↓Rate of respiration Pooling of secretions Impaired gas exchange
Gastrointestinal System	↑Appetite ↑Intestinal tone	Disturbance in appetite Altered protein metabolism Altered digestion and utilization of nutrients
Urinary System	↑Blood flow to kidneys ↑Efficiency in maintaining fluid and acid-base balance ↑Efficiency in excreting body wastes	↑Urinary stasis ↓Risk for renal calculi ↑Bladder muscle tone
Musculoskeletal System	↑Muscle efficiency ↑Coordination ↑Efficiency of nerve impulse transmission	↓Muscle size, tone, and strength ↓Joint mobility, flexibility Bone demineralization ↓Endurance, stability ↑Risk for contracture formation
Metabolic System	↑Efficiency of metabolic system ↑Efficiency of body temperature regulation	↑Risk for electrolyte imbalance Altered exchange of nutrients and gases
Integument	Improved tone, color, turgor, resulting from improved circulation	↑Risk for skin breakdown and formation of decubitus ulcers
Psychological Well-Being	Energy, vitality, general well-being Improved sleep Improved appearance Improved self-concept Positive health behaviors	↑Sense of powerlessness ↓Self-concept ↓Social interaction ↓Sensory stimulation Altered sleep-wake pattern ↑Risk for depression

3. a. Point of origin: Attachment of a muscle to the more stationary bone.
    b. Point of insertion: Attachment of a muscle to the more movable bone.
4. a. The afferent nervous system conveys information from receptors in the periphery of the body to the central nervous system.
    b. Nerve cells called neurons are responsible for conducting impulses from one part of the body to another.
    c. This information is processed by the central nervous system and a response is decided on.
    d. The efferent system conveys the desired response from the CNS to skeletal muscles by way of the somatic nervous system.
5. a. Body alignment or posture: The alignment of body parts that permits optimal musculoskeletal balance and operation and promotes healthy physiologic functioning.
    b. Balance: A body in correct alignment is balanced; its center of gravity is close to the base of support, the line of gravity goes through the base of support, and the object has a wide base of support.
    c. Coordinated body movement: Using major muscle groups rather than weaker ones and taking advantage of the body's natural levers and fulcrums.
6. Sample Answers
    a. Develop a habit of maintaining erect posture and begin activities by broadening the base of support and lowering the center of gravity.
    b. Use the weight of the body as a force for pulling or pushing by rocking on the feet or leaning forward or backward.
    c. Slide, roll, push, or pull an object rather than lift it to reduce the energy needed to lift the weight against the pull of gravity.
    d. Use the weight of the body to push an object by falling or rocking forward, and to pull an object by falling or rocking backward.
7. a. Aerobic exercises (running, swimming, tennis): Sustained muscle movements that increase blood flow, heart rate, and metabolic demand for oxygen over time, thereby promoting cardiovascular conditioning.
    b. Stretching exercises (warm-up and cool-down exercises): Movements that allow muscles and joints to be stretched gently through their full range of motion; increase flexibility.
    c. Strength and endurance exercises (weight training): Weight training, calisthenics, and specific isometric exercises can build both strength and endurance, increase the power of the musculoskeletal system and improve the body.
    d. Activities of daily living (shopping, cleaning): All activities of daily living have an effect on health and provide increased fitness that does not require a gym.
8. Sample Answers
    a. Increased energy, vitality, and general well-being
    b. Improved sleep
    c. Improved self-concept
    d. Increased positive health behaviors

9. a. Pillows: Pillows are used primarily to provide support or to elevate a part. Pillows of different sizes are useful for different body parts.
    b. Mattresses: A mattress should be firm but have sufficient "give" to permit good body alignment to be comfortable and supportive. A well-made and well-supported foam-rubber mattress retains a uniform firmness.
    c. Adjustable bed: The head of an adjustable bed can be elevated to the desired degree and the distance from the floor can be altered to allow the patient to get in and out of bed easier or to allow healthcare workers to give bed care without back strain.
    d. Bed side rails: They help to remind patients that they are not in their usual environment and keep them from falling out of bed.
    e. Trapeze bar: This handgrip suspended from a frame near the head of the bed makes moving and turning considerably easier for many patients and facilitates transfers into and out of bed.
    f. Cradle: A metal frame that keeps the top bedding off the patient's lower extremities while providing privacy and warmth.
    g. Sandbags: Sandbags immobilize an extremity and support body alignment. They are not hard or firmly packed, but should be placed so they do not create pressure on bony prominences.
    h. Trochanter rolls: Used to support the hips and legs so that the femurs do not rotate outward.
    i. Hand/wrist splint: A commercial plastic or aluminum splint is used to hold the thumb in place no matter what position the hand is in.
10. a. Quadriceps drills: Have the patient contract the muscles on the front of the thighs by pulling kneecaps toward hips; hold the position to the count of four; relax muscles for count of four. Frequency: 2–3 times each hour, 4–6 times a day.
    b. Push-ups: Sitting in bed: Instruct patient to lift hips off the bed by pushing down with hands on mattress. Lying on abdomen: Instruct patient to place hands near the outstretched body at shoulder level with palms down on the mattress and elbows bent sharply; then have patient straighten elbows while lifting head and shoulders off bed. Wheelchair: Instruct patient to place hands on arms of chair and raise body up 3–4 times a day.
    c. Dangling: Instruct the patient to sit on the edge of the bed with legs and feet dangling over the side. Rest the patient's feet on the floor or footstool. Have patient assume a marching position. (Remain with patient in case he/she feels faint.)
11. a. Physical assessment: The nurse would assess the following:
    1. General ease of movement: Are body parts fluid and voluntarily movement-controlled and coordinated?
    2. Gait: Is head erect? Are the vertebrae straight, knees and feet forward, and arms swinging freely in alternation with leg swings?
    3. Alignment—in standing position: Can a straight

line be drawn from the ear through the shoulder and hip?

4. Joint structure and function: Are there any joint deformities, limitations in full range of motion?

5. Muscle mass tone and strength: Are they adequate to accomplish movement, work?

6. Endurance: Is patient able to turn in bed, maintain correct alignment when sitting and standing, ambulate, and perform self-care activities?

b. Diagnosis: Activity intolerance related to decreased muscle mass, tone, and strength.

c. Exercise program: Do range-of-motion exercises twice a day to build up muscles and joint capabilities. Use quadriceps drills 2–3 times an hour, 4–6 times a day. Do settings twice a day and push-ups 3–4 times a day.

12. Sample Answers

a. General ease of movement: Normal: Body movements are voluntarily controlled, fluid and coordinated; Abnormal: Involuntary movements, tremors, tics, chorea, etc.

b. Gait and posture: Normal: head erect, vertebrae are straight; Abnormal: spastic hemiparesis, scissors gait.

c. Alignment: Normal: In the standing and sitting position, a straight line can be drawn from the ear through the shoulder and hip, In bed, the head, shoulders, and hips are aligned; Abnormal: Abnormal spinal curvatures, inability to maintain correct alignment independently.

d. Joint structure and function: Normal: Absence of joint deformities, full range of motion; Abnormal: Limitations in the normal range of motion, increased joint mobility.

e. Muscle mass, tone, and strength: Normal: Adequate muscle mass and tone; Abnormal: atrophy, hypotronicity.

f. Endurance: Normal: Ability to turn in bed, maintain correct alignment; Abnormal: weakness, pallor

CHAPTER 38: PATIENT CARE STUDY

1. Objective data are underlined; subjective data are in bold-face.

Robert Witherspoon, a <u>42-year-old university professor,</u> presented for his first "physical" shortly after his father's death. His father died of complications of coronary artery disease. Mr. Witherspoon is <u>5'9" tall, weights 235 lbs,</u> has a decided <u>"paunch,"</u> and reports that **until now he has made no time for exercise because he preferred to utilize his free time reading or listening to classical music.** He enjoys French cuisine, including rich desserts, *and has a cholesterol level of 310 mg/dL (normal is 150–250 mg/dL).* He admits being **frightened by his father's death,** and is appropriately concerned about his elevated cholesterol level. **"I guess I've never given much thought to my health before, but my dad's death changed all that. I know coronary artery disease runs in families and I can tell you that I'm not ready to pack it all in yet. Tell me what I have to do to fight this thing."** He admits that he used to tease a colleague—who lowered his own cholesterol from 290 to 200 mg/dL by diet and exercise alone—

by accusing him of being a fitness freak. **"Now I'm recognizing the wisdom of his health behaviors and wondering if diet and exercise won't do the trick for me. Can you help me design an exercise program that will work?"**

2. Nursing Process Worksheet
Health Problem:

Altered health maintenance; lack of exercise program.

Etiology:

Low value placed on fitness and self-care behaviors in the past.

Signs & Symptoms (Defining Characteristics):

5'9" tall; 235 lbs; until now "no time" for exercise; "I've never given much thought to my health before"; "Tell me what I have to do to fight this thing—can you help me design an exercise program that will work?"

Expected Outcome:

At next visit, 10/27/02, patient will report adherence to the exercise program developed 9/30/02 (additional goals will describe desired changes in weight and cholesterol level).

Nursing Interventions:

1. Explore the patient's fitness goals, interest, skills, exercise opportunities and exercise capacity.

2. Assist the patient in obtaining medical clearance for exercise.

3. Explore feasible exercise activities with the patient, considering health benefits sought, time involved, need for special equipment, precautions, and risk.

4. Develop an exercise program that specifies warm-up and cool-down activities and 3 or 4 major exercise activities from which the patient can choose. Specify frequency, duration, and intensity.

5. Encourage the patient to complement the exercise program with everyday activities that require exercise.

6. Try to identify with the patient potential threats to the exercise program's successful implementation. Plan support strategies.

Evaluative Statement:

10/27/02: Goal partially met—patient reports that the second week into his program his "jogging buddy" got sick, and that without the support of his friend, he stopped exercising regularly; wants to resume. Revision: Explore new strategies to strengthen resolve/adherence.

J. McKeough, RN

3. Patient strengths: Patient is highly motivated to develop new self-care behaviors as a result of his father's death—asking for help.

Personal strengths: Good understanding of the relationship between self-care behaviors (exercise, nutrition) and health; experienced in designing exercise programs; knowledge of benefits/risks associated with exercise; stronginterpersonal/counseling skills.

4. 10/27/02: Whereas the patient left the last session "enthusiastic" about beginning an exercise program, he reported today that he "feels like a failure" since he wasn't faithful to the goals he set for himself. After losing his exercise buddy, he found it easy to "skip runs," and he hasn't found another racquetball partner. We identified and reinforced the progress he has made and developed new expected outcomes that are less dependent on external support.

J. McKeough, RN

Chapter 39

MATCHING
1. g	2. a	3. c	4. h	5. b	6. d
7. f	8. i	9. j	10. c	11. a	12. a
13. d	14. b	5. c, d	16. b	17. d	18. a

CORRECT THE FALSE STATEMENTS
1. True
2. True
3. False—at stage I, NREM sleep
4. False—4–5
5. False—14–20
6. True
7. False—small protein and carbohydrate
8. False—hinders
9. True
10. True
11. False—sleep apnea

MULTIPLE CHOICE
1. b	2. a	3. d	4. b	5. a	6. d
7. c	8. d	9. b	10. c	11. b	12. b

COMPLETION
1. a. Restores physical well-being
   b. Relieves stress and anxiety
   c. Restores the ability to cope and to concentrate on activities of daily living
2. a. Infants: 14–20 hours/day
   b. Growing children: 10–14 hours/day
   c. Adults: 7–9 hours/day
   d. Older adults: May require a longer time to go to sleep and wake earlier and more frequently during the night.
3. a. Physical activity: Activity increases fatigue and promotes relaxation that is followed by sleep. It also increases both REM and NREM sleep.
   b. Psychologic stress: The person experiencing stress tends to find it difficult to obtain the amount of sleep he or she needs and REM sleep decreases.
   c. Motivation: A desire to be wakeful and alert helps overcome sleepiness and sleep or when there is minimal motivation to be awake, sleep generally follows.
   d. Culture: Bedtime rituals, sleeping place, and pattern of sleep may vary according to culture.
   e. Diet: Carbohydrates appear to have an effect on brain serotonin levels and promote feelings of calmness and relaxation; protein may actually increase brain energy alertness and concentration.
   f. Alcohol and caffeine: Alcohol in moderation seems to help induce sleep in some people, however, large quantities limit REM and delta sleep. Caffeine is a CNS stimulant and may interfere with ability to fall asleep.
   g. Smoking: Nicotine has a stimulating effect and smokers usually have a more difficult time falling asleep.
   h. Environmental factors: Most people sleep best in their usual home environments.
   i. Lifestyle: Sleep disorders are the major problem associated with shift work and developing a sleep pattern is especially difficult if the shift changes periodically. Sleep can be affected by watching some types of television shows, participation in stimulating activity, and level of activity or exercise.
   j. Exercise: Moderate exercise is a healthy way to promote sleep, but exercise that occurs within a 2-hour interval before normal bedtime can hinder sleep.
   k. Illness: Illness is a physiologic and psychologic stressor and therefore influences sleep.
   l. Medications: Sleep quality is influenced by certain drugs that may decrease REM sleep.
4. The cause of the sleep disturbance, the related signs and symptoms, when it first began and how often it occurs, how it affects everyday living, the severity of the problem and whether it can be treated independently by nursing, how the patient is coping with the problem, and the success of any treatments attempted.
5. a. Energy level
   b. Facial characteristics
   c. Behavioral characteristics
   d. Data suggestive of potential sleep problems
6. Make sure the patient has a comfortable bed with bottom linen tight and clean. The upper linen should allow freedom of movement and not exert pressure. A quiet and darkened room with privacy, which is properly ventilated and at a comfortable temperature, should be provided.
7. Sample Answers
   a. Sleep Pattern Disturbance: Difficulty remaining asleep related to noise of hospital environment and need for periodic treatment.
   b. Sleep Pattern Disturbance: Excessive daytime sleeping related to effects of biological aging.
   c. Sleep Pattern Disturbance: Altered sleep–wake patterns related to frequent rotations of shift.
   d. Sleep Pattern Disturbance: Premature wakening related to alcohol dependency.
   e. Sleep Pattern Disturbance: Difficulty falling asleep related to worries about family.
8. a. Eyes: dart back and forth quickly
   b. Muscles: small muscle twitching, large muscle immobility
   c. Respirations: Irregular; sometimes interspersed with apnea
   d. Pulse: rapid or irregular
   e. Blood pressure: increases or fluctuates
   f. Gastric secretions: increase
   g. Metabolism: increases; body temperature increases
   h. Sleep cycle: REM sleep enters from stage II of NREM sleep and reenters NREM sleep at stage II; arousal from sleep difficult

9. Sample Answers
   a. Prepare a restful environment.
   b. Offer appropriate bedtime snacks and beverages.
   c. Promote comfort and relaxation.
10. Sample Answers
    a. Usual sleeping and waking times: Do you usually go to bed and wake up around the same time?
    b. Number of hours of undisturbed sleep: Do you have any difficulty falling asleep or wake up during the night?
    c. Quality of sleep: Do you feel rested after the amount of sleep you get?
    d. Number and duration of naps: Do you find yourself falling asleep during the day?
    e. Energy level: Do you feel refreshed after a night's sleep?
    f. Means of relaxing before bedtime: Do you watch television or read before bedtime?
    g. Bedtime rituals: What do you do before going to bed?
    h. Sleep environment: What is your bedroom environment like?
    i. Pharmacologic aids: Do you ever take medications to help you fall asleep?
    j. Nature of a sleep disturbance: What do you think is causing your sleep problem?
    k. Onset of a disturbance: When did you first notice that you had trouble falling asleep?
    l. Causes of a disturbance: Are you doing anything different before bedtime?
    m. Severity of a disturbance: Do you have breathing problems during the night?
    n. Symptoms of a disturbance: Do you grind your teeth at night?
    o. Inteventions attempted and results: What measures have you taken to promote a comfortable sleep environment?

CHAPTER 39: PATIENT CARE STUDY

1. Objective data are underlined; subjective data are in boldface.

   Gina Cioffi, a 23-year-old graduate nurse, has been in her new position as a critical care staff nurse in a large tertiary care medical center for 3 months. "I was so excited about working three 12-hour shifts a week when I started this job, thinking I'd have lots of time for other things I want to do, but I'm not sure anymore. I've been doing extra shifts when we're short-staffed because the money is so good, and right now it seems I'm always tired and all I think about all day long is how soon I can get back to bed. Worst of all when I do finally get into bed, I often can't fall asleep, especially if thing have been busy at work and someone 'went bad.' Does everyone else feel like me?" Looking at Gina, you notice dark circles under her eyes and are suddenly struck by the change in her appearance form when she first started working. At that time, she "bounced into work" looking fresh each morning, and her features were always animated. Now her skin color is pale, her hair and clothes look rumpled, and the "brightness" that was so characteristic of her earlier is strikingly absent. With some gental questioning, you discover that she frequently goes out with new friends she

has made at the hospital when her shift is over, and sometimes goes for 48 hours without sleep. "I know I've gotten myself into a rut. How do I get out of it? I used to think my sleep habits were bad at school, but this is a hundred times worse, because there never seems to be time to crash. I have to just keep on going."

2. Nursing Process Worksheet

Health Problem:

Sleep pattern disturbance: altered sleep-wake patterns.

Etiology:

Twelve-hour shift work and stress of new job.

Signs & Symptoms (Defining Characteristics):

Works three 12-hour shifts plus 2–3 "extra" shifts per week; "right now it seems like I am always tired and all I think about all day long is how soon I can get back to bed; when I do finally get into bed I often can't fall asleep." Dark circles under eyes; pale skin; sometimes goes 48 hours without sleep; reports being less animated.

Expected Outcome:

By this time next month (7/22/02), patient will report she is sleeping soundly for a minimum of 6–7 hours/night at least 6 days a week, as evidenced by her feeling "less fatigued" and more "in control" of sleep situation.

Nursing Interventions:
1. Instruct patient to keep a sleep diary for 7 days and analyze its contents at the end of that week.
2. Counsel patient about the need to reevaluate priorities (e.g., working extra shifts).
3. Develop stress management strategies, including relaxation exercises.
4. Identify and reduce (where possible) factors interfering with sleep.

Evaluative Statement:

10/6/02 Expected outcome met: Sleeping 7–8 hours per night, and generally feels refreshed upon awakening.

N. McLoughlin, RN

3. Patient strengths: Strongly motivated at present to address this problem.
   Personal strengths: Comprehensive knowledge of the physiology of sleep and sleep requirements and patterns; familiarity with the stresses of clinical nursing—especially for the graduate nurse; strong interpersonal skills; creative problem-solver.
4. 10/6/02: Patient "bounced into the office" with a vigor and enthusiasm she displayed when she first started working. Her skin had regained its usual coloring and glow, and her face was animated. She expressed gratitude for my "helping her recover her old self," and reported that she is sleeping 7–8 hours/night, and usually wakes up

refreshed and ready to tackle the new day. On questioning, she expressed an appreciation for the need to balance rest and activity, and appears to have developed a workable plan for ensuring adequate rest.

N. McLoughlin, RN

Chapter 40

MATCHING

1. e	2. k	3. f	4. j	5. a	6. c
7. g	8. b	9. d	10. h	11. d	12. a
13. g	14. b	15. c	16. e	17. c	18. d
19. b	20. a	21. c	22. a	23. b	24. c
25. j	26. b	27. d	28. k	29. a	30. i
31. c	32. f	33. h	34. g		

MULTIPLE CHOICE

1. c	2. d	3. a	4. d	5. a	6. c
7. b	8. d	9. a	10. c	11. d	12. b
13. b	14. d	15. c	16. b	17. c	

COMPLETION

1. See table below.
   Sample Answers
   Situation A: Pain—Acute migraine, related to unrelieved stress as manifested by furrowed brows, nausea and anxiety.
   Situation B: Pain—related to animal scratch and fear, as manifested by pulling back from cat, swelling and redness around scratch, and exaggerated weeping.
   Situation C: Pain—acute postoperative, related to cesarean section as manifested by refusal to move, muscle tension, and rigidity and helplessness.
   Situation D: Chronic pain—related to degenerative joint disease as manifested by grimacing, refusal to walk, increased blood pressure, and exaggerated restlessness.
2. The injured tissue releases chemicals that excite nerve endings. A damaged cell releases histamine, which excites nerve endings. Lactic acid accumulates in tissues injured by lack of a blood supply and is believed to excite nerve endings and cause pain or lower the threshold of nerve endings to other stimuli. Bradykinin, prostaglandins, and substance P are also released.
3. Referred pain can be transmitted to a cutaneous site different from where it originated because afferent neurons enter the spinal cord at the same level as the cutaneous site to which the pain has been referred.

4. The gate control theory states that small-diameter nerve fibers conduct excitatory pain stimuli toward the brain, but nerve fibers of a large diameter inhibit the transmission of pain impulses from the spinal cord to the brain. A gating mechanism is believed to be located in substantia gelatinosa of the dorsal horn of the spinal cord. The "gate" is believed to be capable of comparing the strength of excitatory and inhibitory signals entering this region to determine which impulses will travel toward the brain. When too much information arrives at the gate, certain cells in the spinal cord are believed to interrupt the signal, as if closing the gate.
5. a. Acute pain: Generally rapid in onset, varying in intensity from mild to severe, and lasting from a brief period up to any period of less than 6 months; e.g., surgery pain.
   b. Chronic pain: May be limited, intermittent, or persistent, but lasts for 6 months or longer and interferes with normal functioning; e.g., arthritis pain.
   c. Intractable pain: Pain that is resistant to therapy and persists despite a variety of interventions.
6. Sample Answers
   a. Culture: In one culture it may be acceptable to express pain vocally, whereas in another culture vocal expressions of pain are unacceptable.
   b. Ethnicity: An Italian man may respond to pain with cries, moans, complaints, etc., whereas an Irish man may be calm and unemotional about his pain.
   c. Family, gender, or age: Spouses may reinforce pain behavior in their partners.
   d. Religious beliefs: In some religions, pain is viewed as suffering and as a means of purification to make up for individual or community sin.
   e. Environment and support people: Caring support people can help a patient cope with the strangeness of the healthcare environment.
   f. Anxiety and other stressors: Fear of the unknown may compound anxiety and aggravate pain.
   g. Past pain experience: A child may have no fear of pain because he has never experienced pain.
7. Answers will vary with student's experience.
8. Sample Answers
   a. "You are the authority on your pain experience, and must let your nurse know when you are in pain or when the medication isn't working anymore."
   b. "Physical addiction may occur with chronic opioid use, but this is not the same as the psychologic dependence of addiction. Studies suggest that only half of 1 percent of all individuals with cancer pain and other severe types of pain will become addicted to opioids."

Situation	Behavioral	Physiological	Affective
A	Furrowed brows	Nausea	Anxiety
B	Crying	Swelling and redness on scratched area	Fear
C	Refusal to move	Muscle tension, rigidity	Helplessness
D	Grimacing, refusal to walk	Increased blood pressure	Exaggerated restlessness

c. "Opioid drugs can be used to safely manage your pain as long as we take the appropriate precautions and conscientiously assess any side effects."

9. Sample Answers

a. Duration: "For how long have you been experiencing this pain?"

b. Quantity/intensity: "How frequently do you get these attacks? On a scale of 1–10, how would you rate the intensity of this pain?"

c. Quality: "How would you describe the pain (sharp, intense, dull, throbbing, etc.)?"

d. Physiologic indicators: "Have you noticed any physical changes since you've been experiencing this pain?"

10. Answers will vary with experience of student, and may include the following: If a patient suspects a plot to trick him/her into feeling better, the patient is unlikely to respect or appreciate the good intentions of the physicians and nurses involved.

11. a. Cognitive impairment: Many cognitively impaired patients are unable to verbally report their pain or express concepts; therefore, nurses must rely on their own careful assessments, their empathetic qualities, and the expectation that this patient will experience pain if a verbal patient usually reports this event as painful.

b. 5-year-old child: Children cannot always express their pain; the nurse must observe facial expressions, body positions, crying, and physiologic responses. Communication with parents or guardians is vital for accurate pain assessment.

c. An older patient: Nurses should be aware that there is a fear among older patients that admission of pain may limit independence; boredom, loneliness, and depression may affect an older person's perception of pain and willingness to report it. Also, their choice of terms in describing pain may be deceptive.

CHAPTER 40: PATIENT CARE STUDY

1. Objective data are underlined; subjective data are in boldface.

Tabitha Wilson is a 24-month-old infant with AIDS who is hospitalized this admission with infectious diarrhea. She is well known to the pediatric staff, and there is real concern that she might not pull through this admission. She has suffered many of the complications of AIDS and is no stranger to pain. At the present time, the skin on her buttocks is raw and excoriated, and tears stream down her face whenever she is moved. Her blood pressure also shoots up when she is touched. The severity of her illness has left her extremely weak and listless, and **her foster mother reports that she no longer recognizes her child.** When alone in her crib, she seldom moves, and moans softly. Several nurses have expressed great frustration caring for Tabitha, because they find it hard to perform even simple nursing measures like turning, diapering, and weighing her when they see how much pain these procedures cause.

2. Nursing Process Worksheet

Health Problem:

Pain

Etiology:

Excoriated skin on buttocks and debilitating effects of illness.

Signs & Symptoms (Defining Characteristics):

Tears stream down face when moved, and blood pressure shoots up; moans; skin on buttucks is raw and excoriated.

Expected Outcome:

By 2/15/02, patient's behaviors will indicate that pain is sufficiently relieved for patient to rest comfortably—even during clinical procedures.

Nursing Interventions:

1. Report pain asssessment to MD and collaborate on designing effective pain management program.
2. Ensure that the analgesia administration schedule produces consistent comfort.
3. Collaborate with wound care specialist in implementing program for healing of lesions on buttocks.

Evaluative Statement:

2/15/02: Expected outcome partially met—patient's behavior (absence of tears, decreased moaning, decreased BP) indicate some pain relief, but procedures that involve moving the patient still result in great discomfort. Revision: reconsult with physician.

E. Daniel, RN

3. Patient strengths: Patient and her foster parents are greatly liked by the staff; parents show great willingness to be involved in care.

Personal strengths: Knowledge of pain experience; experience in designing and monitoring pain management regimens; experience with pain management in infants and children; good rapport with wound and skin care specialist; strong interpersonal skills.

4. Tabitha's response to procedures is markedly improved since the new analgesic regimen was implemented. However, while she no longer "tears up" when touched and her blood pressure is more stable during procedures, she continues to cry during her bath and during procedures that involve more movement. Will speak with MD about modifying analgesic regimen.

E. Daniel, RN

Chapter 41

MATCHING

1. a	2. c	3. b	4. a	5. b	6. c
7. a	8. c	9. b	10. b	11. d	12. a
13. j	14. m	15. n	16. b	17. e	18. g
19. h	20. l	21. o	22. i	23. k	24. c

25. d, milk, eggs, nuts
26. a, dairy products
27. g, salt
28. i, seafood
29. e, salt, processed foods
30. k, liver
31. m, fish, tea
32. f, wheat
33. o, liver, whole grains
34. b, milk products, soft drinks
35. h, liver
36. j, oysters
37. l, beans, fruit
38. n, whole grains

39. e	40. a	41. g	42. b	43. i	44. c
45. f	46. d				

MULTIPLE CHOICE

1. d	2. a	3. b	4. c	5. a	6. b
7. b	8. d	9. c	10. a	11. d	12. a
13. b	14. d	15. c	16. b	17. a	18. c
19. b	20. d	21. a			

COMPLETION

1. Nitrogen imbalance is a comparison between catabolism and anabolism and can be measured by comparing nitrogen intake and nitrogen excretion. When catabolism and anabolism are occurring at the same rate; as in healthy adults, the body is in a state of neutral nitrogen balance.

2. a. Saturated fatty acids: Cannot bind additional hydrogen atoms; i.e., their carbon bonds are all saturated. Example: animal fats. Saturated fats raise cholesterol.
   b. Unsaturated fatty acids: Have one or more double bonds between carbon atoms. When double bonds are broken, carbons can bind with additional hydrogen atoms. Example: vegetable fats. Unsaturated fats lower serum cholesterol levels.

3. a. Certain age groups: Infants, adolescents, pregnant and lactating women, and the elderly
   b. Smoking, alcohol abuse, long-term use of certain medications
   c. Chronic illnesses
   d. Poor appetite

4. a. Infancy: The period from birth to 1 year of age is the most rapid period of growth. Nutritional needs per unit of body weight are greater than at any other time in the life cycle.
   b. Toddlers and Preschoolers. During this stage, the decrease in growth is dramatic. Mobility, autonomy, and coordination increase, as do muscle mass and bone density. This age group develops an attitude toward food. Appetite decreases and becomes erratic.
   c. School-aged children: Nutritional implications focus on health promotion. Increasing energy requirements should be balanced with foods of high nutritional value. The appetite improves but may still be irregular.
   d. Adolescents: Nutrient needs increase to support growth. Weight consciousness becomes compulsive in 1 of 100 teenage girls and results in eating disorder.
   e. Adults: Growth ceases and nutritional needs level off.
   f. Pregnant women: Nutrient needs increase to support growth and maintain maternal homeostasis, particularly during the second and third trimester. Caloric needs are higher for lactation than pregnancy.
   g. Older adults: Because of the decreases in BMR and physical activity and loss of lean body mass, energy expenditure decreases. The calorie needs of the body decrease.

5. See table below.

6. Sample Answers
   a. Eat a variety of high-fiber foods daily.
   b. Drink 6–8 glasses of water daily.
   c. Substitute high-fiber foods for lower-fiber foods.
   d. Add bran to diet slowly to decrease likelihood of flatus and distention.

7. a. Anorexia nervosa: Characterized by denial of appetite and bizarre eating patterns; may result in extremely dangerous amount of weight loss; can be fatal. Typical individual is adolescent girl from middle or upper socioeconomic class; competitive; obsessive; distorted body image.

Nutrient	Function	Recommended %
a. Carbohydrates	Supply energy (4 cal/g); also spares protein, helps burn fat efficiently, and prevents ketosis	50%–60%
b. Proteins	Maintain body tissues; support new tissue growth; component of body framework	10%–20%
c. Fats	Important component of cell membranes; synthesis of bile acids; precursor of steroid hormones and vitamin D; most concentrated source of energy (9 cal/g); aids in absorption of fat-soluble vitamins; provides insulation, structure, and body temperature control.	Saturated <10% Unsaturated <30%
d. Vitamins	Metabolism of carbohydrates, protein, and fat	
e. Minerals	Key components of body structures; regulation of body processes	
f. Water	Essential for all biochemical reactions; participates in many biochemical reactions; helps regulate body temperature, helps lubricate body joints; needed for adequate mucous secretions.	1500–3000 mL/day

b. Bulimia: Characterized by episodes of gorging followed by purging. Typical individual is college student who fears gaining weight but is overwhelmed by periods of intense hunger.

8. a. Sex: Men have higher caloric and protein requirements than women because of their larger muscle mass.

b. State of health: The alteration in nutrient requirements that results from illness and trauma varies with the intensity and duration of stress.

c. Alcohol abuse: Alcohol can alter the body's use of nutrients, and thereby its nutrient requirement by numerous mechanisms.

d. Medications: Nutrient absorption may be altered by drugs that change the pH of the gastrointestinal tract, increase gastrointestinal motility, damage the intestinal mucosa, or bind with nutrients, rendering them unavailable to the body.

e. Megadoses of nutrient supplements: An excess of one nutrient can lead to a deficiency of another.

f. Religion: Nurses need to be aware of dietary restrictions associated with religions that might affect a patient's nutritional requirements.

g. Economics: The adequacy of a person's food budget affects dietary choices and patterns.

9. a. Food diaries: The patient records all food and beverages consumed in a specified time period (3–7 days).

b. Diet history: 24-hour recall, food frequency record, plus interview designed to determine past and present food intake and habits.

10. Sample Answer

The nurse should explain diet order to the patient, screen patients at home who are at nutritional risk, observe intake and appetite, evaluate patient's tolerance for specific types of foods, assist the patient with eating, address potential for harmful drug–nutrient interactions, and teach nutrition.

11. Sample Answers

a. Provide simple verbal instruction; include family members when appropriate.

b. Advise the patient to eliminate any foods that are not tolerated.

c. Offer support and encouragement.

12. a. Clear liquid diet: Only foods that are clear liquids at room temperature, including gelatins, fat-free bouillon, ice pops, clear juices, etc.; inadequate in calories, proteins, and most nutrients.

b. Full liquid diet: All liquids that can be poured at room temperature; includes clear liquids plus milk, plain frozen desserts, pasteurized eggs, cereal gruels; high-calorie, high-protein supplements are recommended if used more than 3 days.

c. Soft diet: Regular diets that have been modified to eliminate foods that are hard to digest and chew, including those that are high in fiber and fat; adequate in calories and nutrients and can be used long term.

13. a. Nasogastric feeding tube: Inserted through the nose and into stomach. Advantage: allows stomach to be used as natural reservoir, regulating amount of food that enters intestine. Disadvantage: introduces risk of aspiration of tube feeding solution into lungs.

b. Nasointestinal feeding tube: passed through the nose into the upper portion of the small intestine. Advantage: minimal risk for aspiration. Disadvantage: dumping syndrome may develop.

14. a. Patient's progress toward meeting nutritional goals.

b. Patient's tolerance of and adherence to the diet when appropriate.

c. Patient's level of understanding of the diet and need for further diet instruction.

d. Findings should be communicated to other healthcare team members.

e. Plan should be revised or terminated as needed.

15. A medically supervised VLCD may be used that generally supplies 400–800 calories per day. Supplemental vitamins and minerals should be given, based on patient's laboratory data, and patient should be closely monitored for tolerance, weight loss, and complications.

CHAPTER 41: PATIENT CARE STUDY

1. Objective data are underlined; subjective data are in boldface.

Mr. Church, a 74-year-old white male, is being admitted to the geriatric unit of the hospital for a diagnostic workup. He was diagnosed as having Alzheimer's disease 4 years ago, and just 1 year ago was admitted to a long-term care facility. His wife of 49 years is extremely devoted, and informed the nurse taking the admission history that she instigated his admission to the hospital because **she was alarmed by the amount of weight he was losing.** Assessment revealed a 6-foot tall, emaciated male, who weighed 149 lbs. His wife reported he lost 20 pounds in the last 2 months. The staff at the long-term care facility report that he was eating his meals, and his wife validated that this was the case. No one seemed sure, however, of the caloric content of his diet. His wife nodded her head vigorously when asked if her husband seemed more agitated and hyperactive recently. Mr. Church has dull, sparse hair, pale, dry skin, and dry mucous membranes.

2. Nursing Process Worksheet

Health Problem:

Altered nutrition: Less than body requirements.

Etiology:

Imbalance between energy expenditure and caloric intake.

Signs & Symptoms (Defining Characteristics):

6'0", 149 lbs; appears "emaciated"; 20-lb weight loss over 2 months; is "eating meals"; more "hyperactive and agitated" than usual; dull, sparse hair; pale, dry skin; dry mucous membranes.

Expected Outcome:

In one month (1/20/02), patient will demonstrate signs of ingesting enough calories to meet energy needs, as evidenced by a 5–10 lb weight gain.

Nursing Interventions:

1. Do a 72-hour diet history to determine the average number of calories he ingests daily.
2. Provide whatever assistance he needs with feeding. Add high-calorie snacks to his diet, increasing calories progressively until the pattern of weight loss is replaced by weight gain.
3. Until the desired weight is regained and maintained, weigh the patient daily and keep an accurate fluid I&O and calorie intake record.
4. Explore nursing strategies to reduce agitation and hyperactivity, e.g., music, balance between solitude and social interaction, rest periods, etc.

Evaluative Statement:

1/20/02: Expected outcome met—patient gained 8 lbs over last month and seems to enjoy high-calorie snacks.

M. Bendyna, RN

3. Patient strengths: Patient has a very supportive wife.
   Personal strengths: Sound knowledge of nutrition and of Alzheimer's disease. Experienced in working with persons with Alzheimer's disease and their families. Experienced gerontological nurse.
4. Over the past month, the patient's intake has increased by 2000 cal/day. He enjoys high-calorie snacks of peanut butter and jelly sandwiches, milk shakes, dried fruit and nuts, pasta salads, and an occasional Snickers bar. He has regained 8 of the 20 pounds he lost, and his wife is delighted. He remains hyperactive, but scheduled walks have decreased some of his agitation. Will continue to monitor his nutritonal needs.

M. Bendyma, RN

Chapter 42

MATCHING

1. d	2. a	3. c	4. b	5. c	6. b
7. d	8. a	9. f	10. h	11. k	12. a
13. d	14. c	15. j	16. l	17. e	18. g
19. i	20. d	21. a	22. c	23. c	24. b
25. d					

MULTIPLE CHOICE

1. b	2. c	3. a	4. b	5. d	6. a
7. c	8. d	9. a	10. a	11. b	12. c
13. a	14. d	15. d			

COMPLETION

1. a. Developmental considerations: Infants are born with no urinary control. Most children develop urinary control between the ages of 2 and 5 years. Physiologic changes that accompany normal aging may affect urination in the older adult.
   b. Food and fluid: The kidneys should preserve a careful balance of fluid intake and output. Caffeine-containing beverages have a diuretic effect and increase urine

production. Alcohol produces the same effect by inhibiting the release of antidiuretic hormone. Foods high in water may increase urine production. High-sodium foods and beverages cause sodium and water reabsorption and retention.
   c. Psychologic variables: Individuals experiencing stress often find themselves voiding smaller amounts of urine at more frequent intervals. Stress can also interfere with the ability to relax perineal muscles and the external urethral sphincter.
   d. Activity and muscle tone: Exercise increases metabolism and optimal urine production and elimination. With prolonged periods of immobility, decreased bladder and sphincter tone can result in poor urinary control and urinary stasis.
   e. Pathologic conditions: Certain renal or urologic problems can affect both the quantity and quality of urine produced.
   f. Medication: Medications have numerous effects on urine production and elimination. Nephrotoxic drugs are a grave concern. Abuse of analgesics can result in nephrotoxicity. Certain drugs cause urine to change color.
2. a. The child should be able to hold urine for 1–2 hours.
   b. The child should recognize bladder fullness.
   c. The child should be able to express the need to void and control urination until seated on the toilet.
3. a. Infants and young children: It is important to assess whether the child has achieved bladder control and if a toileting schedule has been established for the child. It is also important to identify the words the child uses to indicate the need to void.
   b. Older adults: Decreased bladder tone may be a problem. The nursing history should note how the person handles these problems and the adequacy of the solution.
   c. Patients with limited or no bladder control/urinary diversions: The procedures and equipment used should be assessed to make sure they follow accepted guidelines and are not predisposing the person to infection or other risk.
4. a. Kidneys: The right kidney may at times be palpated by the nurse by pushing down on the diaphragm as the patient inhales. The left kidney is palpated similarly. The contour and size of the kidneys is noted, as is any tenderness or lumps. A check for costovertebral tenderness should be performed.
   b. Bladder: The bladder cannot be assessed by the nurse when it is empty. When it is distended, the nurse observes the lower abdominal wall, noting any swelling, and palpates the area for tenderness, noting smoothness and roundness of the bladder.
   c. Urethral orifice: This is inspected for any signs of inflammation or discharge. Foul odors should be noted.
   d. Skin integrity and hydration: The skin should be carefully assessed for color, texture, turgor, and the excretion of wastes. The integrity of the skin in the perineal are should also be assessed.
   e. Urine: Each time a patient's urine is handled, it should be assessed for color, odor, clarity, and the presence of sediment. Abnormalities should be noted.

5. Urine is placed in a cylindrical container and the urinometer is inserted in a circular motion without touching the bottom or side of the container. The reading should be made at eye level at the bottom of the meniscus formed by the urine. The density of the urine supports the urinometer. If urine is concentrated, the urinometer will be buoyed high; if urine is dilute, the urinometer will be supported low in the urine.

6. Sample Answers
   a. The patient will produce urine output about equal to fluid intake.
   b. The patient will maintain fluid and electrolyte balance.
   c. The patient will report ease of voiding.
   d. The patient will maintain skin integrity.

7. a. Schedule: Some patients report voiding on demand in no apparent pattern; others have inflexible patterns that have developed over the years and become anxious if these are interrupted.
   b. Privacy: Many adults and children cannot void in the presence of another person; privacy should be offered in the healthcare and home setting.
   c. Position: Helping patients assume normal voiding positions may be all that is necessary to resolve an inability to void.
   d. Hygiene: Patients confined to bed will find it difficult to perform their usual genital hygiene. The nurse should place these patients on a bedpan and pour warm soapy water over the perineal area followed by clear water.

8. Sample Answers
   a. To relieve urinary retention
   b. To obtain a sterile specimen from a woman
   c. To empty the bladder before, during, and after surgery

9. Sample Answers
   a. The patient will explain the cause for the urinary diversion and the rationale for treatment.
   b. The patient will demonstrate self-care behaviors and manage diversion effectively.

CHAPTER 42: PATIENT CARE STUDY

1. Objective data are underlined; subjective data are in boldface.

Mr. Eisenberg, age 84, was hurriedly admitted to a nursing home when his wife of 62 years died. He has two adult children, neither of whom feel prepared to care for him the way his wife did. **"We don't know how mom did it year after year. After he retired from his law practice, he was terribly demanding, and it just seemed nothing she did for him pleased him. His Parkinson's disease does make it a bit difficult for him to get around, but he's able to do a whole lot more than he is letting on. He's always been this way."** You are talking with his son and daughter because the aides have reported to you that he is frequently incontinent of both urine and stool during the day as well as during the night. He is alert and appears capable of recognizing the need to void or defecate and signaling for any assistance. His son and daughter report that this was never a problem at home, that he was able to go into the bathroom with assistance. He has been depressed about his admission to the home and seldom speaks, even when directly approached. He has refused to participate in any of the floor social events since his arrival.

2. Nursing Process Worksheet

Health Problem:

Toileting self-care deficit.

Etiology:

Depression on entering nursing home and decreased will to live.

Signs & Symptoms (Defining Characteristics):

Incontinent of both urine and stool during the day and night (need to determine the frequency); alert and capable of recognizing and signalling the need to void/defecate; able to walk to bathroom with assistance.

Expected Outcome:

Within 2 weeks (6/17/02), patient will communicate the need to void/defecate appropriately, as evidenced by reduction in incontinent episodes to one "accident" daily.

Nursing Interventions:
1. Initiate a regular toileting schedule with the patient in which he is assisted to the bathroom; use these interactions to reinforce the importance of his maintaining his independence.
2. Refrain from using adult incontinent pads or in any way communicating that incontinence is "OK."
3. Call an interdisciplinary conference to develop a strategy to ease his transition to the home.

Evaluative Statement:

6/17/02: Expected outcome partially met—when assisted to the bathroom, the patient voids/defecates; but if the staff neglects to offer their assistance, the patient will not use his call light to request it and incontinent episodes recur (more than one a day on some days). Revision: Continue to counsel regarding transition to the home and importance of independence.

P. Wu, RN

3. Patient strengths: Patient is alert and capable of expressing his needs for assistance. Mobile with assistance.
   Personal strengths: Good knowledge of gerontologic nursing and experience in caring for the elderly. Experienced counselor and teacher of appropriate self-care measures.

4. 6/15/02: A review of the patient's record reveals 3 incontinent episodes in the last 24 hours (2 urine; 1 stool). When asked why he did not ask for assistance to get to the bathroom, the patient refused to answer. Generally he cooperates with the toileting regimen, and when taken to the bathroom voids/defecates as needed. Will continue to counsel regarding the importance of his independently managing his toileting needs. Will reevaluate his ability to recognize the need to void/defecate and ask for assistance.

P. Wu, RN

Chapter 43

MATCHING

1. h	2. a	3. d	4. f	5. c	6. e
7. b	8. g	9. a	10. d	11. c	12. e
13. b, f	14. g	15. a	16. h	17. b	18. d
19. i	20. c	21. e	22. k	23. g	24. f
25. a	26. m	27. h	28. b	29. n	30. c
31. i	32. q	33. o	34. r	35. d	36. l
37. p	38. e	39. k	40. j		

MULTIPLE CHOICE

1. d	2. c	3. c	4. b	5. b	6. a
7. d	8. b	9. c	10. c		

COMPLETION

1. a. Completion of absorption
   b. Manufacture of certain vitamins
   c. Formation of feces
   d. Expulsion of feces from the body
2. a. One is situated in the medulla
   b. A subsidiary center is situated in the spinal cord
3. a. Direct manipulation of the bowel during surgery inhibits peristalsis, causing a condition termed paralytic ileus. This temporary stoppage lasts 24–48 hours.
   b. Inhalation of anesthetic agents inhibit peristalsis by blocking parasympathetic impulses to the intestinal musculature.
4. a. Inspection: The nurse observes the contour of the abdomen, noting any masses or areas of distention.
   b. Auscultation: The nurse uses a warmed stethoscope to listen for bowel sounds in a systematic, clockwise manner in all abdominal quadrants.
   c. Percussion: The nurse percusses all quadrants of the abdomen in a systematic, clockwise manner to identify any masses, fluid or air in the abdomen.
   d. Palpation: Light and deep palpations in each quadrant are performed; tenderness, muscular resistance, enlargement of organs, and masses are noted.
5. a. Developmental considerations: The stool characteristics of an infant depend on whether the infant if being fed breast milk or formula.
   b. Daily patterns: A change in a person's daily routine may lead to constipation.
   c. Food and fluids: Both the type and the amount of foods eaten affect elimination.
   d. Activity and muscle tone: Regular exercise improves gastrointestinal motility.
   e. Lifestyle: A person's daily schedule, occupation, and leisure activities may contribute to a habit of defecating at regular times or to an irregular pattern.
   f. Psychologic variables: In some people anxiety may have a direct effect on gastrointestinal motility, and diarrhea accompanies periods of high anxiety.
   g. Medications: Medications may influence the appearance of the stool, e.g., iron salts result in a black stool from the oxidation of iron.
   h. Diagnostic studies: Patients may need to fast for tests which may alter elimination patterns.

6. Sample Answer
   When were you first diagnosed with diverticular disease? How long have you had the pain? Have you ever had this pain before? How often do you move your bowels? What do your stools look like? Have you noticed any changes in stool lately? What is your regular diet like? Are there any foods you avoid? Any that help relieve the pain?
7. a. Daily fluid intake of 2000–3000 mL
   b. Increased intake of high-fiber foods
   c. Regular exercise
   d. Acceptance of bowel elimination as a normal process of life
8. a. Constipating: processed cheese, lean meat, eggs and pasta
   b. Laxative effect: certain fruits and vegetables, bran, chocolate
   c. Gas-producing: onions, cabbage, beans, cauliflower
9. a. The patient will have a soft, formed bowel movement every 1–3 days without discomfort.
   b. The patient will explain the relation between bowel elimination and dietary fiber, fluid intake and exercise.
   c. The patient will relate the importance of timing, positioning, and privacy to healthy bowel elimination.
10. a. Constipation: Increase high-fiber foods and fluid intake.
    b. Diarrhea: Prepare and store food properly, avoid highly spiced foods or laxative-type foods, increase intake of low-fiber foods, and replace lost fluids.
    c. Flatulence: Avoid gas-producing foods, such as beans, cabbage, onions, cauliflower, and beer.
    d. Ostomies: A low-fiber diet is usually recommended, though patients may experiment with their diet to determine how much fiber they can tolerate.
11. a. Abdominal settings: Lying in a supine position, tighten and hold the abdominal muscles for 6 seconds and then relax them. Repeat several times every waking hour.
    b. Thigh strengthening: Flex and contract the thigh muscles by slowly bringing the knees up to the chest—one at a time—and then lowering them to the bed. Perform several times for each knee, each waking hour.
12. a. To relieve constipation or fecal compaction
    b. To prevent involuntary escape of fecal material during surgical procedures
    c. To promote visualization of the intestinal tract by X-ray film or instrument examination
    d. To help establish regular bowel function during a bowel training program
13. a. Ileostomy: Allows liquid fecal content from the ileum of the small intestine to be eliminated through the stoma.
    b. Colostomy: Permits formed feces from the colon to exit through the stoma.
14. a. Timing: patients should be allowed to heed the natural urge to defecate.
    b. Positioning: The squatting position best facilitates defecation.
    c. Privacy: Most patients consider elimination a private act and nurse should provide privacy for their patients.

d. Nutrition: Patients with elimination problems may need a dietary analysis to determine which foods and fluids are contributing to their problem.

e. Exercise: Regular exercise improves gastrointestinal motility and aids in defication.

CHAPTER 43: PATIENT CARE STUDY

1. Objective data are underlined; subjectve data are in bold-face.

Ms. Elgaresta, <u>age 54, a single, Hispanic woman,</u> is being followed by a cardiologist who monitors her heart arrhythmia. <u>Last month, she was started on a new heart medication.</u> At this visit, she complains to the nurse practitioner who works with the cardiologist: **"Right after I started taking that medication, I got terribly constipated and nothing seems to help. I'm desperate and about ready to try dynamite unless you can think of something else!"** She reports a change in her bowel movements from one soft stool daily to 1–2 hard stools weekly—stools that cause much straining. The nurse practitioner realizes that regulating Ms. Elgaresta's heart is difficult and that her best cardiac response to date has been with the medication that is now causing constipation. Reluctant to suggest substituting another medication too quickly, she asks more questions and discovers the following: **"I've never been much of a drinker. Two cups of coffee in the morning and maybe a glass of wine at night. Water? Almost never. And I don't drink juices or soft drinks."** Analysis of her diet reveals a <u>diet low in fiber:</u> **"I never was one much for vegetables, and they can just keep all this bran stuff that's out on the market! Coffee and a cigarette. That's for me!"** Ms. Elgaresta is a workaholic computer programmer who has little leisure time and spends what little spare she has watching TV. She reports **tiring after walking one flight of stairs,** and states that she avoids all forms of vigorous exercise.

2. Nursing Process Worksheet

Health Problem:

Constipation

Etiology:

New medication, deficient fiber and fluid intake, and insufficient exercise.

Signs & Symptoms (Defining Characteristics):

Change in bowel habits: from one soft, formed stool daily to 1–2 hard stools per week and straining.

Expected Outcome:

One month after new regimen begins (5/4/02), patient reports one soft, formed stool every 1–2 days.

Nursing Interventions:

1. Counsel patient about the relationship between diet (fiber intake and fluids) and bowel elimination, and exercise and bowel elimination.

2. Assess patient's willingness and motivation to make lifestyle changes and develop workable plan.

3. Reinforce importance of continuing medication.

Evaluative Statement:

Expected outcome met—patient now passing soft, formed stool almost every day.

B. Shevorkis, RN

3. Patient strengths: Patient is highly motivated to learn new self-care behaviors.

Personal strengths: Knowledge of the physiology of elimination; experienced patient educator and counselor; excellent role model of healthy self-care behaviors.

4. 5/4/02: Patient in for 1-month follow-up, and expressed delight with effects of new self-care behaviors: (1) decreased fat consumption and increased fiber in diet, (2) increased fluid intake—especially water, (3) increased exercise—four 30-minute periods of aerobic exercise per week. Constipation problem is resolved—passes soft stool almost every day, and reports having much more energy for work. Progress reinforced.

B. Shevorkis, RN

Chapter 44

MATCHING

1. b	2. f	3. i	4. k	5. a	6. e
7. d	8. g	9. h	10. j	11. g	12. j
13. h	14. i	15. e	16. f	17. c	18. a
19. d	20. b	21. d	22. a	23. e	24. b
25. f	26. c	27. e	28. b	29. f	30. a
31. h	32. d	33. a	34. f	35. c	36. b
37. h	38. d	39. e			

MULTIPLE CHOICE

1. d	2. a	3. b	4. d	5. b	6. c
7. c	8. b	9. a	10. d	11. d	12. c
13. b	14. b	15. d	16. a	17. d	18. b
19. d					

COMPLETION

1. a. The integrity of the airway system to transport air to and from the lungs.

   b. A properly functioning alveolar system in the lungs to oxygenate venous blood and remove carbon dioxide from the blood.

   c. A properly functioning cardiovascular system to carry nutrients and wastes to and from body cells.

2. a. Upper airway: The upper airway comprises the nose, pharynx, larynx, and epiglottis. Its main function is to warm, filter, and humidify inspired air.

   b. Lower airway: The lower airway comprises the trachea, right and left main-stem bronchus, segmental bronchi, and terminal bronchioles. The major functions are conduction of air, mucociliary clearance, and production of pulmonary surfactant.

3. According to Boyle's Law, the volume of a gas at a constant temperature varies inversely with the pressure. Pressure in the lungs is lower than atmospheric pressure; this condition facilitates the movement of air into the lungs.

4. a. Any change in the surface area available for diffusion will have a negative effect on diffusion.
   b. Incomplete lung expansion or lung collapse (atelectasis) prevents pressure changes and exchange of gases by diffusion in the lungs.
   c. Any disease or condition that results in thickening of the alveolar–capillary membrane makes diffusion more difficult.
   d. The solubility and molecular weight of the gases are factors in diffusion.

5. a. It is dissolved in plasma.
   b. Most oxygen (97%) is carried in the body by red blood cells in the form of oxyhemoglobin.

6. a. Infant: Respiratory activity is abdominal. The chest wall is so thin that ribs, sternum, and xiphoid process are easily identified.
   b. Preschool and school-age children: Some subcutaneous fat is deposited on the chest wall, so landmarks are less prominent than in an infant; preschool-age child's eustachian tubes, bronchi, and bronchioles are elongated and less angular than in an infant, so the number of routine colds and infections decreases until they enter school.
   c. Older adult: Bony landmarks are more prominent; kyphosis contributes to appearance of leaning forward; barrel chest deformity may result; senile emphysema may be present; power of respiratory and abdominal muscles is reduced.

7. a. Respiratory excursion: This is measured by placing one's hand on the patient's posterior thorax at the level of the 10th rib, with both thumbs almost touching the vertebrae. While patient takes a few deep breaths, the nurse's thumbs should move 5–8 cm symmetrically at maximal inspiration.
   b. Tactile fremitus: The nurse should place his palm's surface on each side of the patient's chest wall, avoiding bony areas; he should detect equal vibrations as the patient says a multisyllabic word.

8. Before: Collect baseline data; instruct patient to remain still.
   During: Observe patient for reactions: any deviation from normal color, pulse and respiratory rates is reported to physician.
   After: Observe patient for changes in respirations; chest X-ray.

9. The inhalation of cigarette smoke increases airway resistance, reduces ciliary action, increases mucus production, causes thickening of the alveolar–capillary membrane, and causes bronchial walls to thicken and lose their elasticity.

10. a. Deep breathing: The nurse instructs the patient to make each breath deep enough to move the bottom ribs. The patient should start slow, inspiring deeply through the nose and expiring slowly through the mouth.
    b. Incentive spirometry: The patient takes a deep breath and observes the results of his/her efforts registered on the spirometry equipment as the patient sustains maximal inspiration.
    c. Abdominal breathing: The patient places one hand on the stomach and the other on the middle of the chest. He/she then breathes slowly in through the nose, letting the abdomen protrude, then out through pursed lips while contracting the abdominal muscles. One hand should be pressing inward and upward on abdomen. These steps should be repeated for 1 minute, followed by a 2-minute rest.

11. a. Avoid open flames in patient's room.
    b. Place "No Smoking" signs in conspicuous places in patient's room.
    c. Check to see that electric equipment is in good working order.
    d. Avoid wearing and using synthetic fabrics that build up static electricity.
    e. Avoid using oils in the area.

12. a. Oropharyngeal/nasophayngeal airway: Semicircular tube of plastic or rubber inserted into the back of the pharynx through the mouth or nose in a spontaneously breathing patient; used to keep the tongue clear of the airway and to permit suctioning of secretions.
    b. Endotracheal tube: Polyvinylchloride tube that is inserted through the nose or mouth into the trachea, using a laryngoscope as guide; used to administer oxygen by mechanical ventilator, to suction secretions easily, or to bypass upper airway obstructions.
    c. Tracheostomy tube: An artificial opening made into the trachea. The curved tracheostomy tube is inserted into this opening to replace an endotracheal tube, provide a method to mechanically ventilate, bypass an upper airway obstruction, or remove tracheobronchial secretions.

13. Airway: Tip the head and check for breathing.
    Breathing: If the victim does not start to breathe spontaneously after the airway is opened, give two slow, full breaths.
    Circulation: Check the pulse. If the victim has no pulse, artificial circulation must be started with breathing.

14. The nurse is responsible for the collection of the baseline data before the examination. Pain medication should be administered before the test if requested. During the procedure the nurse should observe the patient for reactions. The patient's color, pulse, and respiratory rates should be observed, and any deviation from the norm reported to the physician immediately. After the procedure the nurse should observe the patient for changes in respirations. A chest x-ray is usually done to verify the absence of complications.

15. a. Help the patient assume a position that allows free movement of the diaphragm and expansion of the chest wall to promote ease of respiration.
    b. Keep patient's secretions thin by asking the patient to drink 2–3 qt of clear fluids daily.
    c. Provide humidified air.
    d. Perform cupping on the lungs of patient to loosen pulmonary secretions.

e. Use vibration to help loosen respiratory secretions.

f. Provide postural drainage.

g. Help patient maintain good nutrition.

CHAPTER 44: PATIENT CARE STUDY

1. Objective data are underlined; subjective data are in boldface.

Toni is a <u>14-year-old</u> who is in the adolescent mental health unit following a suicide attempt. Her chart reveals that on several occasions when her mother was visiting, she began <u>hyperventilating (respiratory rate of 42 and increased depth)</u>. Gasping for breath on these occasions, she nevertheless pushed away all who approached her to assist. Her mother confided that she and her husband are in the midst of a divorce and that it hasn't been easy for Toni at home. **"I know she's been having a rough time at school, and I guess I've been too caught up in my own troubles to be there for her."** When you attempt to discuss this with Toni and mention her mother's concern, she begins hyperventilating again.

2. Nursing Process Worksheet

Health Problem:

Ineffective breathing patterns.

Expected Outcome:

By her second week in the unit (3/22/02), Toni will demonstrate an effective respiratory rate and rhythm (not to exceed 24) during her mother's visits.

Etiology:

Anxiety

Nursing Interventions:

1. Use interview questions directed to Toni and her mother to determine the nature of the problem, its probable cause, and its effect on her lifestyle.

2. Demonstrate consciously controlled breathing and encourage her to use it during periods of anxiety or activity.

3. Maintain an emotionally "safe" environment. The same nurses should always work with this patient and maintain eye contact during conversations with her.

4. If fear is the cause of her anxiety, encourage her to express concerns. Reduce cause of fear, if feasible.

5. If there is a strong emotional component, discuss with patient the possibility of developing effective coping skills with professional counselling.

Signs & Symptoms (Defining Characteristics):

Periods of hyperventilation (increased RR—42—and increased depth) associated with stressful situations (visits by mother).

Evaluative Outcome:

3/22/02: Expected outcome partially met—on two occasions, Toni remained in control of her breathing during her mother's visits. On at least one occasion, she hyperventilated.

K. O'Leary, RN

3. Patient strengths: The patient's strengths still need to be identified; mother seems to be gaining an appreciation of her needs.

Personal strengths: Good understanding of the effects of stress and experienced in helping patients replace maladaptive coping strategies with adaptive strategies.

4. 3/22/02: This morning, Toni began talking about the difficult situation at home. When asked about her relationship with her mother she began gulping for air, but "caught herself" and quickly reestablished control of her breathing, consciously decreasing her rate and depth. Whereas she has shown no signs of hyperventilation on two of her mother's last visits, she had one episode in which she hyperventilated and totally "lost control," and needed sedation. She stated she feels like she is making progress, but still has a long way to go before she will feel comfortable at home and in control of simple, everyday things, like breathing.

K. O'Leary, RN

Chapter 45

MATCHING

1. b	2. c	3. a	4. a	5. d	6. c
7. b	8. d	9. a	10. c	11. a	12. d
13. b	14. c	15. a	16. g	17. b	18. a
19. i	20. h	21. c	22. e	23. d	24. b
25. a	26. d	27. c	28. c	29. d	30. f
31. b	32. g	33. a	34. e	35. c	36. a
37. c	38. f	39. p	40. b	41. o	42. l
43. h	44. a	45. d	46. e	47. j	48. m
49. n	50. g	51. k			

CORRECT THE FALSE STATEMENTS

1. True
2. False—electrolytes
3. False—hypotonic solution
4. True
5. False—hydrogen
6. False—alkali
7. False—alkaline
8. False—lungs
9. True
10. False—hypernatremia
11. False—disproportionate
12. True

MULTIPLE CHOICE

1. c	2. a	3. b	4. b	5. c	6. d
7. a	8. d	9. b	10. d	11. c	12. a
13. b	14. b				

COMPLETION

1. a. Provides a medium for transporting nutrients to cells and wastes from cells.
   b. Facilitates cellular metabolism and proper cellular chemical functioning.
   c. Acts as a solvent for electrolytes and nonelectrolytes.
   d. Helps maintain normal body temperature.
   e. Facilitates digestion and promotes elimination.
   f. Acts as a tissue lubricant.

2. a. Osmosis: The solvent water passes from an area of lesser solute concentration to an area of greater solute concentration until an equilibrium is established.
   b. Diffusion: The tendency of solutes to move freely throughout a solvent. The solute moves from an area of higher concentration to an area of lower concentration until an equilibrium is established.
   c. Active transport: A process that requires energy for the movement of substances through a cell membrane from an area of lesser concentration to an area of higher concentration.

3. a. Ingested liquids: Fluid intake is regulated by the thirst mechanism and is stimulated by intracellular dehydration and decreased blood volume.
   b. Water in food: The amount of water depends on the food, e.g., melons have a higher water content than bread.
   c. Water from metabolic oxidation: Water is an end product of oxidation that occurs during the metabolism of food.

4. Water is lost through the kidneys as urine, through the skin as perspiration, and through insensible water loss.

5. a. Kidneys: Approximately 170 L of plasma are filtered daily in the adult, while only 1.5 L of urine are excreted. They selectively retain electrolytes and water and excrete wastes.
   b. Cardiovascular system: The heart and blood vessels are responsible for pumping and carrying nutrients and water throughout the body.
   c. Lungs: The lungs regulate oxygen and carbon dioxide levels of the blood.
   d. Thyroid: Thyroxine, released by the thyroid gland, increases blood flow in the body. This in turn increases renal circulation, which results in increased glomerular filtration and urinary output.
   e. Parathyroid glands: The parathyroid glands secrete parathyroid hormone, which regulates the level of calcium in ECF.
   f. Gastrointestinal tract: The GI tract absorbs water and nutrients that enter the body through this route.
   g. Nervous system: The nervous system acts as a switchboard and inhibits and stimulates mechanisms that influence fluid balance.

6. a. Acidosis: Characterized by a high concentration of hydrogen ions in ECF, which causes the pH to fall below 7.35.
   b. Alkalosis: Characterized by a low concentration of hydrogen ions in ECF, which causes the pH to exceed 7.45.

7. a. Respiratory acidosis: An excess of carbonic acid in ECF caused by decreased alveolar ventilation and resulting in the retention of carbon dioxide. The lungs are unable to compensate for the rise in carbonic acid levels. As the carbonic acid concentration increases, the kidneys retain more bicarbonate and increase their excretion of hydrogen.
   b. Respiratory alkalosis: A deficit of carbonic acid in ECF caused by increased alveolar ventilation and resulting in a decrease in carbon dioxide. Respiratory rate and depth increase because carbon dioxide is being excreted faster than normal; depression or cessation of respirations can occur. The kidneys attempt to alleviate this imbalance by increasing bicarbonate excretion and hydrogen retention.
   c. Metabolic acidosis: A deficit of bicarbonate in ECF resulting from an increase in acidic components or an excessive loss of bicarbonate. The lungs attempt to increase the rate of carbon dioxide excretion by increasing the rate and depth of respirations; the kidneys attempt to compensate by retaining bicarbonate and excreting more hydrogen. May result in loss of consciousness and death.
   d. Metabolic alkalosis: An excess of bicarbonate in ECF resulting from loss of acid or ingestion or retention of base. The body attempts to compensate by retaining carbon dioxide. Respirations become slow and shallow, and periods of apnea may occur. The kidneys excrete potassium and sodium along with excess bicarbonate and retain hydrogen within carbonic acid.

8. a. Increased hematocrit: Severe dehydration and shock (when hemoconcentration rises considerably).
   b. Decreased hematocrit: Acute, massive blood loss; hemolytic reaction following transfusion of incompatible blood.
   c. Increased hemoglobin: Hemoconcentration of the blood.
   d. Decreased hemoglobin: Anemia, severe hemorrhage, and following a hemolytic reaction.

9. a. Urine pH and specific gravity: Specific gravity is a measure of kidney's ability to concentrate urine. Normal range: 1.003–1.035. Both may be obtained by dipstick measurement on a fresh voided specimen or through lab analysis.
   b. Serum electrolytes: Indicates plasma levels of select electrolytes.
   c. Arterial blood gases: Indicate the adequacy of oxygenation and ventilation and acid–base status.

10. a. Note the patient's fluid and food intake, and learn what the patient's previous eating and drinking patterns have been.
    b. Note whether thirst is excessive or whether patient experiences little or no thirst.
    c. Note excessive losses of fluid from the body and attempt to prevent losses when possible.
    d. Physiologic changes that accompany the aging process may affect patient's ability to maintain fluid balance.

11. a. Select a vein large enough to accommodate the needle.
    b. Select a site that is naturally splinted by bone, such as the back of the hand or the forearm.

c. Select a site distal to the heart and move proximally, as necessary, to find the appropriate injection site.

d. Select a site while moving toward the heart and away from a damaged vein.

12. Handling all equipment, performing dressing changes, assessing patient for evidence of infection or other complications, and maintaining the supplies necessary to continue home infusion.

13. Metabolic alkalosis

14. Respiratory acidosis with renal compensation

15. Metabolic acidosis with partial respiratory compensation

16. Respiratory alkalosis

17. Respiratory acidosis

18. See table below.

CHAPTER 45: PATIENT CARE STUDY

1. Objective data are underlined; subjective data are in boldface.

Rebecca is <u>a college freshman</u> who, on the night she had her wisdom teeth removed, had an <u>oral temperature of 39.5°C (103.1°F)</u>. She had a sore throat several days prior to the extraction, but neglected to mention this to the oral surgeon. **Because of the soreness in her throat, she reported having greatly decreased both her food and fluid intake.** Friends that night gave her some Tylenol, which brought her temperature down, and encouraged her to drink more fluids. When they checked on her in the morning, <u>her temperature was elevated again</u> and she **said she had felt too weak during the night to drink.** She was brought to the student health service, where the admitting nurse noticed <u>her dry mucous membranes, decreased skin turgor, and rapid pulse.</u> At <u>5'2" and 98 lbs,</u> Rebecca was petite, but she had **lost 4 lbs** in the last week.

pH	PaCO$_2$	HCO$_3$	Nature of Disturbance	Comp. Present? Yes	Comp. Present? No	If Yes Renal	If Yes Respiratory	If Yes Partial	If Yes Complete
7.28	63	25	respiratory acidosis		x				
7.20	40	14	metabolic acidosis		x				
7.52	40	35	metabolic alkalosis		x				
7.48	30	31	resp. & met. alkalosis						
7.16	82	30	respiratory acidosis	x		x		x	
7.36	68	35	respiratory acidosis	x		x			x
7.56	23	26	respiratory alkalosis		x				
7.40	40	26	none						
7.56	23	26	respiratory alkalosis		x				
7.26	70	25	respiratory acidosis		x				
7.52	44	38	metabolic alkalosis		x				
7.32	30	18	metabolic acidosis	x			x	x	
7.49	34	26	respiratory alkalosis		x				
6.98	84	18	resp. & met. alkalosis		x				

2. Nursing Process Worksheet

Health Problem:

Fluid volume deficit.

Etiology:

Decreased fluid intake (sore throat and weakness) and loss of water and electrolytes in fever.

Signs & Symptoms (Defining Characteristics):

Elevated temperature (39.5°C), 4-lb weight loss in 1 week, dry mucous membranes, decreased skin turgor, and rapid pulse.

Expected Outcome:

By 3/19/02, patient will demonstrate corrected fluid volume deficit by (1) balanced fluid intake/output, averaging 2500 mL fluid/day; (2) urine specific gravity within normal range (1.010–1.025); (3) moist mucous membranes and adequate skin turgor; and (4) pulse returned to baseline.

Nursing Interventions:
1. Assess for worsening of fluid volume deficit.
2. Give oral fluids that are nonirritating, as tolerated.
3. If oral fluids are not tolerated, confer with MD regarding IV replacement therapy.
4. Monitor response to fluid therapy; VS, urinary volume, and specific gravity, increased skin turgor, moist mucous membranes, increased body weight.

J. Barclay, RN

Evaluative Statement:

3/19/02: Goals met—patient has corrected fluid volume deficit; fluid intake and output average 2700 mL fluid/day; pulse returned to baseline; skin turgor improved; mucous membranes are moist.

J. Barclay, RN

3. Patient strengths: Previously healthy; concerned friends; highly motivated to correct deficit.
   Personal strengths: Strong knowledge of fluid, electrolyte and acid–base balance; good interpersonal skills.
4. 3/19/02: Patient tolerating oral replacement fluids and understands importance of increasing fluids until the deficit is corrected. Friends remind her to drink at frequent intervals. Pulse returned to baseline. Yesterday's fluid intake was 2900 mL fluid; output, 2500 mL. Improved skin turgor and moist mucous membranes. Gained 2 lbs.

J. Barclay, RN